This book is dedicated with love

to my best friend, colleague, and husband, Julius A. Gylys
and
to my children, Regina Maria and Julius A., II
and
to Andrew, Julia, and Caitlin

—BAG

to my mother, best friend, mentor and co-author, Barbara A. Gylys
and
to my father, Julius A. Gylys
and
to my husband, Bruce Masters, and my children, Andrew, Julia, and Caitlin. All of whom have given me continuous encouragement and support.

—RMM

Preface

The second edition of *Medical Terminology Simplified: A Programmed Learning Approach by Body Systems* reflects current trends and new approaches to teaching medical terminology. It remains a self-instructional book that can also be used in the classroom. The book is designed to provide individuals entering the healthcare profession with skills to learn medical terminology easily and quickly. Full color has been incorporated as a pedagogic tool in both the text and figures. Prefixes are highlighted in pink and suffixes are highlighted in blue for easier recognition. Full color in the figures enables the student to see a true representation of the body system or pathological condition. To develop a contemporary teaching and learning package, the authors have implemented a number of insightful suggestions from numerous educators and students. Each body system unit includes:

- A summary of major combining forms related to the body system covered in the unit
- A pathology section that provides a more comprehensive understanding of pathological conditions
- Additional medical records and evaluations

The authors not only updated but also incorporated new features in the textbook and *Instructor's Guide*. Additionally, they have provided supplemental teaching aids, including an *Interactive Medical Terminology CD-ROM* program.

As we prepare to enter the new millennium, the computer revolution in education is exerting an increasing influence on teachers and students in all levels of education. Educators are being challenged to integrate the latest technology into the learning process in order to promote commitment to excellence in education and a high level of performance of future professionals. New alternative learning systems, one of which is distance education, are being developed to meet student needs. To help instructors prepare for these new learning systems, the authors have provided a variety of teaching aids. Descriptions and illustrations of the entire learning package for *Medical Terminology Simplified* are enumerated below.

Supplementary Teaching Materials

Audiocassette Tapes. Two audiocassette tapes are included with each textbook.* Medical terms covered in a body system's unit are summarized at the end of the unit and identified with the corresponding frame from which they originate. Thus additional information can be obtained and reviewed as the pronunciation of the terms is given on the tape.

Interactive CD-ROM. The instructor may choose to adopt the book with a multimedia *Interactive Medical Terminology CD-ROM* program. The competency-based software is self-paced and includes graphics, audio, a pull-down dictionary based on *Taber's* 18th edition, and help menus, along with numerous interactive activities designed at a 90 percent competency level that provide immediate feedback. A printout of student's progress is also available.

Instructor's Guide. A comprehensive *Instructor's Guide* is available to instructors who adopt the second edition of *Medical Terminology Simplified*. The *Instructor's Guide* helps the teacher make

---

*The instructor may choose to adopt: (1) the book with the two shrink-wrapped audiocassettes or
(2) the book with the two shrink-wrapped audiocassettes and a multimedia *Interactive Medical Terminology CD-ROM* program, designed at a 90 percent competency level.

the best possible use of the textbook and provides a variety of supplementary teaching aids. Some of the special features include the following:

- A *CyberTest*™ computerized test bank provides a means to create custom or random-selected quizzes or quick tests as well as comprehensive midsemester and final exams. A hard copy of all of the multiple-choice test questions is included in the *Instructor's Guide*.
- Suggested course outlines that can be used to teach a 10- or 15-week course.
- Suggestions to develop a contemporary learning package that integrates the latest technological tools for a self-paced distance learning course. Current distance learning websites include general information about the course, course requirements, a course syllabus, an interactive chat room with bulletin-board-type discussions, and direct e-mail access between the instructor and students enrolled in the course. The distance learning technology available at your school or institution will determine the implementation of the latest technological teaching tools.
- Additional medical records reports, evaluations, and dictionary exercises.
- Crossword puzzles and solutions.
- Master copies of selected figures from each unit to produce transparencies.

How to Use This Book

This self-instructional book is designed to provide you with skills to learn medical terminology easily and quickly. The following distinctive features are included in this learning package:

- The programmed learning approach presents a word-building method for developing a medical vocabulary in an effective and interesting manner. It can be used in a traditional classroom setting or with an instructor of an independent study.
- The workbook-text format is designed to guide you through exercises that teach and reinforce medical terminology.
- Numerous activities in each unit are designed to enable you to be mentally and physically involved in the learning process. With this method you not only understand but also remember the significant concepts of medical word building.
- You learn by active participation. You write answers in response to blocks of information, complete review exercises, and analyze medical reports. After the review exercises, reinforcement frames will direct you, if you are not satisfied with your level of comprehension, to go back and rework the corresponding informational frames. You can also make flash cards for the word elements in the unit. Use the cards to reinforce your retention of the word elements. First, compile the cards for the word elements included in the review you are completing, and review those elements. Then complete and correct the review. If you are not satisfied with the score, review the flash cards again before retaking the review. Follow this procedure each time you are ready to complete a review. The flash cards can also be used before you complete the Unit Exercises at the end of each unit.
- The audiocassette tapes provide reinforcement of pronunciation, definitions of medical words, and spelling practice.
- Pronunciation keys for all the medical words are included in the frame answer boxes. The pronunciation guidelines on pages ix and x show you how to interpret these keys.
- The extensive *Interactive Medical Terminology CD-ROM* software program includes graphics, audio, and various drill and practice exercises to help you master and achieve a minimum 90 percent competency level in medical terminology.
- The special features of the appendixes at the back of the book are useful for study, review, and reference as you begin your career in the allied health field. The appendixes include:

Appendix A: Index of Medical Word Elements. Alphabetically lists medical word elements with corresponding pronunciations and meanings. This appendix employs two methods for word-element indexing—first by medical word element, then by English term.
Appendix B: Answer Key. Provides answers to labeling and unit exercises.
Appendix C: Diagnostic Procedures. Includes clinical, radiographic, and laboratory procedures that are used to establish a diagnosis and determine a type of treatment.
Appendix D: Drug Classifications. Provides prescription and nonprescription agents that are used for the treatment of various medical conditions.

Appendix E: Abbreviations. Lists a summary of commonly used medical abbreviations and their meanings.

Appendix F: Medical Specialties. Provides a summary and description of medical specialties.

Taber's Cyclopedic Medical Dictionary, 18th edition, is a highly recommended companion reference, because it provides etymologies for nearly all of the main entries presented in this book.

What You Will Learn from This Book

When you have completed *Medical Terminology Simplified: A Programmed Learning Approach by Body Systems, second edition*, you will be able to do the following:

1. Identify the organs and structures of the body systems.
2. Explain the main functions of the body systems.
3. Define the word roots and combining forms used to describe the organs and structures.
4. Define suffixes and prefixes in medical words.
5. Build and analyze thousands of medical words.
6. Understand the meaning of new medical words by defining the elements.
7. Master pronunciation and spelling of medical terms by using the pronunciation guides and audiocassette tapes.

Use the textbook as a reference. Besides the invaluable information, illustrations, and diagrams in each unit, the appendixes include a wealth of information that can be applied in a medical setting.

Pronunciation Guidelines

Although medical words generally follow rules that govern the pronunciation of English words, they may be difficult to pronounce when you first encounter them. The guides provided throughout this book will make this task much easier. In order to master the pronunciation, study the basic rules of pronunciation, listen to the audiocassettes, and repeat words after your instructor has introduced them.

Here are some rules that will be of great help to you:

- **ae** and **oe**, pronounce only the second vowel.
  Examples: burs**ae**, pleur**ae**, r**oe**ntgen.
- **c** and **g** are given the soft sound of s and j, respectively, before e, i, and y in words of both Greek and Latin origins.
  Examples: **c**erebrum, **c**ircumcision, **c**ycle, **g**el, **g**ingivitis, **g**iant, **g**yrate.
- **c** and **g** have a hard sound before other letters.
  Examples: **c**ardiac, **c**ast, **g**astric, **g**onad.
- **e** and **es**, when forming the final letter or letters of a word, are often pronounced as separate syllables.
  Examples: syncop**e**, systol**e**, nar**es**.
- **ch** is sometimes pronounced like *k*.
  Examples: **ch**olesterol, **ch**olera, **ch**olemia.
- **i** at the end of a word (to form a plural) is pronounced *eye*.
  Examples: bronch**i**, fung**i**, nucle**i**.
- **pn** at the beginning of a word is pronounced with only the *n* sound.
  Examples: **pn**eumonia, **pn**eumotoxin.
- **pn** in the middle of a word is pronounced with a hard *p* and a hard *n*.
  Examples: ortho**pn**ea, hyper**pn**ea.
- **ps** is pronounced like *s*.
  Examples: **ps**ychology, **ps**ychosis.
- All other vowels and consonants have ordinary English sounds.

Most medical words in this textbook are spelled phonetically. Pronunciations are included in each unit, using diacritical marks to indicate most of the long and short vowels. Diacritics are marks over or under vowels. In this text, only two diacritics are used:

The macron (¯) indicates the long sound of vowels, as in the following:
a in rāte
e in rēbirth
i in īsle
o in ōver
u in ūnite

The breve (˘) indicates the short sound of vowels, as in the following:
a in ăpple
e in ĕver
i in ĭt
o in nŏt
u in cŭt

Capitalization is used to indicate stress on certain syllables, as in LET-ter.

Acknowledgments

The authors express special and sincere appreciation for the effort of the following individuals who, through their professionalism and skill, improved the second edition of the textbook:

- Leslie Ann Arrigo, AFB-MA, BS
  Instructor
  Mercyhurst College
  McAuley Division
  Erie, Pennsylvania
- Nina Thierer, CMA
  Faculty
  Ivy Tech State College
  Medical Assistant Department
  Fort Wayne, Indiana

The authors also thank the following individuals who reviewed the first edition of the textbook:

- Rachel C. Allstatter, CMA
  Director of Medical Programs
  Cincinnati Metropolitan College
  Cincinnati, Ohio
- Leslie Ann Arrigo, BS, AFB in MA
  Instructor
  Mercyhurst College
  McAuley Division
  Erie, Pennsylvania
- Ronald G. Beckett, MED, RRT
  Program Director
  Respiratory Therapy Department
  Quinnipiac College
  Toledo, Ohio
- Marty Hitchcock, CMA, AS
  Program Director/Instructor
  Medical Assisting Department
  Gwinnett Technical Institute
  Lawrenceville, Georgia
- Shirley Montgomery, MA
  Professor, Medical Assisting
  Lively Area Vocational-Technical Institute
  Tallahassee, Florida
- Nina Thierer, CMA
  Faculty
  Ivy Tech State College
  Medical Assistant Department
  Fort Wayne, Indiana
- Sue Wambold, MEd, RN, RDCS
  Director of Cardiovascular Technology Program
  Health & Human Services Department
  University of Toledo
  Toledo, Ohio

Also, Julius A. Gylys, PhD; Judith A. Shook, CMT, AD, Pathology Department, Toledo Hospital; Heather Doll, Team Leader, Health Information Services, Riverside Hospital, Toledo, Ohio; and Michael S. Applebaum, MD.

We also thank the editors and production staff of F. A. Davis Company, especially:

- Jean-François Vilain, Publisher, Health Professions, who oversaw the entire production process.
- Marianne Fithian, Developmental Editor, who edited several drafts of the manuscript, helping it along at every stage.
- Stephen D. Johnson, Production Editor, for his thoroughness and diligence in successfully completing the project.
- Herbert J. Powell, Jr., Director of Production, and Robert Butler, Assistant Director of Production, whose hard work, patience, and expertise made the production of this book possible.

Contents

Introduction to Programmed Terminology and Medical Word Building

INSTRUCTIONS: In the first few pages, you will learn the most efficient use of this self-instructional programmed learning approach.

First remove the sliding card and cover the colored answer column with it.

1-1 Programmed learning is made up of teaching units called frames. Each frame presents information and calls for an answer on your part. For example, complete the sentence below by writing the appropriate word on the blank line.

A frame consists of a block of information and a blank line on which you will

answer

write an _____ .

Slide the card down to see the correct answer.

After you correct the answer, read the next frame.

1-2 A frame consists of information and a blank line. The information

frame

presented after 1–1 and 1–2 is called a _____ .

Slide the card down to see the correct answer.

1-3 It is important to keep the answer column covered until you write your

answer

_____ .

1-4 This text is designed to help you learn medical terminology effectively. The principal technique used throughout the book is known as programmed learning, which consists of a series of teaching units called frames.

Several methods are employed in this book to help you master medical terminol-

learning

ogy, but the main technique used is called programmed _____ .

answer(s)

1–5 After you write your answer, it is important to verify its correctness. To do this, compare your answer with the one listed in the answer column.

To obtain immediate feedback on your responses, you must verify your

_____ .

INSTRUCTION FRAME: Study the frames in sequence because each frame builds on the previous one. Words will be reviewed and repeated throughout the textbook to reinforce your learning. Consequently, you do not need to memorize every word that is presented.

one

1–6 The number of blank lines in a frame determines the number of words you write for your answer. Review the number of blank lines in Frame 1–5. It has

_____ blank line(s). Therefore, the answer requires one word.

---

two, lines

1–7 A frame that requires two answers will have _____ blank _____ .

1–8 In some frames you will be asked to write the answer in your own words. In these instances, there will be one or more blank lines across the entire frame.

List at least two reasons why you want to learn medical terminology. Keep these objectives in mind as you work through the textbook.

_____

_____

INSTRUCTION FRAME: Do not peek at the answer column before you write your response and do not look ahead in a unit. Progress in developing a medical vocabulary depends on your ability to learn the material presented in each frame.

frame

1–9 Completing one frame at a time is the most effective method of learning. To achieve your goal of learning medical terminology, complete one

_____ at a time.

---

back

1–10 Whenever you make an error, it is important to go back and review the previous frame(s). You need to determine why you wrote the wrong answer before proceeding to the next frame.

You may always go _____ and review information you have forgotten. Just remember do not look ahead.

---

correct, check, or verify

1–11 Do not be afraid of making a mistake. In programmed learning, you will learn and profit by your mistakes if you correct them immediately.

Always _____ your answer immediately after you write it.

---

answer

1–12 Because accurate spelling is essential in the field of medicine, correct all misspelled words immediately. Do this by comparing your answer with the one in

the left-hand _____ column.

| correctly or accurately | **1–13** Correct spelling in a medical record can be a critical element in determining the validity of evidence presented in a lawsuit. A physician can lose a lawsuit simply because words were misspelled in a medical record.

Medical words must be spelled _____ in a medical record. |

BASIC ELEMENTS OF A MEDICAL WORD

| suffix, prefix | **1–14** To analyze medical words, you need to understand four elements that are used to form words. These four elements are the *word root*, the *combining form*, the *suffix*, and the *prefix*.

The four elements that form a medical word are the word root, combining form, _____ , and _____ . |

| elements or parts | **1–15** Medical terminology is not difficult to learn once you understand how the word elements are combined to form a word.

To develop a medical vocabulary, you must understand the _____ that form medical words. |

Word Roots

| teach | **1–16** A word root is the main part or foundation of a word; all words have at least one word root.

In the words **teach**er, **teach**es, **teach**ing, the word root is _____ . |

| speak | **1–17** In the words **speak**er, **speak**s, **speak**ing, the word root is _____ . |

| | **1–18** Identify the roots in the following words: |

	Word	*Root*
read	reader	_____
spend	spender	_____
play	player	_____

INFORMATIVE FRAME: A word root may be used alone or combined with other elements to form a complete word. Some examples are listed below.

Root as a Complete Word	*Root as a Part of a Word*
speak	**speak**er
alcohol	**alcohol**ism
insulin	**insulin**emia
lump	**lump**ectomy
sperm	**sperm**icidal

alcohol	**1–19** Throughout the textbook, a slash is used to separate word elements, as shown in the following examples. Identify the root in the examples.
dent	alcohol/ic _____
lump	dent/ist _____
insulin	lump/ectomy _____
gastr	insulin/ism _____
	gastr/itis _____

cardi	**1–20** In medical words, the root usually indicates a body part. For example, the root in cardi/al, cardi/ac, and cardi/o/gram is _____, and it means heart.

electr, cardi, -gram	**1–21** Electr/o/cardi/o/gram has two roots and a suffix. The two roots are _____ and _____. The suffix is _____ .

dent/al	**1–22** You will find that the roots in medical words are usually derived from Greek or Latin. Some examples are **dent** in the word dent/ist, **pancreat** in the word pancreat/itis, and **dermat** in the word dermat/o/logist.
pancreat/itis	Underline the roots in the following words:
dermat/o/logist	dent/al
	pancreat/itis
	dermat/o/logist

part	**1–23** In Frame 1–22, the root **dent** means tooth, **pancreat** means pancreas, and **dermat** means skin. All three roots indicate a body _____ .

Combining Forms

INFORMATIVE FRAME: The difficulty of pronouncing certain combinations of word roots requires the insertion of a vowel. For example, gastr/o/enter/itis; instead of joining the two word roots **gastr** and **enter** directly, insert the vowel **o** and say gastr/o/enter/itis. The word is now easy to pronounce.
　　Word roots and combining forms that stand alone are listed in bold throughout the frames in the textbook.

combining form	**1–24** When you take a word root and add a vowel (usually an **o**), the new word element is called a *combining form*.
	A word root plus a vowel is known as a _____ _____ .

combining form	**1–25** The vowel is called a *combining vowel*; the word root plus a vowel is called a _____ _____ .

therm/o	**1–26** The combining form in therm/o/meter is _____ / _____ .

combining form dent, o	**1-27** **Dent/o** is an example of a _____ _____ . The root in **dent/o** is _____ ; the combining vowel is _____ .

o
o
o
	1-28 List the combining vowel in each of the following elements.
	    arthr/o _____
	    phleb/o _____
	    lith/o _____

<u>therm</u>/o, <u>abdomin</u>/o,
  <u>nephr</u>/o
	1-29 Underline the word root in the following combining forms.
	    therm/o
	    abdomin/o
	    nephr/o

1-30 Use the combining vowel **o** to change the following roots to combining forms, and separate the elements with a slash.

	Root	*Combining Form (Root + Vowel)*
cyst/o	**cyst**	_____
arthr/o	**arthr**	_____
leuk/o	**leuk**	_____
gastr/o	**gastr**	_____

o	**1-31** Usually the combining vowel is an **o**, although other vowels may be encountered occasionally. The combining vowel in a word is usually an _____ .

1-32 Instead of joining the two word roots **speed** and **meter** directly, we add the combining vowel **o** to form the word speed/o/meter. Add a vowel to each of the word elements listed here. Recall that the vowel makes the word easier to pronounce.

	speed-meter becomes	speed/o/meter
micr/o/film (MĪ-krō-fīlm) phon/o/graph (FŌ-nō-graf) micr/o/scope (MĪ-krō-skōp)	micr-film becomes phon-graph becomes micr-scope becomes	_____ / ____ / _____ _____ / ____ / _____ _____ / ____ / _____

vowel	**1-33** Words in frame 1-32 are easy to pronounce because you added the combining vowel **o** to the root. To make a word easier to pronounce, add a combining _____ to the root.
elements or parts	**1-34** Even though you may or may not know the meaning of the words in this unit, you have already started to learn the word-building system by identifying the basic _____ of a medical word.

medical	**1–35** Using the word-building system to learn medical terminology will even help you understand complex medical terms. By identifying the basic elements of a medical word, you are on your way to learning _____ terminology using the word-building system.
micr micr/o	**1–36** In the word micr/o/scope, the root is _____ . The combining form is _____ / _____ .

INFORMATIVE FRAME: When a word has more than one root, a combining vowel is used to link the roots to each other. The roots in oste/o/arthr/itis are **oste** (bone) and **arthr** (joint). These two roots are linked together with the combining vowel **o.**

o	**1–37** In the word gastr/o/enter/itis, the roots **gastr** (stomach) and **enter** (intestine) are linked together with the combining vowel _____ .
leuk, cyt -penia	**1–38** The roots in leuk/o/cyt/o/penia are _____ and _____ . The suffix is _____ .
leuk/o, cyt/o	**1–39** Identify the combining forms in leuk/o/cyt/o/penia: _____ / _____ and _____ / _____ .
electr/o, cardi/o	**1–40** List the combining forms in electr/o/cardi/o/gram: _____ / _____ and _____ / _____ .
back	**1–41** You are now using the programmed learning method. If you are having difficulty writing the correct answers, go back to Frame 1–1 and rework the frames. To master material that has been covered, you can always go _____ to review the frames.

Suffixes

suffix	**1–42** A *suffix* is added to the end of a word root or combining form to modify its meaning. When a suffix stands alone throughout this textbook, it is highlighted in blue. The element that follows a word root and changes its meaning is a _____ .

play/er
read/er
speak/er
	1–43 **Play, read**, and **speak** are complete words and also roots. Add the suffix -er (meaning "one who") to each root to modify its meaning.
	    Play becomes _____ / _____ .
	    Read becomes _____ / _____ .
	    Speak becomes _____ / _____ .

1-44 By adding the suffix -er ("one who"), we create nouns that mean the following:

Play / er means one who plays.

one who

one who

Read / er means _____ _____ reads.

Speak / er means _____ _____ speaks.

1-45 If we were to add the suffix -able (meaning "capable of being"), we would create adjectives that mean the following:

capable of being

capable of being

capable of being

Play / able means _____ ____ _____ played.

Speak / able means _____ ____ _____ spoken.

Read / able means _____ ____ _____ read.

1-46 A combining vowel *is* used to link a root to a suffix that begins with a consonant. The awkwardness of pronunciation necessitates the insertion of a combining vowel.

Here are some examples:

scler / o / derma

mast / o / dynia

arthr / o / plasty

Scler-derma becomes _____ / ____ / _____ .

Mast-dynia becomes _____ / ____ / _____ .

Arthr-plasty becomes _____ / ____ / _____ .

1-47 A combining vowel is *not* used before a suffix that begins with a vowel.

Here are some examples:

tonsill / itis
(tŏn-sĭl-Ĭ-tĭs)
scler / osis
(sklĕ-RŌ-sĭs)
gastr / ectomy
(găs-TRĔK-tō-mē)
arthr / itis
(ăr-THRĪ / tĭs)

Tonsill-itis becomes _____ / _____ .

Scler-osis becomes _____ / _____ .

Gastr-ectomy becomes _____ / _____ .

Arthr-itis becomes _____ / _____ .

1-48 Changing the suffix changes the meaning of the word. In the word

root, suffix

dent / al, **dent** is the word _____ and -al is the _____ .

1-49 A dent / ist is a specialist in teeth. Dent / al means "pertaining to teeth." Simply changing the suffix has given the word a new meaning.

-ist

-al

The suffix in dent / ist is _____ . It means specialist.

The suffix in dent / al is _____ . It means pertaining to.

1-50 Throughout the textbook, whenever a suffix stands alone, it will be preceded with a hyphen, as in -oma (tumor). This indicates that another word part needs to be placed in front of the hyphen before a complete word is formed.

hyphen

A suffix that stands alone will be preceded with a _____ .

dent /<u>ist</u>
(DĔN-tĭst)
arthr /o /<u>centesis</u>
(ăr-thrō-sĕn-TĒ-sĭs)
polyp /<u>oid</u>
(PŎL-ē-poyd)
angi /<u>oma</u>
(ăn-jē-Ō-mă)
gastr /<u>ic</u>
(GĂS-trĭk)
nephr /<u>itis</u>
(nĕf-RĪ-tĭs)
scler /o /<u>derma</u>
(sklĕr-ō-DĔR-mă)

1–51 Underline the suffixes in the following words.

dent / ist

arthr /o /centesis

polyp /oid

angi /oma

gastr /ic

nephr /itis

scler /o /derma

---

arthr /o

scler /o

dent, polyp

angi, gastr, nephr

1–52 The element preceding a suffix can be either a word root or a combining form. Review Frame 1–51 and identify the following.

The combining forms that precede the suffixes: _____ / _____

and _____ / _____ .

The roots that precede the suffixes: _____ , _____ ,

_____ , _____ , _____ .

1–53 Analyze the following words by identifying their elements. The first one is completed for you.

Word	Combining Form	Root	Suffix
arthr /o /scop /ic	**arthr /o**	**scop**	-ic
dermat /itis	_____	_____	_____
append /ix	_____	_____	_____
vagin /itis	_____	_____	_____
oste /o /arthr /itis	_____	_____	_____
gastr /o /enter /itis	_____	_____	_____
orth /o /ped /ic	_____	_____	_____

The answers to this frame are in Appendix B, page 469.

---

suffixes

1–54 From the examples in Frame 1–53, you see that medical words can be formed by various combinations of combining forms, roots, and

_____ .

therm/o/meter
(thĕr-MŎM-ĕ-tĕr)
speed/o/meter
(spē-DŎM-ĕt-ĕr)
micr/o/scope
(MĪ-krō-skōp)

oste/o/arthr/itis
(ŏs-tē-ō-ăr-THRĪ-tĭs)

1–55   Recall that a combining vowel is used to link one word root to another word root.

Therm-meter becomes _____ / _____ / _____ .

Speed-meter becomes _____ / _____ / _____ .

Micr-scope becomes _____ / _____ / _____ .

Oste-arthr/itis becomes

_____ / _____ / _____ / _____ .

---

gastr/o/scope
(GĂS-trō-skōp)
men/o/rrhea
(mĕn-ō-RĒ-ă)
angi/o/rrhexis
(ăn-jē-ŏr-ĔK-sĭs)
ureter/o/lith
(ū-RĒ-tĕr-ō-lĭth)

1–56   Recall that a combining vowel is used before a suffix that begins with a consonant.

gastr-scope becomes _____ / _____ / _____ .

men-rrhea becomes _____ / _____ / _____ .

angi-rrhexis becomes _____ / _____ / _____ .

ureter-lith becomes _____ / _____ / _____ .

---

consonant

1–57   The suffixes -scope, -rrhexis, and -rrhea begin with a consonant. A combining vowel *is* used before a suffix that begins with

_____ .

---

leuk/emia
(loo-KĒ-mē-ă)
cephal/algia
(sĕf-ă-LĂL-jē-ă)
gastr/itis
(găs-TRĪ-tĭs)
append/ectomy
(ăp-ĕn-DĔK-tō-mē)

1–58   A combining vowel is *not* used before a suffix that begins with a vowel.

Leuk-emia becomes _____ / _____ .

Cephal-algia becomes _____ / _____ .

Gastr-itis becomes _____ / _____ .

Append-ectomy becomes _____ / _____ .

---

combining vowel,

combining form

1–59   The suffixes -algia, -edema, and -uria begin with a vowel. A _____ _____ or _____ _____ is *not* used before a suffix that begins with a vowel.

INFORMATIVE FRAME: The following two rules will help you write medical words correctly. Remember, however, that there are some exceptions to the rules. You will learn the exceptions as you progress through the units.

Rule 1: A combining vowel *is* used to link one root to another root, and before a suffix that begins with a consonant.
Rule 2: A combining vowel is *not* used before a suffix that begins with a vowel.

enter / o / cyst / o / plasty
(ĕn-tĕr-ō-SĬS-tō-plăs-tē)
Rule 1

leuk / o / cyt / o / penia
(loo-kō-sī-tō-PĒ-nē-ă)
Rule 1

erythr / o / cyt / osis
(ĕ-rĭth-rō-sī-TŌ-sĭs)
Rules 1, 2

oste / o / arthr / itis
(ŏs-tē-ō-ăr-THRĪ-tĭs)
Rules 1, 2

1-60 Here are some examples applying the two rules.

enter-cyst-plasty becomes

_____ / _____ / _____ / _____ / _____ .

(Rule(s) _____)

leuk-cyt-penia becomes

_____ / _____ / _____ / _____ / _____ .

(Rule(s) _____)

erythr-cyt-osis becomes

_____ / _____ / _____ / _____ .

(Rule(s) _____)

oste-arthr-itis becomes

_____ / _____ / _____ / _____ .

(Rule(s) _____)

---

root, suffix

1-61 You may or may not already know the meaning of the suffixes listed in this unit. It is not necessary for you to know what they mean yet. These terms and definitions will be reviewed in later units. What is important now is that you understand how to divide words into their component parts (prefix, root, combining form, suffix). For example, in the term pancreat / itis, **pancreat** is the

_____ ; -itis is the _____ .

---

cardi / o / gram
(KĂR-dē-ō-grăm)

A combining vowel is used before a suffix that begins with a consonant.

1-62 Form a word with cardi-gram.

_____ / _____ / _____

(root)   (suffix)

Summarize the rule that applies.

_____

_____ .

---

carcin / oma
(kăr-sĭ-NŌ-mă)

A combining vowel is not used before a suffix that begins with a vowel.

1-63 Form a word with carcin-oma. _____ / _____

(root)   (suffix)

Summarize the rule that applies.

_____

_____ .

---

suffix

1-64 Suffixes added to word roots indicate which part of speech the word is. A word can be changed from a noun to an adjective simply by changing the suffix.

To alter the part of speech of a word, you change the _____ .

-ic -ist -ia	**1–65** List the suffixes in the following words. gastr/ic _____ (adjective ending) dent/ist _____ (noun ending) pneumon/ia _____ (noun ending)

Prefixes

impatient implant	**1–66** A *prefix* is a syllable or syllables placed before a word or word root to alter its meaning or create a new word. If we place the prefix im- before **patient** and **plant**, we create new words that have different meanings. Patient becomes _____ / _____ . Plant becomes _____ / _____ .
prefix	**1–67** Recall that a word element located at the beginning of a word is known as a _____ .

SUMMARY FRAME: Throughout the frames in the textbook, prefixes that stand alone are highlighted in pink; word roots and combining forms that stand alone are highlighted in bold; and suffixes that stand alone are highlighted in blue.

intra- post- peri- pre-	**1–68** Intra/muscul/ar, post/nat/al, peri/card/itis, and pre/operative are medical terms that have prefixes. Determine the prefix for each word in this frame. _____ _____ _____ _____
prefix root suffix	**1–69** Recall that whenever a prefix stands alone, it will be identified with a hyphen after it, as in hyper-, and will be highlighted pink. When it is part of a word, the prefix will not be highlighted but a slash will separate it from the next element. Analyze hyper/insulin/ism by identifying the elements. hyper- is a _____ . insulin is a _____ . -ism is a _____ .
prefixes	**1–70** Hypo-, intra-, super-, and homo- are examples of _____ .
after	**1–71** Pre/operative designates the time before a surgery. By changing the prefix, you change the meaning of the word. Because pre- means before, can you guess what post- in post/operative means? _____

post-, after after	**1–72** You will recognize many prefixes in medical terms because they are the same prefixes used in ordinary English. In the term, post/mortem, the prefix is _____ and means _____ . Post/mortem means _____ death.

pre-, before, before	**1–73** In the term pre/mature, the prefix is _____ and means _____ . Pre/mature means _____ maturity.

INFORMATIVE FRAME: Some words can also be used as suffixes. For example, mature and sex are both words that are used as suffixes in the words pre/mature and uni/sex. Other words might consist of just a prefix and a word root, as in pre/test and dis/charge.

	1–74 Use the following word roots with the adjective ending -al to form words that mean **pertaining to**. The first word is completed for you.

	Word Root	*Word*	*Meaning*	
	rect	rect/al	pertaining to the rectum	
dent/al, pertaining to	**dent**	_____ / ____	_____ _____ the teeth	
gastr/al, pertaining to	**gastr**	_____ / ____	_____ _____ the stomach	
intestin/al, pertaining to	**intestin**	_____ / ____	_____ _____ the intestines	

SUMMARY FRAME: Combinations of four elements are used to form medical words. These four elements are the word root, combining form, suffix, and prefix. Some words can also be used as suffixes. Other words may consist of just a prefix and a word root.

Review A

Identify the basic elements of each word in the appropriate box. Write the suffix first. Then write the element(s) in the first part(s) of the word. Remember, it is not important for you to know the meaning of the words in this unit, but you should understand how to divide them into their basic elements. The first word is completed for you.

| Medical Word and Meaning | BASIC ELEMENTS OF A MEDICAL WORD | | | |
	Prefix	Combining Form(s) (root + vowel)	Word Roots(s)	Suffix
p e r i / d e n t / al around teeth pertaining to (pĕr-ĭ-DĔN-tăl)	peri-		dent	-al
a b / n o r m / a l away usual pertaining to from normal (ăb-NŎR-măl)				
h e p a t / i t i s liver inflammation (hĕp-ă-TĪ-tĭs)				
s u p r a / r e n / a l above kidney pertaining to (SOO-pră-RĒ-năl)				
t r a n s / v a g i n /a l across vagina pertaining to (trăns-VĂJ-ĭn-ăl)				
g a s t r / o / i n t e s t i n /a l stomach intestine pertaining to (găs-trō-ĭn-TĔS-tĭ-năl)				
m a c r o /c e p h a l / i c large head pertaining to (măk-rō-sĕf-ĂL-ĭk)				
r e n / o / p a t h y kidney disease (rē-NŎP-ă-thē)				
t h e r m / o / m e t e r heat instrument to measure (thĕr-MŎM-ĕ-tĕr)				
h e p a t / o / m e g a l y liver enlargement (hĕp-ă-tō-MĔG-ă-lē)				
s u b / s t e r n / a l under sternum pertaining to below (sŭb-STĔR-năl)				
h y p o / i n s u l i n / i s m under insulin condition below (hī-pō-ĬN-sū-lĭn-ĭzm)				
g a s t r / o / e n t e r / o / p a t h y stomach intestine disease (găs-trō-ĕn-tĕr-Ŏ-pă-thē)				

| | BASIC ELEMENTS OF A MEDICAL WORD | | | |
Medical Word and Meaning	Prefix	Combining Form(s) (root + vowel)	Word Roots(s)	Suffix
arteri/o/scler/ osis artery hardening abnormal condition (ăr-tē-rē-ō-sklĕ-RŌ-sĭs)				
hypo/derm/ic under skin pertaining to (hī-pō-DĔR-mĭc)				

Check your answers with Review A Answer Key, page 469.

Review B

Use the basic elements in the Review A Answer Key, page 469, to form words. The first word is completed for you.

peridental _____

_____

_____

_____

_____

_____

_____

_____

_____

_____

_____

_____

_____

Check your answers with Review B Answer Key, page 469.

REINFORCEMENT FRAME: If you are not satisfied with your level of comprehension, go back to 1–1 and rework the frames.

FORMING ADJECTIVE, NOUN, DIMINUTIVE, AND PLURAL SUFFIXES

The following suffixes are added to word roots to indicate either a part of speech or a singular or plural form of a word.

Adjective Suffixes

The adjective suffixes that mean "pertaining to" and/or "relating to," or both, are:

Adjective Suffix	Example
-ac*	cardi/ac heart
-al	neur/al nerve
-ar	muscul/ar muscle
-ary	saliv/ary saliva
-eal	mening/eal meninges
-ic	hypo/derm/ic under skin
-ical[†]	med/ical medicine
-ory	audit/ory hearing
-ous[‡]	cutane/ous skin
-tic	acous/tic sound

* -ac ending is rarely used
[†] -ical is a combination of -ic and -al
[‡] -ous also means composed of, producing

Noun Suffixes

The suffixes added to word roots to indicate a noun are:

Noun Suffix	Meaning	Example
-ia	condition (of)	pneumon/ia lung
-iatry	treatment, medicine	pod/iatry foot
-is	forms the noun from the root	pelv/is pelvis
-ism	condition (of)	alcohol/ism alcohol
-ist	specialist	uro/log/ist urology study (of)
-y	condition (of)	path/y disease

Diminutive Suffixes

A diminutive ending forms a word designating a small version of an object indicated by the word root.

Diminutive Suffix	Meaning	Example
-ole -icle -ula -ule	small, minute	arteri/ole artery part/icle piece mac/ula spot ven/ule vein

Plural Suffixes

The rules for forming plural words from singular words are listed below.

Singular Form	Plural Form	Rule	EXAMPLE Singular	Plural
a	ae	Retain the a and add e	pleura	pleurae
ax	aces	Drop the x and add ces	thorax	thoraces
en	ina	Drop en and add ina	lumen	lumina
is	es	Drop the is and add es	diagnosis	diagnoses
ix ex	ices	Drop the ix or ex and add ices	appendix apex	appendices apices
on	a	Drop on and add a	ganglion	glanglia
um	a	Drop um and add a	bacterium	bacteria
us	i	Drop us and add i	bronchus	bronchi
y	ies	Drop y and add ies	deformity	deformities
ma	mata	Retain the ma and add ta	carcinoma	carcinomata

Review C

Write the plural form for each of the following words and state the rule that applies.

Singular	Plural	Rule
1. sarcoma	sarcomata	Retain the *ma* and add *ta*
2. thrombus	_____	_____
3. appendix	_____	_____
4. diverticulum	_____	_____
5. ovary	_____	_____
6. diagnosis	_____	_____
7. lumen	_____	_____
8. vertebra	_____	_____
9. thorax	_____	_____
10. spermatozoon	_____	_____

Check your answers with Review C Answer Key, page 469.

Digestive System

The digestive system is also referred to as the alimentary or gastrointestinal (GI) tract. It consists of organs and glands whose purpose is to break down food products that can be used by the body as a source of energy and to eliminate solid waste substances.

The GI tract forms a tube that begins at the mouth, where food enters the body. It ends at the anus, where solid waste substances are eliminated from the body (Fig. 2–1).

The combining forms related to the digestive system are summarized here. Review this information before you begin to work the frames.

COMBINING FORMS

Oral Cavity

Combining Form	Meaning	Example	Pronunciation
or/o	mouth	or/al pertaining to	ŎR-ăl
stomat/o		stomat/itis inflammation	stō-mă-TĪ-tĭs
gloss/o	tongue	gloss/ectomy excision	glŏs-ĔK-tō-mē
lingu/o		lingu/al pertaining to	LĬNG-gwăl
dent/o	teeth	dent/ist specialist	DĔN-tĭst
odont/o		orth/odont/ist straight specialist	ŏr-thō-DŎN-tĭst
gingiv/o	gum(s)	gingiv/itis inflammation	jĭn-jĭ-VĪ-tĭs

Pharynx and Esophagus

Combining Form	Meaning	Example	Pronunciation
esophag/o	esophagus	esophag/o/scope instrument to examine	ē-SŎF-ă-gō-skōp
gastr/o	stomach	gastr/o/scopy visual examination	găs-TRŎS-kō-pē
pharyng/o	pharynx	pharyng/itis inflammation	făr-ĭn-JĪ-tĭs
pylor/o	pylorus	pylor/o/tomy incision, cut into	pī-lŏr-ŎT-ō-mē

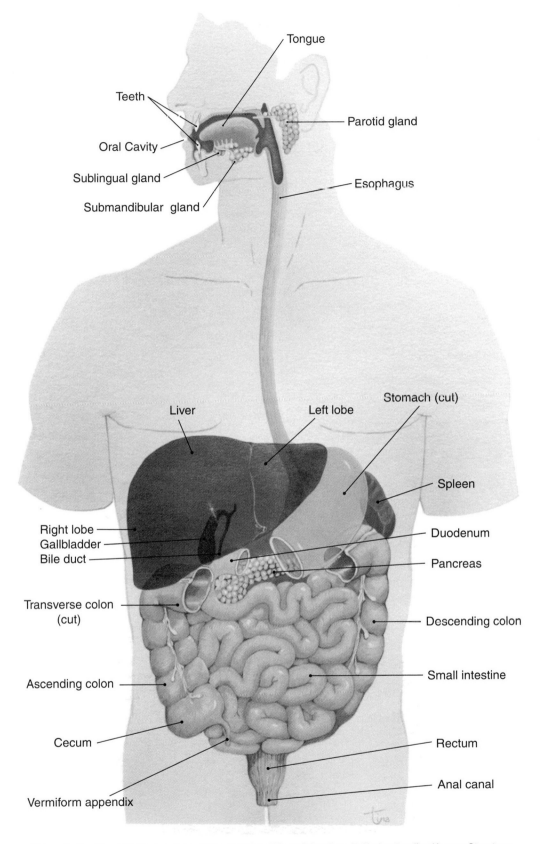

Figure 2–1. The digestive system. (From Scanlon, VC, and Sanders, T: Understanding Human Structure and Function. FA Davis, Philadelphia, 1997, p 285, with permission.)

Small Intestine and Colon (Large Intestine)

Combining Form	Meaning	Example	Pronunciation
an/o	anus	anal pertaining to	Ā-nŭs
append/o		append/ectomy excision	ăp-ĕn-DĔK-tō-mē
appendic/o	appendix	appendic/itis inflammation	ă-pĕn-dĭ-SĪ-tĭs

col/o
colon/o
	colon	col/o/centesis
		    puncture
		colon/o/scope
		    instrument to view or
		    examine
			kō-lō-sĕn-TĒ-sĭs
			
			kō-LŎN-ō-skōp

duoden/o	duodenum	duoden/o/stomy
		    forming an opening
		    (mouth)
			doo-ŏd-ĕn-ŎS-tō-mē

enter/o	intestines (usually small intestine)	enter/o/pathy disease	ĕn-tĕr-ŎP-ă-thē
ile/o	ileum	ile/o/stomy forming an opening (mouth)	ĭl-ē-ŎS-tō-mē
jejun/o	jejunum	jejun/o/rrhaphy suture	jē-joo-NŎR-ă-fē
proct/o	anus, rectum	proct/o/logist specialist in the study (of)	prŏk-TŎL-ō-jĭst
rect/o	rectum	rect/o/cele hernia, swelling	RĔK-tō-sēl
sigmoid/o	sigmoid colon	sigmoid/o/scopy visual examination	sĭg-moy-DŎS-kō-pē

DIGESTIVE TRACT

Oral Cavity

2–1 Examine the Index of Medical Word Elements, Part A of Appendix A, and use it to find the meanings of the following word elements that are used in this unit. Write the meaning of each element in the appropriate blank.

Medical Word Element	Meaning
-al	_____
-algia	_____
-dynia	_____
-ic	_____
stomat/o	_____
or/o	_____

2–2 Examine the Index of Medical Word Elements, Part B of Appendix A. Use it to learn the medical word element for each of the following English terms that are used in this unit.

English Term	*Medical Word Element*
flow, discharge	_____
jaw	_____
through	_____

2–3 The chemical and mechanical process of digestion begins in the **(1) oral cavity** or **mouth**, when food is chewed to make it easier to swallow.

Label the oral cavity in Figure 2–2.

stomat/o

or/o

2–4 The combining forms for the mouth are **or/o** and **stomat/o**. From stomat/itis, construct the combining form for mouth:

_____ / _____ .

From or/al, construct a combining form for mouth: _____ / _____ .

stomat/itis

2–5 The suffix -itis refers to inflammation. It is used in all body systems to describe an inflammation of a particular organ. Combine **stomat/o** and -itis to form a word meaning inflammation of the mouth:

_____ / _____ .

A combining vowel is not used to link a suffix that begins with a vowel.

2–6 Recall the reason you used the word root rather than the combining form before the suffix -itis. Briefly state the rule.

_____

_____

stomat/al
(STŌ-mă-tăl)

or/al
(ŎR-ăl)

2–7 Two adjective suffixes that mean pertaining to are -ic and -al.

Combine **stomat/o** and -al to form a word meaning pertaining to the mouth:

_____ / _____

Combine **or/o** and -al to form a word meaning pertaining to the mouth:

_____ / _____

A combining vowel is not used to link a suffix that begins with a vowel.

2–8 Recall why, in the word or/al, you used the word root (**or**) rather than the combining form (**or/o**) before the suffix -al. Briefly, state the rule.

_____

_____

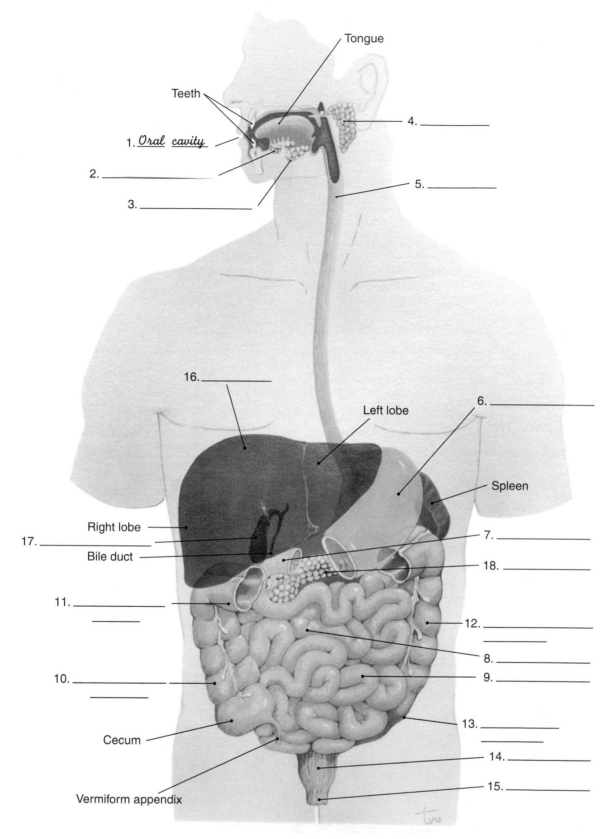

Tongue

Teeth

1. *Oral cavity*

2. _____

3. _____

4. _____

5. _____

16. _____

Left lobe

6. _____

Spleen

Right lobe

17. _____

Bile duct

7. _____

18. _____

11. _____
_____

12. _____
_____

8. _____

10. _____
_____

9. _____

Cecum

13. _____
_____

14. _____

Vermiform appendix

15. _____

Figure 2–2. The digestive system. (Adapted from Scanlon, VC, and Sanders, T: Understanding Human Structure and Function. FA Davis, Philadelphia, 1997, p 285, with permission.)

stomat, mouth	**2–9** A medical word may be simply a word root, or it may be various combinations of elements. In the words stomat/al, stomat/itis, and stomat/ic the word root is _____ . It refers to the _____ .
pain, mouth **pain, mouth**	**2–10** The suffixes -dynia and -algia refer to pain. Stomat/o/dynia is a _____ in the _____ . Stomat/algia is a _____ in the _____ .
combining vowel or combining form	**2–11** The suffixes -dynia and -algia are used interchangeably. Because -algia begins with a vowel, a combining vowel is *not* used to link the suffix to the word root. Because -dynia begins with a consonant, a _____ _____ *is* used to link the suffix.
stomat/o/dynia (stō-mă-tō-DĬN-ē-ă) **stomat/algia** (stō-mă-TĂL-jē-ă)	**2–12** Use **stomat/o** to develop a word meaning pain in the mouth: _____ / _____ / _____ or _____ / _____
sial/o	**2–13** During the chewing process, the salivary glands secrete saliva. These juices begin the chemical breakdown of food. The combining form **sial/o** refers to saliva or the salivary glands. From sial/ic (pertaining to saliva), construct the combining form for saliva or salivary gland: _____ / _____
sial/itis	**2–14** Use **sial/o** + -itis to form a word meaning an inflammation of a salivary gland: _____ / _____
-rrhea	**2–15** The suffix -rrhea is used in words to mean flow or discharge. From sial/o/rrhea, write the element that means flow or discharge: _____ .
saliva **discharge**	**2–16** Sial/o/rrhea is a condition in which there is an excessive flow of saliva. Analyze sial/o/rrhea by defining the elements. **Sial/o** refers to the salivary glands or _____ . -rrhea refers to flow or _____ .
through **flow or discharge**	**2–17** Dia- is a prefix meaning through. Dia/rrhea is a frequent passage of watery bowel movements. Analyze dia/rrhea by defining the elements. dia- means _____ . -rrhea means _____ or _____ .

dia/rrhea (dī-ă-RĒ-ă)	**2–18** A person with an irritable bowel may experience a frequent passage of watery bowel movements or _____ / _____ .

dia/rrhea (dī-ă-RĒ-ă)	**2–19** Some foods, such as prunes, are likely to cause _____ / _____ .

2–20 Use the Index of Medical Word Elements in Part A of Appendix A as a guide to complete this frame. It is a handy reference to use whenever you are in doubt about a word element or need help to recall a definition. Another useful reference is Appendix E, which provides a list of abbreviations.

Medical Word Elements	Meaning
-ary	_____
gastr/o	_____
lingu/o	_____
myc/o	_____
peri-	_____
sub-	_____

2–21 There are three pairs of salivary glands: the **(2) sublingual**, the **(3) submandibular** or **submaxillary**, and the **(4) parotid glands**. Saliva is secreted by these glands into the oral cavity by way of narrow ducts.

Label the salivary glands in Figure 2–2.

tongue	**2–22** The combining form **lingu/o** refers to the tongue; the prefix sub- means under. Sub/lingu/al means pertaining to under the _____ .

jaw	**2–23** The combining form **maxill/o** refers to the jaw. Sub/maxill/ary means pertaining to under the _____ .

-ary	**2–24** From sub/maxill/ary, determine the element that means pertaining to: _____

pertaining to	**2–25** The suffixes -ary, -al , and -ic are adjective endings meaning _____ _____ .

below below above	**2–26** Refer to Figure 2–1 and use the directional words "below" or "above" to complete this frame. The sub/lingu/al gland is located _____ the tongue. The sub/maxill/ary, also known as the sub/mandibul/ar gland is located _____ the jaw. The tongue is located _____ the esophagus.

| lingu/o | **2–27** From sub/lingu/al, construct the combining form for tongue:

_____ / _____ . |

INFORMATIVE FRAME: When defining a medical word, first define the suffix. Second, define the beginning of the word; finally, define the middle of the word. Take the example of sub/maxill/ary:

(2) (3)   (1)

1. Define the suffix first; -ary means "pertaining to."
2. Define the beginning of the word; sub- means "under" or "below."
3. Define the middle of the word; **maxill** means "jaw."

| suffix

beginning

last | **2–28** The element that is defined first is the _____ .

The element that is defined next is the _____ of the word.

The middle or rest of the word is defined _____ . |

| -al

sub-

lingu | **2–29** Use the technique described in the previous informative frame to define sub/lingu/al:

Write the element that is defined first: _____

Write the element that is defined next: _____

Write the element that is defined last: _____ |

| pertaining to,

tongue | **2–30** Lingu/o/dent/al means _____ _____ the

_____ and teeth. |

| dent | **2–31** From lingu/o/dent/al, determine the word root for teeth: _____ |

| abnormal condition,

mouth | **2–32** The suffix -osis refers to an abnormal condition. Stomat/osis literally means an _____ _____ of the

_____ . |

| stomat/osis

stomat/itis | **2–33** Use **stomat/o** to form medical words meaning an abnormal condition of the mouth: _____ / _____

inflammation of the mouth: _____ / _____ |

| myc | **2–34** Stomat/o/myc/osis is an abnormal condition of a mouth fungus. From stomat/o/myc/osis, identify the root meaning fungus: _____ . |

| abnormal
condition, fungus | **2–35** Myc/osis literally means an _____

_____ of a _____ . |

abnormal condition fungus	**2–36** Whenever you see -osis in a word, you will know it means an _____ _____ . Whenever you see **myc/o** in a word, you will know it refers to a _____ .
specialist	**2–37** Recall that medical words are defined by reading first the back, then the front of the word. The noun ending suffix -ist refers to a specialist. A dent/ist is a _____ in teeth.
dent/o	**2–38** From dent/ist, construct the combining form for teeth: _____ / _____ .
-logist	**2–39** The combining form **log/o** means "study of." Combine **log/o** and -ist to form a new suffix meaning specialist in the study of: _____
specialist specialist	**2–40** Two noun suffixes that you will often use to form medical words are: -logy study of -logist specialist in the study of A cardi/o/logist is a _____ in the study of the heart. A gastr/o/logist is a _____ in the study of the stomach.
gastr/o	**2–41** From gastr/o/logist, determine the combining form for stomach: _____ / _____ .
gastr/o/logy (găs-TRŎL-ō-jē) cardi/o/logy (kăr-dē-ŎL-ō-jē)	**2–42** Refer to Frame 2–40 to form medical words meaning study of the stomach: _____ / _____ / _____ study of the heart: _____ / _____ / _____
stomach (STŬM-ăk)	**2–43** A gastr/o/logist treats diseases of the _____ .
gastr/o/logist (găs-TRŎL-ō-jĭst)	**2–44** The specialist who determines that a person has a stomach disorder is a _____ / _____ / _____ .
gastr/o/intestin/al (găs-trō-ĭn-TĔS-tĭn-ăl) cancer (KĂN-sĕr)	**2–45** Refer to Appendix E: Abbreviations, to complete this frame. GI means _____ / _____ / _____ / _____ . CA means _____ .

dent / o	**2–46** The combining form for teeth is _____ / ___ .

pain, tooth odont / algia (ō-dŏn-TĂL-jē-ă)	**2–47** Another combining form for teeth is **odont / o**. Odont / algia literally means _____ in a _____ . A toothache is another word for odont / o / dynia or _____ / _____ .

specialist, teeth	**2–48** **Orth / o** refers to straight. Orth / odont / ist literally means _____ in straight _____ .

odont orth -ist	**2–49** From orth / odont / ist, determine the following word root for teeth: _____ word root for straight: _____ element meaning specialist: _____

orth / odont / ist (ŏr-thō-DŎN-tĭst)	**2–50** A person who has crooked teeth should see the specialist known as an _____ / _____ / _____ .

orth / odont / ist (ŏr-thō-DŎN-tĭst)	**2–51** A person who needs braces to straighten his or her teeth should see a specialist known as an _____ / _____ / _____ .

	2–52 Use the Index of Medical Word Elements in Part A of Appendix A to define peri / odont / itis. (Use the index whenever you need help to work the frames.) -itis refers to _____ . (suffix) peri- refers to _____ . (prefix) **odont** refers to _____ . (root)

dent / o, odont / o	**2–53** The two combining forms for teeth are _____ / ___ and _____ / ___ .

gingiv / o	**2–54** Gingiv / itis is a general term for inflammation of the gums. It is usually caused by an accumulation of food particles in the crevices between the gum and teeth. From gingiv / itis, construct the combining form for gums: _____ / ___ .

gingiv / itis (jĭn-jĭ-VĪ-tĭs)	**2–55** Form a word that means an inflammation of the gums. _____ / _____

inflammation, teeth inflammation, gums	**2–56** One of the primary symptoms of gingiv/itis is bleeding of the gums. This condition can lead to a more serious disorder, peri/odont/itis. Gingiv/itis is best prevented by correct brushing of the teeth and proper gum care. Peri/odont/itis is an _____ around the _____ . Gingiv/itis is an _____ of the _____ .

-osis
 	
-ist
 	
-logist
	2–57 Three suffixes introduced in this unit were -osis , and -ist , and -logist . Identify the suffix that means
	
	    abnormal condition: _____
	
	    specialist: _____
	
	    specialist in the study of: _____

gingiv/osis
(jĭn-jĭ-VŌ-sĭs)
dent/ist
 	
orth/odont/ist
(ŏr-thō-DŎN-tĭst)
	2–58 Develop words to mean
	
	    an abnormal condition of the gums: _____ / _____
	
	    specialist in teeth: _____ / _____
	
	    specialist in straightening teeth: _____ / _____ / _____

tooth pain, tooth	**2–59** Dent/algia is a toothache. Literally, it means pain in a _____ . Dent/o/dynia also means _____ in a _____ .

Review

Select the medical word element(s) that match(es) the meaning.

dent/o	-al	dia-
gastr/o	-algia	peri-
gingiv/o	-ary	sub-
lingu/o	-dynia	
maxill/o	-ist	
myc/o	-itis	
odont/o	-osis	
or/o	-rrhea	
orth/o		
sial/o		
stomat/o		

a. _____ abnormal condition

b. _____ pertaining to (adjective)

c. _____ around

d. _____ below, under

e. _____ flow, discharge

f. _____ fungus

g. _____ gums

h. _____ jaw

i. _____ mouth

j. _____ pain

k. _____ saliva, salivary glands

l. _____ stomach

m. _____ specialist

n. _____ straight

o. _____ teeth

p. _____ through

q. _____ tongue

Check your answers with the Review Answer Key on the following page.

Review Answer Key

a. -osis

b. -al, -ary

c. peri-

d. sub-

e. -rrhea

f. myc/o

g. gingiv/o

h. maxill/o

i. or/o, stomat/o

j. -algia, -dynia

k. sial/o

l. gastr/o

m. -ist

n. orth/o

o. dent/o, odont/o

p. dia-

q. lingu/o

REINFORCEMENT FRAME: If you are not satisfied with your level of comprehension, go back to Frame 2–1 and rework the frames. **You can also make flash cards on 3 by 5 index cards for the word elements in the unit. Use the cards to reinforce your retention of the word elements. First, compile the cards for the word elements included in the review you are completing, and review those elements. Then complete and correct the review. If you are not satisfied with the score, review the flash cards again before retaking the review. Follow this procedure each time you are ready to complete a review. The flash cards can also be used before you complete the Unit Exercises at the end of each unit.**

Pharynx, Esophagus, Stomach

2-60 Food continues its descent down the **(5) esophagus** to the stomach. In the **(6) stomach**, undigested food is mixed with gastric juices to further break it down into a liquid mass called **chyme**. Label Figure 2–2 to learn the parts of the digestive system.

---

esophagus
(ē-SŎF-ă-gŭs)
chyme
(KĬM)

2-61 Identify the tube that transports food from the mouth to the stomach:

_____ .

Gastr/ic juices break down food into a liquid mass called _____ .

---

gastr/o

2-62 From gastr/ic (pertaining to the stomach), construct the combining form for stomach: _____ / _____ .

---

esophag/o

2-63 Esophag/itis can be caused by excessive acid production in the stomach. From esophag/itis, construct the combining form for esophagus:

_____ / _____ .

---

gastr/itis
(găs-TRĪ-tĭs)

2-64 Combine **gastr/o** and **-itis** to form a word meaning an inflammation of the stomach. Remember to drop the combining vowel because the suffix begins with a vowel. _____ / _____ .

---

gastr/itis
(găs-TRĪ-tĭs)

2-65 A gastr/ic ulcer (Fig. 2–3) resembles a punched-out round sore, which may cause gastr/itis and ulcers. An important factor of a gastric ulcer is oversecretion of stomach acids, but alcoholic beverages and smoking are also related to an increased incidence of ulcers.

Build a medical word meaning inflammation of the stomach:

_____ / _____ .

---

gastr/algia
(găs-TRĂL-jē-ă)

2-66 Gastr/o/dynia is the medical term for pain in the stomach.

Form another word that means pain in the stomach: _____ / _____ .

---

inflammation

stomach, esophagus

2-67 Gastr/o/esophag/itis is an _____ of the

_____ and _____ .

-rrhea

2-68 Gastr/o/rrhea is an excessive secretion of gastric juice. The element in this word that means "flow" or "discharge" is _____ .

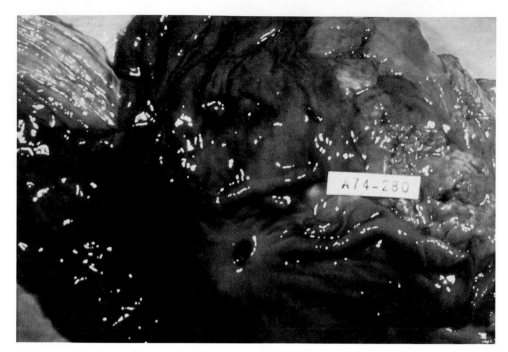

Figure 2–3. Gastric ulcer. (From WRS Group, with permission.)

gastr/itis
(găs-TRĪ-tĭs)

2–69 Build a medical word meaning an inflammation of the stomach:

_____ / _____ .

2–70 Use your medical dictionary to define *lesion*.

_____

_____

duoden/al
(dū-ō-DĒ-năl)
gastr/ic
(GĂS-trĭk)

2–71 Peptic ulcers are lesions. They are found in the lining of the stomach or first part of the small intestine. Peptic ulcers that occur in the small intestine are known as duoden/al ulcers; peptic ulcers that occur in the stomach are known as gastr/ic ulcers (Fig. 2–3).

Build medical words meaning

pertaining to the duodenum: _____ / _____

pertaining to the stomach: _____ / _____

surgery

2–72 Surgery is a branch of medicine that treats diseases, injuries, and deformities by manual or operative methods. The branch of medicine that is concerned with operative procedures is known as _____ .

mouth

2–73 The surgical suffix -plasty is used in words to mean surgical repair. Stomat/o/plasty is a surgical repair of the _____ .

esophag/o/plasty (ē-SŎF-ă-gō-plăs-tē) gastr/o/plasty (GĂS-trō-plăs-tē)	**2–74** Form medical words meaning surgical repair of the esophagus: _____ / ____ / _____ surgical repair of the stomach: _____ / ____ / _____

INFORMATIVE FRAME: The surgical suffixes that refer to cutting are listed here. Use this information to complete Frames 2–75 through 2–84.

Surgical Suffix	*Meaning*
-ectomy	excision, removal
-tomy	incision, cut into
-tome	instrument to cut

esophagus (ē-SŎF-ă-gŭs)	**2–75** Whenever you see a suffix or word with **tom** in it, relate it to cutting. An esophag/o/tome is an instrument to cut the _____ .
esophag/o/tome (ē-SŎF-ă-gō-tōm)	**2–76** When a surgeon wants to cut or incise the esophagus, the physician will ask for the instrument called an _____ / ____ / _____ .
-ectomy	**2–77** Partial or total gastr/ectomy is often performed for stomach cancer. From gastr/ectomy, identify the element meaning excision or removal: _____ .
gastr/ectomy (găs-TRĔK-tō-mē)	**2–78** The surgical procedure for removal of the stomach is called a _____ / _____ .
gastr -ectomy	**2–79** Partial or total gastr/ectomy is often performed for stomach cancer. From gastr/ectomy, identify the element meaning stomach: _____ excision or removal: _____
gastr/ectomy (găs-TRĔK-tō-mē)	**2–80** A perforated (punctured) stomach ulcer may also require a partial _____ / _____ .
stomach	**2–81** A gastr/o/tome is an instrument to cut or incise the _____ .

gastr / o / tome (GĂS-trō-tōm)	**2–82** When there is a need to cut or incise the stomach, the physician will use an instrument called a _____ / _____ / _____ .
esophagus (ē-SŎF-ă-gŭs)	**2–83** An esophag / o / tomy is an incision of the _____ .
gastr / o / tomy (găs-TRŎT-ō-mē)	**2–84** Develop a word meaning incision of the stomach: _____ / _____ / _____
carcin / o	**2–85** Whenever **carcin / o** is used in a word it means cancer. From carcin / oma, construct the combining form for cancer: _____ / _____ .
-ous	**2–86** Cancer / ous means pertaining to cancer. Identify the adjective element meaning pertaining to: _____ .
cancerous or malignant -oma	**2–87** A carcin / oma is a tumor that is _____ . Determine the element meaning tumor: _____

cancer
tumor
	2–88 Often, a patient has an organ removed because of a carcin / oma. Analyze carcin / oma by defining the elements.
	    carcin / o refers to _____ .
	    -oma refers to _____ .

cancer	**2–89** CA is an abbreviation for cancer. When you see CA in a medical chart, you will know it means _____ .

gastr / itis
(găs-TRĪ-tĭs)
epi / gastr / ic
(ĕp-ĭ-GĂS-trĭk)
	2–90 A prefix meaning above or upon is epi-. An epi / gastr / ic pain may result from an acute form of gastr / itis.
	Identify the words in this frame meaning
	    inflammation of the stomach: _____ / _____
	    pertaining to above the stomach: _____ / _____ / _____

2–91 **Hemat/o** refers to blood. A person suffering from acute gastr/itis may vomit blood (hemat/emesis), belch, or experience a loss of appetite.

Determine the words in this frame that mean

hemat/emesis
(hĕm-ăt-ĔM-ĕ-sĭs)
gastr/itis
(găs-TRĪ-tĭs)

vomiting blood: _____ / _____

inflammation of the stomach: _____ / _____

REMINDER FRAME: Use the Index of Medical Words Elements, in Appendix A, or your medical dictionary when you need help to work a frame.

hyper/emesis
(hī-pĕr-ĔM-ĕ-sĭs)

2–92 Besides being used as a suffix, **emesis** is a word that means vomiting. Combine hyper- (excessive) + -emesis to form a word meaning excessive vomiting: _____ / _____ .

hemat/o

2–93 From hemat/emesis, build a combining form that means blood:

_____ / _____ .

hemat/emesis
(hĕm-ăt-ĔM-ĕ-sĭs)

2–94 Bleeding in the stomach may be due to a gastric ulcer, and the patient may vomit blood. This condition is known as _____ / _____ .

above, upon
stomach
pertaining to

2–95 The most common symptom of gastr/ic disease is epi/gastr/ic pain. Analyze epi/gastr/ic by defining the elements.

epi- means _____ or _____ .

gastr/o means _____ .

-ic means _____ _____ .

-pepsia
dys-

2–96 Dys/pepsia literally means painful or difficult digestion and is a form of gastric indigestion. It is not a disease in itself but may be symptomatic of other diseases or disorders. Determine the elements in this frame that mean

digestion: _____

bad, painful, or difficult: _____

dys/pepsia
(dĭs-PĔP-sē-ă)

2–97 Over-the-counter antacids (agents that neutralize acidity) usually provide prompt relief of pain from _____ / _____ .

dys/phagia
(dĭs-FĀ-jē-ă)

2–98 The suffix -phagia means swallow or eat. Use dys- and -phagia to form a word meaning difficult or painful swallowing: _____ / _____ .

bad, painful, difficult swallow(ing), eat(ing)	**2–99** Dys/phagia is a symptom that is often caused by the use of tobacco. Analyze dys/phagia by defining the elements. dys- means _____ , _____ , or _____ . -phagia means _____ or _____ .
aer/o	**2–100** A person who has aer/o/phagia swallows air. From aer/o/phagia, determine the combining form for air: _____ / _____ .
aer/o/phagia (ĕr-ō-FĀ-jē-ă)	**2–101** Infants have a tendency to swallow air as they suck milk from a bottle. This condition is called _____ / _____ / _____ .

Review

Select the medical word element(s) that match(es) the meaning.

aer/o	-algia	-pepsia	dys-
carcino/o	-dynia	-phagia	epi-
esophag/o	-ectomy	-rrhea	
gastr/o	-emesis	-tome	
hemat/o	-itis	-tomy	
	-oma		

a. _____ above, upon

b. _____ air

c. _____ bad, painful, difficult

d. _____ blood

e. _____ cancer

f. _____ digestion

g. _____ esophagus

h. _____ excision, removal

i. _____ inflammation

j. _____ incision, cut into

k. _____ instrument to cut

l. _____ flow, discharge

m. _____ pain

n. _____ stomach

o. _____ swallow, eat

p. _____ tumor

q. _____ vomiting

Check your answers with the Review Answer Key on the following page.

Review Answer Key

a. epi-

b. aer/o

c. dys-

d. hemat/o

e. carcin/o

f. -pepsia

g. esophag/o

h. -ectomy

i. -itis

j. -tomy

k. -tome

l. -rrhea

m. -dynia, -algia

n. gastr/o

o. -phagia

p. -oma

q. -emesis

REINFORCEMENT FRAME: If you are not satisfied with your level of comprehension, go back to Frame 2–60 and rework the frames. **You can also make flash cards on 3 by 5 index cards for the word elements in the unit. Use the cards to reinforce your retention of the word elements. First, compile the cards for the word elements included in the review you are completing, and review those elements. Then complete and correct the review. If you are not satisfied with the score, review the flash cards again before retaking the review. Follow this procedure each time you are ready to complete a review. The flash cards can also be used before you complete the Unit Exercises at the end of each unit.**

Small Intestine and Colon

2–102 Examine the Index of Medical Word Elements in Part A of Appendix A. Use it to find the meaning of the elements that are used in this unit.

Medical Word Element	*Meaning*
-ectomy	_____
enter/o	_____
-rrhaphy	_____
-stenosis	_____
-stomy	_____
-tomy	_____

2–103 The small intestine consists of three parts: the **(7) duodenum**, the **(8) jejunum**, and the **(9) ileum**.

Label the parts of the small intestine in Figure 2–2.

duodenum
(dū-ō-DĒ-nŭm)

jejunum
(jē-JŪ-nŭm)

ileum
(ĬL-ē-ŭm)

2–104 **duoden/o** refers to the first part of the small intestine. This is called the

_____ .

jejun/o refers to the second part of the small intestine. This is called the

_____ .

ile/o refers to the third part of the small intestine. This is called the

_____ .

excision or removal

duodenum

2–105 A duoden/ectomy is a surgical procedure meaning

_____ of the

_____ .

excision or removal

jejunum

2–106 A jejun/ectomy is a surgical procedure meaning

_____ of the

_____ .

excision or removal

ileum

2–107 An ile/ectomy is a surgical procedure meaning

_____ of the

_____ .

2–108 List the three parts of the small intestine and their combining forms.

Part	*Combining Form*
1. _____	_____
2. _____	_____
3. _____	_____

duodenum, duoden/o
(dū-ō-DĒ-nŭm)
jejunum, jejun/o
(jē-JŪ-nŭm)
ileum, ile/o
(ĬL-ē-ŭm)

---

duodenum
(dū-ō-DĒ-nŭm)

2–109 The surgical procedure duoden/o/stomy is the formation of a new opening into the _____ .

-stomy

2–110 Identify the element in Frame 2–109 that means forming a new opening. _____

---

opening, jejunum
(jē-JŪ-nŭm)

2–111 The surgical procedure jejun/o/stomy means forming a new _____ into the _____ .

---

opening

ileum
(ĬL-ē-ŭm)

2–112 Often the colon is removed in colon cancer (Fig. 2–4) and an ile/o/stomy is made. The person must wear an ile/o/stomy bag to collect the fecal material from the ileum.

The surgical procedure ile/o/stomy means forming a new _____ into the _____ .

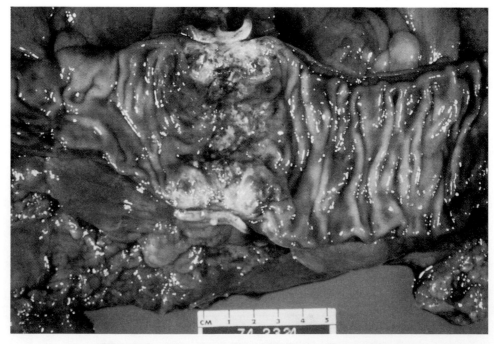

Figure 2–4. Colon cancer. (From WRS Group, with permission.)

-stomy	**2–113** The suffix meaning forming a new opening is _____ . It also means mouth because the opening is shaped like a mouth.

-tomy jejun/o/tomy (jē-jū-NŎT-ō-mē)	**2–114** For people who cannot eat by mouth, a jejun/al (pertaining to the jejunum) feeding tube is often placed through a jejun/o/tomy incision. The surgical suffix meaning incision or cut into is _____ . An incision of the jejunum is known as a _____ / o / _____ .

duoden/o/tomy (dū-ŏd-ĕ-NŎT-ō-mē)	**2–115** An incision of the duodenum is known as a _____ / o / _____ .

ile/o/tomy (ĭl-ē-ŎT-ō-mē)	**2–116** An incision of the ileum is known as an _____ / o / _____ .

ileum (ĬL-ē-ŭm) suture	**2–117** The surgical suffix -rrhaphy refers to suture (sew). An ile/o/rrhaphy is performed to surgically repair the ileum. Analyze ile/o/rrhaphy by defining the elements. **ile/o** means _____ . -rrhaphy means _____ .

duoden/ectomy (dū-ō-dĕn-ĔK-tō-mē) duoden/o/rrhaphy (dū-ō-dĕ-NŎR-ă-fē)	**2–118** In a bleeding duoden/al (pertaining to the duodenum) ulcer, a sewing over of the bleeding portion of the duodenum can often prevent a duoden/ectomy. Develop surgical words meaning excision of the duodenum: _____ / _____ suture of the duodenum: _____ / o / _____

jejun/o/rrhaphy (jē-jū-NŎR-ă-fē) ile/o/rrhaphy (ĭl-ē-ŎR-ă-fē)	**2–119** Form surgical words meaning suture of the jejunum: _____ / o / _____ suture of the ileum: _____ / o / _____

new opening mouth	**2–120** Recall that -stomy means forming a _____ _____ or _____ .

stomach, duodenum (dū-ō-DĒ-nŭm)	**2–121** A gastr/o/duoden/o/stomy is the formation of a new opening between the _____ and _____ .

stomach, ileum (ĬL-ē-ŭm)	**2–122** A gastr / o / ile / o / stomy is the formation of a new opening between the _____ and _____ .
ileum (ĬL-ē-ŭm)	**2–123** Most of the absorption of food takes place in the third part of the small intestine, which is the _____ .
inflammation, ileum (ĬL-ē-ŭm)	**2–124** Crohn's disease, a chronic inflammation of the ileum, may affect any part of the intestinal tract. It is distinguished from closely related bowel disorders by its inflammatory pattern; it is also called regional ile / itis. Ile / itis is an _____ of the _____ .
enter / o	**2–125** Enter / al is a word meaning pertaining to the intestine (usually the small intestine). From enter / al, construct the combining form for intestine: _____ / _____ .
inflammation intestine(s)	**2–126** Enter / itis is a(n) _____ of the _____ .
enter / ectomy (ĕn-tĕr-ĔK-tō-mē)	**2–127** A surgical procedure, excision of the intestine is known as a(n) _____ / _____ .
enter / o / rrhaphy (ĕn-tĕr-ŌR-ă-fē)	**2–128** Suture of the intestine (intestinal wound) is a surgical procedure called _____ / o / _____ .
enter / itis (ĕn-tĕr-Ī-tĭs)	**2–129** Crohn's disease is distinguished from closely related bowel disorders by its inflammatory pattern. It is also known as regional enter / itis. Form a word meaning inflammation of the intestine: _____ / _____ .

2–130 The colon, also called the large intestine, extends from the ileum of the small intestine to the anus. The colon consists of three parts: **(10) ascending, (11) transverse,** and **(12) descending colon**.

Label the three parts of the colon in Figure 2–2.

2–131 The combining form **col/o** is used in words to mean colon.

Form medical words to mean

col/ectomy
(kō-LĔK-tō-mē)
col/itis
(kō-LĪ-tĭs)
col/o/tomy
(kō-LŎT-ō-mē)

excision of the colon: _____ / _____

inflammation of the colon: _____ / _____

incision into the colon: _____ / o / _____

2–132 A patient with colon cancer (see Fig. 2–4) may require a col/o/stomy. Write the surgical term meaning
forming a new opening or mouth into the colon:

col/o/stomy
(kō-LŎS-tō-mē)
col/o/rrhaphy
(kō-LŎR-ă-fē)

_____ / _____ / _____

suture of the colon: _____ / _____ / _____

2–133 The absorption of water by the colon changes the intestinal contents from a fluid to a more solid consistency known as feces or stool.

Use your medical dictionary to define *feces*.

_____

_____

2–134 Locate and name the three main parts of the colon in Figure 2–2.

ascending, transverse,

descending

_____ , _____ ,

and _____ .

2–135 The **(13) sigmoid colon** is S shaped and extends from the descending colon into the **(14) rectum**.

Label Figure 2–2 to identify the sigmoid colon and rectum.

2–136 The surgical procedure sigmoid/ectomy is an excision of all or part of the sigmoid colon.

From sigmoid/ectomy, determine the root for the sigmoid colon:

sigmoid
(SĬG-moyd)

_____ .

2–137 Formulate a term meaning inflammation of the sigmoid colon:

sigmoid/itis
(sĭg-moyd-Ī-tĭs)

_____ / _____

2–138 The rectum terminates in the lower opening of the gastrointestinal tract, the **(15) anus**.

Label the anus in Figure 2–2.

inflammation, rectum (RĔK-tŭm)	**2–139** The combining form **rect/o** refers to the rectum. Rect/itis is a(n) _____ of the _____ .

inflammation, rectum (RĔK-tŭm) colon (KŌ-lŏn)	**2–140** Rect/o/col/itis is a(n) _____ of the _____ and _____ .

pain	**2–141** Rect/algia is a _____ in the rectum.

surgical repair rectum (RĔK-tŭm)	**2–142** Rect/o/plasty is a _____ _____ of the _____ .

pertaining to rectum (RĔK-tŭm)	**2–143** Rect/o/vagin/al means _____ _____ the _____ and vagina.

VALIDATION FRAME: Check your labeling of Figure 2–2 with the answers in Appendix B, Answer Key.

stenosis (stĕ-NŌ-sĭs) stenosis (stĕ-NŌ-sĭs)	**2–144** Besides being used as a suffix, stenosis is a word that means narrowing or stricture of a passage or orifice, which may result in an obstruction. A narrowing or stricture of the pylorus is called pyloric _____ . A narrowing or stricture of any of the orifices leading into the heart is called cardiac _____ .

rect/o
 	
-stenosis
	2–145 Rect/o/stenosis is a stricture or narrowing of the rectum.
	Determine the elements in this frame meaning
	    rectum: _____ / _____
	    stricture or narrowing: _____

proct/itis (prŏk-TĪ-tĭs)	**2–146** The combining form **proct/o** refers to the rectum and anus. Locate the rectum and anus in Figure 2–2. An inflammation of the rectum and anus is known as _____ / _____ .

rectum (RĔK-tŭm) anus (Ā-nŭs)	**2–147** Proct / o / dynia is a pain in the _____ and _____ .
proct / algia (prŏk-TĂL-jē-ă)	**2–148** Use -algia to form another word meaning pain in the rectum and anus: _____ / _____
rectum (RĔK-tŭm) rectum, anus (RĔK-tŭm), (Ā-nŭs)	**2–149** Spasm is a word that is also used as a suffix, and it means involuntary contraction or twitching. A rect / o / spasm is a spasm of the _____ . A proct / o / spasm is a spasm of the _____ and _____ .
proct / o / scopy (prŏk-TŎS-kō-pē) colon (KŌ-lŏn)	**2–150** The suffix -scope is used in words to mean an instrument to view; the suffix -scopy is used in words to mean a visual examination. Visual examination of the rectum and anus is called _____ / ____ / _____ . A physician uses a sigmoid / o / scope to view the sigmoid _____ .
sigmoid colon (SĬG-moyd KŌ-lŏn) visual examination	**2–151** Sigmoid / o / scopy is used to screen for colon cancer (see Fig. 2–4). The American Cancer Society recommends a first sigmoid / o / scopy after the age of 50. It is done sooner if there is a family history (FH) of colon cancer. Analyze sigmoid / o / scopy by defining the elements. **sigmoid / o** means _____ _____ . -scopy means _____ _____ .
sigmoid / o / scopy (sĭg-moy-DŎS-kō-pē)	**2–152** To assess an abnormality in the colon, the physician performs a visual examination of the sigmoid colon called _____ / ____ / _____ .
sigmoid / o / scope (sĭg-MOY-dō-skōp)	**2–153** A sigmoid / o / scope, which is a flexible fiberoptic tube (permits transmission of light to visualize images around curves and corners), is placed through the anus to visualize part of the gastro / intestin / al tract. When the physician examines the colon, the physician uses a _____ / ____ / _____ .

sigmoid/ectomy
(sĭg-moyd-ĔK-tō-mē)
carcin/oma
(kăr-sĭ-NŌ-mă)

2–154 The sigmoid colon is **S** shaped and is the last part of the colon. Sigmoid/ectomy is most often performed for carcin/oma of the sigmoid colon.

Identify the words in this frame that mean

excision of the sigmoid colon: _____ / _____

tumor (of) cancer: _____ / _____

---

examination, colon
                (KŌ-lŏn)

2–155 A col/o/scopy is commonly referred to as a colon/o/scopy. Both terms mean a visual _____ of the _____ .

---

colon/itis
(kō-lŏn-Ī-tĭs)
colon/o/scope
(kō-LŎN-ō-skōp)
colon/o/scopy
(kō-lŏn-ŎS-kō-pē)

2–156 Use **colon/o** to form medical words meaning

inflammation of the colon: _____ / _____

instrument to examine the colon: _____ / _____ / _____

visual examination of the colon: _____ / _____ / _____

---

enter/o/scopy
(ĕn-tĕr-ŎS-kō-pē)

2–157 Enter/o/scopy is used to assess the intestines. A visual examination of the intestines is known as a(n) _____ / _____ / _____ .

---

enter/o/scope
(ĔN-tĕr-ō-skōp)

2–158 When there is a need to view the intestine, the physician uses a(n) _____ / _____ / _____ .

---

duoden/o/scopy
(dū-ŏd-ĕ-NŎS-kō-pē)

sigmoid/o/scopy
(sĭg-moy-DŎS-kō-pē)
gastr/o/scopy
(găs-TRŎS-kō-pē)

2–159 Use -scopy to form medical words meaning

visual examination of the duodenum: _____ / _____ / _____

visual examination of sigmoid colon:

_____ / _____ / _____

visual examination of the stomach: _____ / _____ / _____

Review

Select the medical word element(s) that match(es) the meaning.

col/o
colon/o
duoden/o
enter/o
jejun/o
ile/o
proct/o
rect/o
sigmoid/o

-algia
-dynia
-ectomy
-rrhaphy
-scope
-scopy
-spasm
-stomy
-stenosis
-tome
-tomy

a. _____ colon

b. _____ duodenum

c. _____ excision, removal

d. _____ forming a new opening

e. _____ incision, cut into

f. _____ instrument to cut

g. _____ intestine(s)

h. _____ jejunum

i. _____ ileum

j. _____ pain

k. _____ rectum

l. _____ rectum, anus

m. _____ sigmoid colon

n. _____ stricture, narrowing

o. _____ suture

p. _____ twitching

q. _____ visual examination

Check your answers with the Review Answer Key on the following page.

Review Answer Key

a. col/o, colon/o

b. duoden/o

c. -ectomy

d. -stomy

e. -tomy

f. -tome

g. enter/o

h. jejun/o

i. ile/o

j. -dynia, -algia

k. rect/o

l. proct/o

m. sigmoid/o

n. -stenosis

o. -rrhaphy

p. -spasm

q. -scopy

REINFORCEMENT FRAME: If you are not satisfied with your level of comprehension, go back to Frame 2–102 and rework the frames. **You can also make flash cards on 3 by 5 index cards for the word elements in the unit. Use the cards to reinforce your retention of the word elements. First, compile the cards for the word elements included in the review you are completing, and review those elements. Then complete and correct the review. If you are not satisfied with the score, review the flash cards again before retaking the review. Follow this procedure each time you are ready to complete a review. The flash cards can also be used before you complete the Unit Exercises at the end of each unit.**

REMINDER FRAME: Define medical words by first defining the suffix and then the first part(s) of the word. Refer to the informative frame on page 27 to review this method.

AUDIOCASSETTE EXERCISE

The audiocassette tape helps you master the pronunciation of medical words. Listen to the tape for instructions to complete this exercise. You may also use this exercise without the audiotape to practice correct pronunciation and spelling of the terms.

Frame	Word	Pronunciation	Spelling Exercise
2–101	[] aerophagia	(ĕr-ō-FĀ-jē-ă)	_____
2–96	[] antacids	(ănt-ĂS-ĭds)	_____
2–149	[] anus	(Ā-nŭs)	_____
2–86	[] cancerous	(KĂN-sĕr-ŭs)	_____
2–154	[] carcinoma	(kăr-sĭ-NŌ-mă)	_____
2–40	[] cardiologist	(kăr-dē-ŌL-ō-jĭst)	_____
2–42	[] cardiology	(kăr-dē-ŌL-ō-jē)	_____
2–61	[] chyme	(KĪM)	_____
2–131	[] colectomy	(kō-LĔK-tō-mē)	_____
2–131	[] colitis	(kō-LĪ-tĭs)	_____
2–156	[] colonoscope	(kō-LŎN-ō-skōp)	_____
2–156	[] colonoscopy	(kō-lŏn-ŎS-kō-pē)	_____
2–132	[] colorrhaphy	(kō-LŎR-ă-fē)	_____
2–155	[] coloscopy	(kō-LŎS-kō-pē)	_____
2–132	[] colostomy	(kō-LŎS-tō-mē)	_____
2–131	[] colotomy	(kō-LŎT-ō-mē)	_____
2–144	[] Crohn's disease	(KRŌNZ dĭ-ZĒZ)	_____
2–59	[] dentalgia	(dĕn-TĂL-jē-ă)	_____
1–51	[] dentist	(DĔN-tĭst)	_____
2–59	[] dentodynia	(dĕn-tō-DĬN-ē-ă)	_____
2–18	[] diarrhea	(dī-ă-RĒ-ă)	_____
2–118	[] duodenectomy	(dū-ō-dĕn-ĔK-tō-mē)	_____
2–118	[] duodenorrhaphy	(dū-ō-dĕ-NŎR-ă-fē)	_____
2–159	[] duodenoscopy	(dū-ŏd-ĕ-NŎS-kō-pē)	_____
2–109	[] duodenostomy	(dū-ŏd-ĕ-NŎS-to-me)	_____
2–115	[] duodenotomy	(dū-ŏd-ĕ-NŎT-ō-mē)	_____
2–104	[] duodenum	(dū-ō-DĒ-nŭm)	_____
2–97	[] dyspepsia	(dĭs-PĔP-sē-ă)	_____
2–98	[] dysphagia	(dĭs-FĀ-jē-ă)	_____
2–92	[] emesis	(ĔM-ĕ-sĭs)	_____
2–125	[] enteral	(ĔN-tĕr-ăl)	_____
2–127	[] enterectomy	(ĕn-tĕr-ĔK-tō-mē)	_____
2–129	[] enteritis	(ĕn-tĕr-Ī-tĭs)	_____
2–128	[] enterorrhaphy	(ĕn-tĕr-ŎR-ă-fē)	_____
2–158	[] enteroscope	(ĔN-tĕr-ō-skōp)	_____
2–157	[] enteroscopy	(ĕn-tĕr-ŎS-kō-pē)	_____
2–90	[] epigastric	(ĕp-ĭ-GĂS-trĭk)	_____
2–63	[] esophagitis	(ē-sŏf-ă-JĪ-tĭs)	_____

Frame	Word	Pronunciation	Spelling Exercise
2–74	[] esophagoplasty	(ē-SŎF-ă-gō-plăs-tē)	_____
2–76	[] esophagotome	(ē-SŎF-ă-gō-tōm)	_____
2–83	[] esophagotomy	(ē-sŏf-ă-GŎT-ō-mē)	_____
2–61	[] esophagus	(ē-SŎF-ă-gŭs)	_____
2–133	[] feces	(FĒ-sēz)	_____
2–153	[] fiberoptic	(fī-bĕr-ŎP-tĭk)	_____
2–66	[] gastralgia	(găs-TRĂL-jē-ă)	_____
2–78	[] gastrectomy	(găs-TRĔK-tō mē)	_____
2–70	[] gastric	(GĂS-trĭk)	_____
2–64	[] gastritis	(găs-TRĪ-tĭs)	_____
2–121	[] gastroduodenostomy	(găs-trō-dū-ō-dĕ-NŎS-tō-mē)	_____
2–66	[] gastrodynia	(găs-trō-DĪN-ē-ă)	_____
2–67	[] gastroesophagitis	(găs-trō-ē-sŏf-ă-JĪ-tĭs)	_____
2–122	[] gastroileostomy	(găs-trō-ĭl-ē-ŎS-tō-mē)	_____
2–45	[] gastrointestinal	(găs-trō-ĭn-TĔS-tĭn-ăl)	_____
2–44	[] gastrologist	(găs-TRŎL-ō-jĭst)	_____
2–42	[] gastrology	(găs-TRŎL-ō-jē)	_____
2–74	[] gastroplasty	(găs-TRŌ-plăs-tē)	_____
2–68	[] gastrorrhea	(găs-trō-RĒ-ă)	_____
2–159	[] gastroscopy	(găs-TRŎS-kō-pē)	_____
2–82	[] gastrotome	(GĂS-trō-tōm)	_____
2–84	[] gastrotomy	(găs-TRŎT-ō-mē)	_____
2–55	[] gingivitis	(jĭn-jĭ-VĪ-tĭs)	_____
2–58	[] gingivosis	(jĭn-jĭ-VŌ-sĭs)	_____
2–91	[] hematemesis	(hĕm-ăt-ĔM-ĕ-sĭs)	_____
2–94	[] hyperemesis	(hī-pĕr-ĔM-ĕ-sĭs)	_____
2–107	[] ileectomy	(ĭl-ē-ĔK-tō-mē)	_____
2–119	[] ileorrhaphy	(ĭl-ē-ŎR-ă-fē)	_____
2–112	[] ileostomy	(ĭl-ē-ŎS-tō-mē)	_____
2–116	[] ileotomy	(ĭl-ē-ŎT-ō-mē)	_____
2–104	[] ileum	(ĬL-ē-ŭm)	_____
2–114	[] jejunal	(jē-JŪ-năl)	_____
2–106	[] jejunectomy	(jē-jū-NĔK-tō-mē)	_____
2–119	[] jejunorrhaphy	(jē-jū-NŎR-ă-fē)	_____
2–111	[] jejunostomy	(jē-jū-NŎS-tō-mē)	_____
2–114	[] jejunotomy	(jē-jū-NŎT-ō-mē)	_____
2–104	[] jejunum	(jē-JŪ-nŭm)	_____
2–30	[] linguodental	(lĭng-gwō-DĔN-tăl)	_____
2–35	[] mycosis	(mī-KŌ-sĭs)	_____
2–47	[] odontalgia	(ō-dŏn-TĂL-jē-ă)	_____
2–7	[] oral	(ŎR-ăl)	_____
2–50	[] orthodontist	(ŏr-thō-DŎN-tĭst)	_____
2–21	[] parotid	(pă-RŎT-ĭd)	_____

Frame	Word	Pronunciation	Spelling Exercise
2–56	[] periodontitis	(pĕr-ē-ō-dŏn-TĪ-tĭs)	_____
2–148	[] proctalgia	(prŏk-TĂL-jē-ă)	_____
2–146	[] proctitis	(prŏk-TĪ-tĭs)	_____
2–147	[] proctodynia	(prŏk-tō-DĬN-ē-ă)	_____
2–150	[] proctoscopy	(prŏk-TŎS-kō-pē)	_____
2–149	[] proctospasm	(PRŎK-tō-spăzm)	_____
2–141	[] rectalgia	(rĕk-TĂL-jē-ă)	_____
2–139	[] rectitis	(rĕk-TĪ-tĭs)	_____
2–140	[] rectocolitis	(rĕk-tō-kō-LĪ-tĭs)	_____
2–142	[] rectoplasty	(RĔK-tō-plăs-tē)	_____
2–149	[] rectospasm	(RĔK-tō-spăzm)	_____
2–145	[] rectostenosis	(rĕk-tō-stĕn-Ō-sĭs)	_____
2–143	[] rectovaginal	(rĕk-tō-VĂJ-ĭ-năl)	_____
2–139	[] rectum	(RĔK-tŭm)	_____
2–13	[] salivary	(SĂL-ĭ-vĕr-ē)	_____
2–13	[] sialic	(sī-ĂL-ĭc)	_____
2–14	[] sialitis	(sī-ă-LĪT-tĭs)	_____
2–15	[] sialorrhea	(sī-ă-lō-RĒ-ă)	_____
2–154	[] sigmoidectomy	(sĭg-moyd-ĔK-tō-mē)	_____
2–137	[] sigmoiditis	(sĭg-moyd-Ī-tĭs)	_____
2–153	[] sigmoidoscope	(sĭg-MOY-dō-skōp)	_____
2–152	[] sigmoidoscopy	(sĭg-moy-DŎS-kō-pē)	_____
2–149	[] spasm	(SPĂZM)	_____
2–7	[] stomatal	(STŌ-mă-tăl)	_____
2–12	[] stomatalgia	(stō-mă-TĂL-jē-ă)	_____
2–9	[] stomatic	(stō-MĂT-ĭk)	_____
2–5	[] stomatitis	(stō-mă-TĪ-tĭs)	_____
2–12	[] stomatodynia	(stō-mă-tō-DĬN-ē-ă)	_____
2–34	[] stomatomycosis	(stō-mă-tō-mī-KŌ-sĭs)	_____
2–73	[] stomatoplasty	(STŌ-mă-tō-plăs-tē)	_____
2–32	[] stomatosis	(stō-mă-TŌ-sĭs)	_____
2–22	[] sublingual	(sŭb-LĬNG-gwăl)	_____
2–22	[] submaxillary	(sŭb-MĂK-sĭ-lĕr-ē)	_____

2–160   Use the Index of Medical Word Elements in Part A of Appendix A to define word elements that are used in this unit.

Medical Word Elements	Meaning
chol/e	_____
cholecyst/o	_____
choledoch/o	_____
cyst/o	_____
hepat/o	_____
pancreat/o	_____

2–161   Examine the Index of Medical Word Elements in Part B of Appendix A. Use it to write the following elements that are used in this unit.

English Term	Medical Word Element
excision, removal	_____
pain	_____ or _____
stone, calculus	_____ or _____ / ____
surgical repair	_____
suture	_____
vomiting	_____

Accessory Organs of Digestion: Liver, Gallbladder, and Pancreas

The combining forms related to the accessory organs of digestion are summarized below. Review this information before you begin to work the frames.

Combining Form	Meaning	Example
cholangi/o	bile vessel	cholangi/ole small
cholecyst/o	gallbladder	cholecyst/o/gram record
chol/e	bile, gall	chol/emia blood
choledoch/o	bile duct	choledoch/o/lith stone, calculus
hepat/o	liver	hepat/oma tumor
pancreat/o	pancreas	pancreat/itis inflammation
sial/o	saliva, salivary glands	sial/o/lith stone, calculus

2–162   Even though food does not pass through the **(16) liver,** **(17) gallbladder,** and **(18) pancreas**, these organs play a vital role in the proper digestion and absorption of nutrients. Label the accessory organs in Figure 2–2.

---

hepat / o

cholecyst / o

pancreat / o

2–163   From hepat / itis (inflammation of the liver), construct the combining form for liver: _____ / _____ .

From cholecyst / itis (inflammation of the gallbladder), construct the combining form for the gallbladder: _____ / _____ .

From pancreat / itis (inflammation of the pancreas), construct the combining form for pancreas: _____ / _____ .

---

hepat / itis
(hĕp-ă-TĪ-tĭs)

2–164   Hepat / itis may be caused by a variety of agents, including viral infections.

An inflammation of the liver is called _____ / _____ .

---

hepat / ectomy
(hĕp-ă-TĔK-tō-mē)
hepat / o / dynia
(hĕp-ă-tō-DĬN-ē-ă)
hepat / algia
(hĕp-ă-TĂL-jē-ă)
hepat / o / rrhaphy
(hĕp-ă-TŎR-ă-fē)

2–165   Form medical words meaning

excision of the liver: _____ / _____

pain in the liver: _____ / _____ / _____ or

_____ / _____

suture of the liver: _____ / _____ / _____

---

liver

gallbladder, pancreas

2–166   The three accessory organs of digestion are: _____ ,

_____ , and _____ .

2–167   The **(1) hepatic, (2) cystic,** and **(3) pancreatic ducts** join the **(4) common bile duct**, which carries digestive juices into the **(5) duodenum**.

Label the structures in Figure 2–5.

---

cyst / o

2–168   From cyst / itis (inflammation of the bladder), construct the combining form meaning bladder: _____ / _____ .

---

hepat / ic
(hĕ-PĂT-ĭk)
cyst / ic
(SĬS-tĭk)
pancreat / ic
(păn-krē-ĂT-ĭk)

2–169   Use the suffix -ic to form medical words meaning

pertaining to the liver: _____ / _____

pertaining to the bladder: _____ / _____

pertaining to the pancreas: _____ / _____

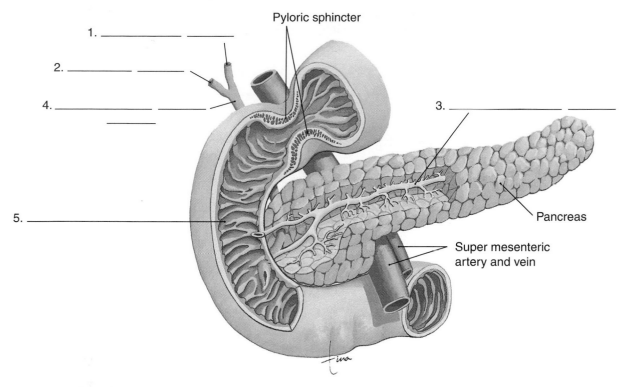

1. _____ _____

2. _____ _____

Pyloric sphincter

4. _____ _____
_____

3. _____ _____

Pancreas

5. _____

Super mesenteric
artery and vein

Figure 2–5. The pancreas, sectioned to show the pancreatic ducts. (Adapted from Scanlon, VC, and Sanders, T: Understanding Human Structure and Function. FA Davis, Philadelphia, 1997, p 295, with permission.)

VALIDATION FRAME: Check your labeling of Figure 2–5 by looking at the Answer Key in Appendix B.

hepat/ic, cyst/ic (hĕ-PĂT-ĭk), (SĬS-tĭk) pancreat/ic (păn-krē-ĂT-ĭk)	**2–170** Refer to Frame 2–167 to write the names of the ducts that transport juices that aid in digestion: _____ / _____ , _____ / _____ , _____ / _____ , and the common bile duct.
vomiting	**2–171** The combining form **chol/e** refers to bile or gall. Chol/emesis means _____ bile.
chol/e/cyst/o	**2–172** Bile or gall is a bitter secretion produced by the liver and stored in the gallbladder. It passes into the small intestine via the bile ducts when needed for digestion. Combine **chol/e** and **cyst/o** to develop a new combining form meaning gallbladder: _____ / ____ / _____ / ____ .
gallbladder	**2–173** Cholecyst/itis is an inflammation of the _____ .
e	**2–174** So far you have used **o** as the combining vowel, but on occasion you may find that another vowel is used. For example, the combining form **chol/e** is an exception to the rule. In this case, the combining vowel is an ____ .

bile, gall vomit	**2–175** When a person vomits bile, the condition is called chol/emesis. Analyze chol/emesis by defining the elements. **chol/e** refers to _____ or _____ . -emesis refers to _____ .

liver	**2–176** The suffix -lith is used in words to mean stone or calculus. A hepat/o/lith is a stone or calculus in the _____ .

pancreat/o/lith (păn-krē-ĂT-ō-lĭth) cholecyst/o/lith (kō-lē-SĬS-tō-lĭth) hepat/o/lith (hĕp-Ă-tō-lĭth)	**2–177** Form medical words meaning stone in the pancreas: _____ / _____ / _____ stone in the gallbladder: _____ / _____ / _____ calculus in the liver: _____ / _____ / _____

chol/e	**2–178** A chol/e/lith is a gallstone. Unless a gallstone obstructs a biliary duct, the stones may or may not cause symptoms. Figure 2–6 shows an inflamed gallbladder packed full of gallstones. The exact cause of gallstones is unknown, but they occur more frequently in women, elderly people, and obese persons. From chol/e/lith, determine the combining form meaning bile or gall: _____ / _____ .

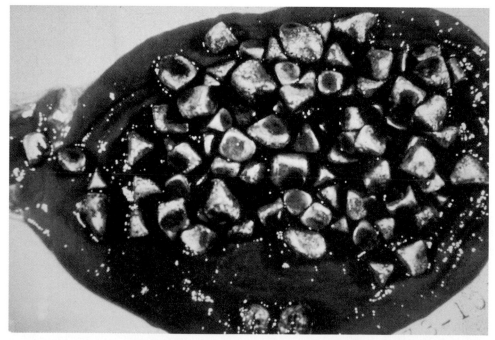

Figure 2–6. Inflamed gallbladder with gallstones. Patients may suffer from a variety of attacks characterized by belching, bloating, and severe abdominal pains, which may be knifelike and radiate from the right upper abdomen through to the back. Attacks of gallbladder pain are classically caused by the movement of a stone into the duct draining bile from the gallbladder. (From WRS Group, with permission.)

DIGESTIVE SYSTEM • 59

stone, calculus (KĂL-kū-lŭs)	**2–179** Recall that -lith means _____ or _____ .

chol/e/lith (KŌL-lē-lĭth)	**2–180** The most common type of gallstone contains cholesterol. These stones or calculi are formed in the gallbladder or bile ducts. The medical name for gallstone is _____ / _____ / _____ .

bile duct	**2–181** **Choledoch/o** is a combining form for bile duct. A choledoch/o/lith is a stone in the _____ _____ .

bile duct	**2–182** **Choledoch/o** refers to the common bile duct (see Fig. 2–5), and means _____ _____ .

choledoch/itis (kō-lē-dō-KĪ-tĭs) choledoch/o/rrhaphy (kō-lĕd-ō-KŎR-ă-fē) choledoch/o/plasty (kō-LĔD-ō-kō-plăs-tē)	**2–183** Use **choledoch/o** to develop medical words meaning inflammation of the bile duct: _____ / _____ suture of the bile duct: _____ / _____ / _____ surgical repair of the bile duct: _____ / _____ / _____

superior superior inferior	**2–184** The terms "inferior" (below) and "superior" (above) are used to designate positions in the human anatomy. Refer to Figure 2–1 and use "inferior" or "superior" to work this frame. The tongue is _____ to the esophagus. The rectum is _____ to the anus. The common bile duct is _____ to the cystic bile duct.

stone, calculus bile duct	**2–185** Choledoch/o/lith is a _____ or _____ in the common _____ _____ .

choledoch/o/lith (kō-LĔD-ō-kō-lĭth) choledoch/o/rrhaphy (kō-lĕd-ō-KŎR-ă-fē) choledoch/o/tomy (kō-lĕd-ō-KŎT-ō-mē)	**2–186** When a stone is trapped in the common bile duct, the duct is incised to remove the stone, and then the duct is sutured. Form medical words meaning a stone in the bile duct: _____ / _____ / _____ suture of the bile duct: _____ / _____ / _____ incision of the bile duct: _____ / _____ / _____

gallbladder	**2–187** Locate the gallbladder, also called **cholecyst**, in Figure 2–1. This pouchlike structure is used to store bile, which is produced by the liver. Cholecyst is the medical name for the _____ .

cholecyst/itis (kō-lē-sĭs-TĪ-tĭs)	**2–188** An inflammation of the gallbladder may be caused by the presence of gallstones. Formulate a word meaning an inflammation of the gallbladder. _____ / _____
gallstone	**2–189** A chole/lith is a _____ .
stone, calculus (KĂL-kū-lŭs)	**2–190** The pancreat/ic duct transports pancreatic juices to the duodenum to help the digestive process. A pancreat/o/lith is a _____ or _____ within the pancreas.
pancreat/o -lith	**2–191** From pancreat/o/lith, identify combining form for pancreas: _____ / _____ element meaning stone or calculus: _____
hepat/itis hepat/osis hepat/oma hepat/o/lith (hĕp-ă-TĪ-tĭs), (hĕp-ă-TŌ-sĭs), (hĕp-ă-TŌ-mă), (hĕp-Ă-tō-lĭth)	**2–192** Hepatitis B, the most common infectious hepatitis seen in hospitals, is transferred by blood and body secretions. Hospital personnel are usually vaccinated as a preventative measure. Use a diagonal line (slash) to divide the following words into the basic elements. h e p a t i t i s h e p a t o s i s h e p a t o m a h e p a t o l i t h
stone, calculus (KĂL-kū-lŭs)	**2–193** **Lith/o** is also used in words as a combining form meaning stone or calculus. Whenever you see -lith or **lith/o**, you will know that both elements mean _____ or _____ .
stone calculus (KĂL-kū-lŭs)	**2–194** The suffixes -osis and -iasis are used to indicate an abnormal condition or diseased condition. The difference between the two suffixes is that -osis is used as a common suffix to denote a disorder but usually does not indicate the specific cause of the abnormal condition. In contrast, the suffix -iasis is attached to a word root to identify an abnormal condition that is produced by something that is specified.* For example, lith/iasis is an abnormal condition produced by a _____ or _____ .

*There are a few exceptions to this rule.

liver	**2–195** Hepat/osis is an abnormal or diseased condition of the _____ . The cause of the abnormality is not specified and could be the result of any number of liver diseases.

2–196 When you form a word meaning an abnormal condition of stones or calculi, use -iasis because the abnormal or diseased condition is produced by something specified (stones).

Construct medical words that mean

lith/iasis
(lĭth-Ī-ă-sĭs)

an abnormal condition of stones: _____ / _____

an abnormal condition of pancreat/ic stones:

pancreat/o/lith/iasis
(păn-krē-ă-tō-lĭ-THĪ-ă-sĭs)

_____ / ____ / _____ / _____

2–197 Chol/e/lith/iasis (see Fig. 2–6) is most common in obese women who are older than 40 years of age. A person who has an abnormal or diseased

chol/e/lith/iasis
(kō-lē-lĭ-THĪ-ă-sĭs)

condition of gallstones suffers from _____ / ____ / _____ / _____ .

INFORMATIVE FRAME: In some instances, you will find that -osis and -iasis are interchangeable. Whenever you are in doubt about which suffix to use, refer to your medical dictionary.

2–198 Acute cholecyst/itis often leads to infection of the gallbladder and duct. Analyze cholecyst/itis by defining the elements.

inflammation

-itis refers to _____ .

gallbladder

cholecyst/o refers to the _____ .

2–199 The majority of acute cholecyst/itis cases are the result of gallstones lodged in the bile ducts, which causes pain. Form medical words meaning

cholecyst/o/dynia
(kō-lē-sĭs-tō-DĬN-ē-ă)

pain in the gallbladder: _____ / ____ / _____

cholecyst/algia
(kō-lē-sĭs-TĂL-jē-ă)

or _____ / _____

abnormal condition of gallbladder stone(s):

cholecyst/o/lith/iasis
(kō-lē-sĭs-tō-lĭ-THĪ-ă-sĭs)

_____ / ____ / _____ / _____

2–200 Sometimes the gallbladder is removed because the presence of gallstones causes a severe inflammation. The surgical procedure to excise the

cholecyst/ectomy
(kō-lē-sĭs-TĔK-tō-mē)

gallbladder is known as _____ / _____ .

2–201 Because of its critical function of producing insulin and digestive enzymes, a complete excision of the pancreas it almost never performed. However, when an excision of the pancreas is dictated, the surgeon performs a

pancreat/ectomy
(păn-krē-ă-TĔK-tō-mē)

_____ / _____ .

pancreat/ectomy (păn-krē-ă-TĔK-tō-mē)	**2–201** Pancreat/ic cancer is an extremely lethal cancer, and surgery is performed for relief, but it is not a cure for the cancer. When the surgeon removes either part or all of the pancreas, the surgeon performs a _____ / _____ .
cholecyst/ectomy (kō-lē-sĭs-TĔK-tō-mē)	**2–202** Because the gallbladder performs no function except storage, it is not essential for life. When the surgeon removes a gallbladder, the surgical procedure is called a _____ / _____ .
-plasty	**2–203** Plastic surgery is the surgical specialty for the restoration, repair, or reconstruction of body structures. Determine the suffix for surgical repair: _____ .
esophag/o/plasty (ē-SŎF-ă-gō-plăs-tē) choledoch/o/plasty (kō-LĔD-ō-kō-plăs-tē)	**2–204** Develop medical words meaning surgical repair of the esophagus: _____ / ____ / _____ surgical repair of the bile duct: _____ / ____ / _____
flow, discharge	**2–205** The suffix -rrhea refers to _____ or _____ .
dia/rrhea (dī-ă-RĒ-ă)	**2–206** A person who has frequent passage of watery bowel movements has a condition called _____ / _____ .
therm/o	**2–207** A dia/therm/y treatment generates heat through (tissues). From dia/therm/y, construct the combining form meaning heat: _____ / ____ .
through heat	**2–208** Analyze dia/therm/y by defining the elements. dia- means _____ . **therm** means _____ . -y is a noun-ending suffix.
heat	**2–209** In Unit 1 you learned how to identify the elements in therm/o/meter. Now you know that **therm/o** is the combining form that refers to _____ .
heat	**2–210** Whenever you see **therm/o** in a word, you will know it means _____ .

tox tox/o	**2-211** Even though you have not reviewed the word tox/ic, determine the word root for poison: _____ The combining form that refers to poison is _____ / _____ .

abnormal condition poison toxic/o	**2-212** Toxic/osis literally means an _____ _____ of _____ . The combining form for poison is _____ / _____ .

poisonous	**2-213** When a person swallows a tox/ic substance, it means he or she has swallowed a substance that is _____ .

REMINDER FRAME: Whenever you have difficulty completing a frame, use the Index of Medical Word Elements in Appendix A. You can also refer to the Summary of Medical Word Elements at the end of each unit or a medical dictionary. Do not feel that you must remember everything that is covered. The important thing to remember is to look up information to complete the frame.

gallbladder	**2-214** The suffix -gram is used in words to mean record; the suffix -graphy is used in words to mean the process of recording. A cholecyst/o/gram is an x-ray picture (record) of the _____ .

gallbladder	**2-215** Cholecyst/o/graphy is the process of examining the _____ by x-ray study.

gallbladder	**2-216** Cholecyst/o/gram literally means record of the _____ .

recording gallbladder	**2-217** Cholecyst/o/graphy literally means the process of _____ the _____ .

cholecyst/o/gram (kō-lē-SĬS-tō-grăm) cholecyst/o/graphy (kō-lē-sĭs-TŎG-ră-fē)	**2-218** Develop medical words meaning record (x-ray picture) of the gallbladder: _____ / _____ / _____ process of recording (taking an x-ray of) the gallbladder: _____ / _____ / _____

enlarged	**2-219** **Megal/o** means enlargement. A word containing **megal/o** will mean that a body structure is _____ .

noun	**2–220** Recall that a -y suffix makes a word a noun. Hepat / o / megal / y is a (noun, adjective) _____ .
enlarged or enlargement	**2–221** The suffix -megaly is used in words to mean _____ .
hepat / o / megaly (hĕp-ă-tō-MĔG-ă-lē)	**2–222** Alcoholics usually suffer from hepat / o / megaly. When people have enlarged livers, they are diagnosed with _____ / _____ / _____ .
gastr / o / megaly (găs-trō-MĔG-ă-lē)	**2–223** Form a word meaning enlargement of the stomach: _____ / _____ / _____
stomach	**2–224** Gastr / o / megaly and megal / o / gastr / ia both mean enlargement of the _____ .
megal / o / gastr / ic (mĕg-ă-lō-GĂS-trĭk)	**2–225** In megal / o / gastr / ia the suffix -ia is a noun ending that denotes condition. Use -ic to change this word to an adjective. _____ / _____ / _____
enlarged enlarged	**2–226** Define the following terms: Megal / o / esophagus is an esophagus that is _____ . Megal / o / gastr / ia is a condition of a stomach that is _____ .

Review

Select the medical word element(s) that match(es) the meaning.

chol/e   -algia   -lith   dia-
cholecyst/o   -dynia   -megaly
choledoch/o   -ectomy   -osis
cyst/o   -emesis   -plasty
esophag/o   -gram   -rrhaphy
hepat/o   -graphy   -rrhea
pancreat/o   -iasis   -stomy
therm/o
toxic/o

a. _____ abnormal condition

b. _____ abnormal condition (produced by something specified)

c. _____ bile duct

d. _____ bile, gall

e. _____ bladder

f. _____ enlargement

g. _____ esophagus

h. _____ excision, removal

i. _____ flow, discharge

j. _____ forming a new opening, mouth

k. _____ gallbladder

l. _____ heat

m. _____ liver

n. _____ pain

o. _____ pancreas

p. _____ poison

q. _____ process of recording

r. _____ record

s. _____ stone, calculus

t. _____ surgical repair

u. _____ suture

v. _____ through

w. _____ vomiting

Check your answers with the Review Answer Key on the following page.

Review Answer Key

a. -osis

b. -iasis

c. choledoch/o

d. chol/e

e. cyst/o

f. -megaly

g. esophag/o

h. -ectomy

i. -rrhea

j. -stomy

k. cholecyst/o

l. therm/o

m. hepat/o

n. -algia, -dynia

o. pancreat/o

p. toxic/o

q. -graphy

r. -gram

s. -lith

t. -plasty

u. -rrhaphy

v. dia-

w. -emesis

REINFORCEMENT FRAME: If you are not satisfied with your level of comprehension, go back to Frame 2–160 and rework the frames. **You can also make flash cards on 3 by 5 index cards for the word elements in the unit. Use the cards to reinforce your retention of the word elements. First, compile the cards for the word elements included in the review you are completing, and review those elements. Then complete and correct the review. If you are not satisfied with the score, review the flash cards again before retaking the review. Follow this procedure each time you are ready to complete a review. The flash cards can also be used before you complete the Unit Exercises at the end of each unit.**

Additional Pathological Conditions

anorexia (ăn-o-RĔK-sē-ă): lack of appetite (-orexia = appetite).

ascites (ă-SĪ-tēz): accumulation of fluid in the abdomen.

borborygmus (bŏr-bō-RĬG-mŭs): gurgling or rumbling sound heard over the large intestine, caused by gas moving through the intestines.

bulimia (bū-LĬM-ē-ă): eating disorder that is characterized by recurrent binge eating, purging of the food with laxatives and/or vomiting, and persistent overconcern with body shape and weight.

cirrhosis (sĭ-RŌ-sĭs): a chronic disease of the liver.

dysentery (DĬS-ĕn-tĕr-ē): a term applied to a number of intestinal disorders, especially of the colon, characterized by inflammation of the mucous membrane.

hematochezia (hĕm-ă-tō-KĒ-zē-ă): passage of stools containing red blood rather than tarry stools.

hemorrhoid (HĔM-ō-royd): a mass of enlarged, twisted varicose veins in the mucous membrane inside or just outside the rectum. Also known as "piles."

hernia (HĔR-nē-ă): protrusion or projection of an organ or a part of an organ through the wall of the cavity that normally contains it.

inflammatory bowel disease (IBD): ulceration of mucosa of the colon. Also known as *ulcerative colitis*.

irritable bowel syndrome: a disturbance of intestinal function of unknown cause. The symptoms usually include an alteration in bowel activity and abdominal discomfort. Also called *spastic colon*.

jaundice (JAWN-dĭs): condition characterized by yellowness of skin, whites of eyes, mucous membranes, and body fluids owing to deposition of bile pigment resulting from excess bilirubin in the blood (hyperbilirubinemia).

ulcer (ŬL-sĕr): an open sore or lesion of the skin or mucous membrane, accompanied by sloughing of inflamed necrotic tissue.

volvulus (VŎL-vū-lŭs): a twisting of the bowel upon itself, causing obstruction. Usually requires surgery to untwist the loop of bowel.

Medical Record

The reports that follow are related to the medical specialty called gastroenterology. A gastroenterologist specializes in diagnosing and treating diseases and disorders of the stomach and intestines.

MEDICAL RECORD 2–1. Rectal Bleeding

Dictionary Exercise

This exercise will help you master the terminology in the medical record. Underline the following terms in the reading exercise and use a medical dictionary to define the words. The pronunciations of medical terms in this report are included in the audiocassette exercise on pages 73–75.

angulation _____

anorectal _____

appendectomy _____

carcinoma _____

colonic _____

constipation _____

diarrhea _____

distress _____

diverticulum _____

dysphagia _____

emesis _____

enteritis _____

hematemesis _____

ileostomy _____

nausea _____

polyp _____

postprandial _____

regional _____

scope _____

sigmoidoscopy _____

Word Element Exercise

Break down the following words into their basic elements. The first one is completed for you.

dys/phagia   appendectomy
diarrhea   sigmoidoscopy
hematemesis   anorectal
enteritis   rectal
colonic   carcinoma
ileostomy

VALIDATION FRAME: Check your answers in Appendix B, Answer Key.

Reading Exercise

Read the case study out loud.

This 50-year-old white male has lost approximately 40 pounds since his last examination. The patient says he has had no dysphagia or postprandial distress, and there is no report of diarrhea, nausea, emesis,

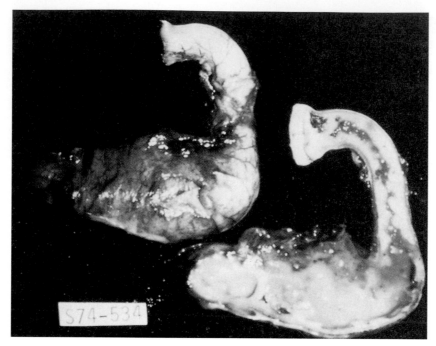

Figure 2–7. Appendicitis. (From WRS Group, with permission.)

hematemesis, or constipation. The patient has had a history of regional enteritis, appendicitis (Fig. 2–7), and colonic bleeding. The regional enteritis resulted in an ileostomy with appendectomy about 6 months ago. On 5/30/XX a sigmoidoscopy using a 10-cm scope showed no evidence of bleeding at the anorectal area. A 25-cm scope was then inserted to a level of 13 cm. At this point, angulation prevented further passage of the scope. No abnormalities had been encountered, but there was dark blood noted at that level. My impression is that the rectal bleeding could be due to a polyp, bleeding diverticulum (Fig. 2–8), or rectal carcinoma.

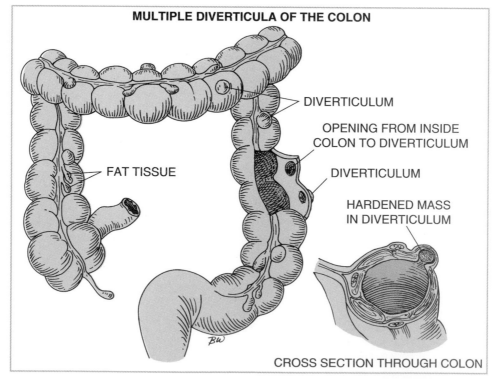

Figure 2–8. Diverticula of the colon. (From Taber's Cyclopedic Medical Dictionary, ed 18. FA Davis, Philadelphia, 1997, p 565, with permission.)

MEDICAL RECORD EVALUATION 2–1. Rectal Bleeding

1. What is the patient's symptom that made him seek medical help?

2. What surgical procedures were performed on the patient for his regional enteritis?

3. What abnormality was found with the sigmoidoscopy?

4. What is causing the rectal bleeding?

5. Write the plural form of diverticulum.

MEDICAL RECORD 2–2. Carcinosarcoma of the Esophagus

Dictionary Exercise

This exercise will help you master the terminology in the medical record. Underline the following terms in the reading exercise and use a medical dictionary to define the words. The pronunciations of medical terms in this report are included in the audiocassette exercise on pages 73–75.

aortic arch _____

barium _____

biopsy _____

carcinosarcoma _____

cm _____

dysphagia _____

esophagus _____

esophagoscopy _____

friable _____

intraluminal _____

lymph node _____

mediastinal _____

malignant _____

OR _____

polypoid _____

resection _____

reanastomosis _____

Word Element Exercise

Break down the following words into their basic elements.

carcinosarcoma   pathology
dysphagia   polypoid
esophagoscopy   esophageal

VALIDATION FRAME: Check your answers in Appendix B, Answer Key.

Reading Exercise
Read the case study out loud.

Admitting Diagnosis: Carcinosarcoma of the esophagus.

Discharge Diagnosis: Carcinosarcoma of the esophagus.

History of Present Illness: Patient had been complaining of dysphagia over the last 4 months with a worsening in symptoms recently.

Surgery: Esophagoscopy was performed and a small friable biopsy was obtained. Pathology tests confirmed it to be malignant. A barium x-ray study revealed polypoid, intraluminal, esophageal obstruction. Surgical findings revealed an infiltrating tumor of the middle third of the esophagus with intraluminal, friable, polypoid masses, each 3 cm in diameter. A resection of the esophagus was performed with reanastomosis of the stomach at the aortic arch. An adjacent mediastinal lymph node was excised. There were no complications during the procedure. Patient left the OR in stable condition.

MEDICAL RECORD EVALUATION 2–2. Carcinosarcoma of the Esophagus

1. What surgery was performed on this patient?

2. What diagnostic testing confirmed malignancy?

3. Where was the carcinosarcoma located?

4. Why was the adjacent lymph node excised?

ABBREVIATIONS

Abbreviations Related to Diagnostic Tests

BA	barium	FBS	fasting blood sugar
BaE	barium enema	GTT	glucose tolerance test
CA	cancer	IBD	inflammatory bowel disease
cm	centimeter	HCl	hydrochloric acid
CT scan, CAT scan	computerized tomography scan	IVC	intravenous cholangiography
Dx	diagnosis	SGOT, SGPT	liver function enzyme tests
EGD	esophagogastroduodenoscopy	UGI	upper gastrointestinal
GI	gastrointestinal		

Other Abbreviations Related to the Gastrointestinal System

BM	bowel movement	PE	physical examination
HAV	hepatitis A virus	RUQ	right upper quadrant
HBV	hepatitis B virus		

Audiocassette Exercise

The audiocassette tape helps you master the pronunciation of medical words. Listen to the tape for instructions to complete this exercise. You may also use this list without the audiotape to practice correct spelling and pronunciation of the terms.

Frame	Word	Pronunciation	Spelling Exercise
Reading Exercise	[] angulation	(ăng-ū-LĀ-shŭn)	_____
Reading Exercise	[] anorectal	(ā-nō-RĔK-tăl)	_____
Additional Pathological Conditions	[] anorexia	(ăn-ō-RĔK-sē-ă)	_____
Reading Exercise	[] appendectomy	(ăp-ĕn-DĔK-tō-mē)	_____
Additional Pathological Conditions	[] ascites	(ă-SĪ-tēz)	_____
Additional Pathological Conditions	[] borborygmus	(bŏr-bō-RĬG-mŭs)	_____
Additional Pathological Conditions	[] bulimia	(bū-LĬM-ē-ă)	_____
2–179	[] calculus	(KĂL-kū-lŭs)	_____
Reading Exercise	[] carcinoma	(kăr-sĭ-NŌ-mă)	_____
Reading Exercise	[] carcinosarcoma	(kăr-să-nō-săr-KŌM-ă)	_____
2–187	[] cholecyst	(KŌ-lē-sĭst)	_____
2–199	[] cholecystalgia	(kō-lē-sĭs-TĂL-jē-ă)	_____
2–188	[] cholecystitis	(kō-lē-sĭs-TĪ-tĭs)	_____
2–199	[] cholecystodynia	(kō-lē-sĭs-tō-DĬN-ē-ă)	_____
2–218	[] cholecystogram	(kō-lē-SĬS-tō-grăm)	_____
2–218	[] cholecystography	(kō-lē-sĭs-TŎG-ră-fē)	_____
2–177	[] cholecystolith	(kō-lē-SĬS-tō-lĭth)	_____
2–197	[] cholecystolithiasis	(kō-lē-sĭs-tō-lĭ-THĪ-ă-sĭs)	_____
2–183	[] choledochitis	(kō-lē-dō-KĪ-tĭs)	_____
2–186	[] choledocholith	(kō-LĔD-ō-kō-lĭth)	_____
2–183	[] choledochoplasty	(kō-LĔD-ō-kō-plăs-tē)	_____
2–183	[] choledochorrhaphy	(kō-lĕd-ō-KŌR-ă-fē)	_____
2–186	[] choledochotomy	(kō-lĕd-ō-KŎT-ō-mē)	_____
2–180	[] cholelith	(KŌ-lē-lĭth)	_____
2–197	[] cholelithiasis	(kō-lē-lĭ-THĪ-ă-sĭs)	_____
2–171	[] cholemesis	(kō-LĔM-ĕ-sĭs)	_____
Additional Pathological Conditions	[] cirrhosis	(sĭ-RŌ-sĭs)	_____
Reading Exercise	[] colonic	(kō-LŎN-ĭk)	_____
Reading Exercise	[] constipation	(kŏn-stĭ-PĀ-shŭn)	_____
2–169	[] cystic	(SĬS-tĭk)	_____
2–168	[] cystitis	(SĬS-TĪ-tĭs)	_____
2–206	[] diarrhea	(dī-ă-RĒ-ă)	_____
2–207	[] diathermy	(DĪ-ă-thĕr-mē)	_____
Reading Exercise	[] diverticulum	(dī-vĕr-TĬK-ū-lŭm)	_____

Frame	Word	Pronunciation	Spelling Exercise
Additional Pathological Conditions	[] dysentery	(DĬS-ĕn-tĕr-ē)	_____
2–97	[] dyspepsia	(dĭs-PĔP-sē-ă)	_____
Reading Exercise	[] dysphagia	(dĭs-FĀ-jē-ă)	_____
Reading Exercise	[] emesis	(ĔM-ĕ-sĭs)	_____
Reading Exercise	[] enteritis	(ĕn-tĕr-Ī-tĭs)	_____
Reading Exercise	[] esophageal	(ē-sŏf-ă-JĒ-ăl)	_____
2–204	[] esophagoplasty	(ē-SŎF-ă-gō-plăs-tē)	_____
Reading Exercise	[] esophagoscopy	(ē-SŎF-ă-gŏs-kō-pē)	_____
2–223	[] gastromegaly	(găs-trō-MĔG-ă-lē)	_____
Reading Exercise	[] hematemesis	(hĕm-ăt-ĔM-ĕ-sĭs)	_____
Additional Pathological Conditions	[] hematochezia	(hĕm-ă-tō-KĒ-zē-ă)	_____
Additional Pathological Conditions	[] hemorrhoid	(HĔM-ō-royd)	_____
2–165	[] hepatalgia	(hĕp-ă-TĂL-jē-ă)	_____
2–165	[] hepatectomy	(hĕp-ă-TĔK-tō-mē)	_____
2–169	[] hepatic	(hĕ-PĂT-ĭk)	_____
2–164	[] hepatitis	(hĕp-ă-TĪ-tĭs)	_____
2–192	[] hepatitis B	(hĕp-ă-TĪ-tĭs BĒ)	_____
2–165	[] hepatodynia	(hĕp-ă-tō-DĬN-ē-ă)	_____
2–177	[] hepatolith	(hĕp-Ă-tō-lĭth)	_____
2–192	[] hepatoma	(hĕp-ă-TŌ-mă)	_____
2–222	[] hepatomegaly	(hĕp-ă-tō-MĔG-ă-lē)	_____
2–165	[] hepatorrhaphy	(hĕp-ă-TŎR-ă-fē)	_____
2–192	[] hepatosis	(hĕp-ă-TŌ-sĭs)	_____
Additional Pathological Conditions	[] hernia	(HĔR-nē-ă)	_____
Reading Exercise	[] ileostomy	(ĬL-ē-ŏs-tō-mē)	_____
Additional Pathological Conditions	[] inflammatory bowel disease (IBD)		_____
Additional Pathological Conditions	[] irritable bowel syndrome		_____
Reading Exercise	[] intraluminal	(ĭn-tră-LŪ-mĭ-năl)	_____
Additional Pathological Conditions	[] jaundice	(JAWN-dĭs)	_____
Reading Exercise	[] malignant	(mă-LĬG-nănt)	_____
Reading Exercise	[] mediastinal	(mē-dē-ăs-TĪ-năl)	_____
2–226	[] megaloesophagus	(mĕg-ă-lō-ē-SŎF-ă-gŭs)	_____
2–224	[] megalogastria	(mĕg-ă-lō-GĂS-trē-ă)	_____
2–225	[] megalogastric	(mĕg-ă-lō-GĂS-trĭk)	_____
Reading Exercise	[] nausea	(NĂW-sē-ă)	_____
2–162	[] pancreas	(PĂN-krē-ăs)	_____
2–201	[] pancreatectomy	(păn-krē-ă-TĔK-tō-mē)	_____
2–169	[] pancreatic	(păn-krē-ĂT-ĭk)	_____

Frame	Word	Pronunciation	Spelling Exercise
2–163	[] pancreatitis	(păn-krē-ă-TĪ-tĭs)	_____
2–177	[] pancreatolith	(păn-krē-ĂT-ō-lĭth)	_____
2–197	[] pancreatolithiasis	(păn-krē-ă-tō-lĭ-THĪ-ă-sĭs)	_____
Reading Exercise	[] polyp	(PŎL-ĭp)	_____
Reading Exercise	[] postprandial	(pōst-PRĂN-dē-ăl)	_____
Reading Exercise	[] regional	(RĒ-jŭn-ăl)	_____
Reading Exercise	[] sigmoidoscopy	(sĭg-moy-DŎS-kō-pē)	_____
2–209	[] thermometer	(thĕr-MŎM-ĕ-tĕr)	_____
2–211	[] toxic	(TŎKS-ĭk)	_____
2–212	[] toxicosis	(tŏks-ĭ-KŌ-sĭs)	_____
Additional Pathological Conditions	[] ulcer	(ŬL-sĕr)	_____
Additional Pathological Conditions	[] volvulus	(VŎL-vū-lŭs)	_____

Unit Exercises

DEFINITIONS

Review the Unit Summary on pages 83–85. You can also make your own flash cards to reinforce your learning of the medical word elements presented in this unit. Write the definition for each element.

SUFFIXES, PREFIXES, AND ABBREVIATIONS

Element	Meaning
SURGICAL SUFFIXES	
1. -ectomy	_____
2. -plasty	_____
3. -rrhaphy	_____
4. -stomy	_____
5. -tomy	_____
OTHER SUFFIXES	
6. -algia, -dynia	_____
7. -emesis	_____
8. -gram	_____
9. -graphy	_____
10. -iasis	_____
11. -itis	_____
12. -lith	_____
13. -megaly	_____
14. -oma	_____
15. -osis	_____
16. -pepsia	_____
17. -phagia	_____
18. -rrhea	_____
19. -scope	_____
20. -scopy	_____
21. -spasm	_____
22. -stenosis	_____
PREFIXES AND ABBREVIATIONS	
23. dia-	_____
24. dys-	_____
25. epi-	_____
26. hypo-	_____
27. peri-	_____
28. sub-	_____
29. GI	_____
30. CA	_____

COMBINING FORMS RELATED TO THE GASTROINTESTINAL SYSTEM

31. dent/o, odont/o   _____

32. col/o, colon/o   _____

33. duoden/o   _____

34. enter/o   _____

35. esophag/o   _____

36. gastr/o   _____

37. gingiv/o   _____

38. ile/o   _____

39. jejun/o   _____

40. lingu/o   _____

41. maxill/o   _____

42. proct/o   _____

43. rect/o   _____

44. sial/o   _____

45. sigmoid/o   _____

OTHER COMBINING FORMS IN UNIT 2

46. aer/o   _____

47. carcin/o   _____

48. hemat/o   _____

49. myc/o   _____

50. orth/o   _____

VALIDATION FRAME: Correct your answers using Index of Medical Word Elements, Appendix A. If you scored less than _____%,* review Unit 2 Digestive System Summary (pages 83–85) and retake this exercise.

    To obtain a percentage score, multiply the number of correct answers times 2.

Number of Correct Answers: _____   **Percentage Score:** _____

*Enter the percentage required by your instructor to complete this course.

Vocabulary

Match the medical word(s) below with the definitions in the numbered list.

alimentary canal	dysphagia	rectoplasty
cholecystectomy	friable	salivary glands
cholecystogram	gastroscopy	sigmoid colon
choledoch	hematemesis	sigmoidotomy
cholelithiasis	hepatomegaly	stomach
duodenotomy	ileostomy	stomatalgia
dyspepsia	linguogingival	

1. _____ A visual examination of the stomach.

2. _____ Bad, painful, difficult digestion.

3. _____ Vomiting blood.

4. _____ Record of the gallbladder.

5. _____ Glands that secrete saliva.

6. _____ Another term for the GI system.

7. _____ Pain in the mouth.

8. _____ An incision of the duodenum.

9. _____ Enlargement of the liver.

10. _____ Painful swallowing.

11. _____ Removal of the gallbladder.

12. _____ Pertaining to the tongue and gums.

13. _____ Incision of the sigmoid colon.

14. _____ Surgical repair of the rectum.

15. _____ Organ to which the esophagus transports food.

16. _____ Formation of a new opening (mouth) into the ileum.

17. _____ Abnormal condition of gallstones.

18. _____ Easily broken or pulverized.

19. _____ Bile duct.

20. _____ The S-shaped lower end of the colon.

VALIDATION FRAME: Check your answers in the Answer Key, Appendix B. If you scored less than _____%, review the vocabulary and retake this exercise.

To obtain a percentage score, multiply the number of correct answers times 5.

Number of Correct Answers: _____   **Percentage Score:** _____

PATHOLOGICAL CONDITIONS

Match the medical word(s) below with the definitions in the numbered list.

anorexia
ascites
bolus
borborygmus
bulimia
cirrhosis

Crohn's disease
dysentery
hematochezia
hemorrhoids
hernia

inflammatory bowel disease (IBD)
irritable bowel syndrome
jaundice
ulcer
volvulus

1. _____ A twisting of the bowel upon itself causing obstruction.

2. _____ Protrusion or projection of an organ or a part of an organ through the wall of the cavity that normally contains it.

3. _____ A lack of appetite.

4. _____ A chronic liver disease.

5. _____ Red blood in stools.

6. _____ Accumulation of fluid in the abdomen.

7. _____ Eating disorder with a psychosomatic basis.

8. _____ Gurgling, rumbling sounds caused by movement of gas through the intestines.

9. _____ Open sore or lesion of skin tissue.

10. _____ Yellow discoloration of the skin caused by abnormally high levels of bilirubin in the blood.

11. _____ Intestinal function disturbance that includes an alteration in bowel activity and abdominal discomfort.

12. _____ Painful, inflamed intestines, especially the colon.

13. _____ Enlarged, twisted varicose veins in the rectal region.

14. _____ Ulceration of mucosa of the colon. Also called *ulcerative colitis*.

15. _____ Chronic inflammation of the intestinal tract, most commonly the ileum. Also called *regional enteritis*.

VALIDATION FRAME: Check your answers in the Answer Key, Appendix B. If you scored less than _____%, review the vocabulary and retake this exercise.

To obtain a percentage score, multiply the number of correct answers times 6.67.

Number of Correct Answers: _____

Percentage Score: _____

UNIT SUMMARY

COMBINING FORMS RELATED TO THE DIGESTIVE SYSTEM

Form	Pronunciation	Meaning
chol/e	kō-lē	bile, gall
cholecyst/o	kō-lē-sĭs-tō	gallbladder
choledoch/o	kō-lē-dō-kō	bile duct
col/o colon/o	kō-lō kō-lŏn-ō	colon (large intestine)
dent/o odont/o	dĕnt-ō ō-dŏn-tō	teeth
duoden/o	dū-ŏd-ē-nō	duodenum (first part)
enter/o	ĕn-tĕr-ō	intestine (usually small)
esophag/o	ē-sŏf-ă-gō	esophagus
gastr/o	găs-trō	stomach
gingiv/o	jĭn-jĭ-vō	gum
hepat/o	hĕp-ă-tō	liver
ile/o	ĭl-ē-ō	ileum (third part)
jejun/o	jē-jū-nō	jejunum (second part)
lingu/o	lĭng-gwō	tongue
or/o stomat/o	ŏr-ō stō-mă-tō	mouth
pancreat/o	păn-krē-ăt-ō	pancreas
proct/o	prŏk-tō	rectum, anus
rect/o	rĕk-tō	rectum
sial/o	sī-ăl-tō	saliva, salivary glands
sigmoid/o	sĭg-moy-dō	sigmoid colon

OTHER COMBINING FORMS IN UNIT 2

Form	Pronunciation	Meaning
aer/o	ĕr-ō	air
carcin/o	kăr-sĭn-ō	cancer
hemat/o	hĕm-ă-tō	blood
lith/o	lĭth-ō	stone, calculus
maxill/o	măk-sĭ-lō	jaw
myc/o	mī-kō	fungus
orth/o	ŏr-thō	straight
therm/o	thĕr-mō	heat

Form	Pronunciation	Meaning
tox/o toxic/o	tŏk-sō ⎫ tŏks-ĭ-kō ⎭	poison
vagin/o	vă-jĭn-ō	vagina

SUFFIXES AND PREFIXES

Suffix (Prefix)	Pronunciation	Meaning
ADJECTIVE-ENDING SUFFIXES		
-al -ar -ary -ic	ăl ⎫ ăr ⎪ ĕr-ē ⎬ ĭk ⎭	pertaining to
NOUN-ENDING SUFFIXES		
-ia	ē-ă	condition
-ist	ĭst	specialist
SURGICAL SUFFIXES		
-ectomy	ĕk-tō-mē	excision, removal
-plasty	plăs-tē	surgical repair
-rrhaphy	ră-fē	suture
-tome	tōm	instrument to cut
-tomy	tō-mē	incision, cut into
OTHER SUFFIXES		
-algia -dynia	ăl-jē-ă ⎫ dĭn-ē-ă ⎭	pain
-emesis	ĕm-ĕ-sĭs	vomit
-gram	grăm	record
-graphy	gră-fē	process of recording
-iasis	ī-ă-sĭs	abnormal condition (produced by something specified)
-itis	ī-tĭs	inflammation
-lith	lĭth	stone, calculus
-logist	lō-jĭst	specialist in the study of
-logy	lō-jē	study of
-megaly	mĕg-ă-lē	enlargement
-oma	ō-mă	tumor
-osis	ō-sĭs	abnormal condition
-pepsia	pĕp-sē-ă	digestion
-phagia	fā-jē-ă	swallow, eat

Suffix (Prefix)	Pronunciation	Meaning
-rrhea	rē-ă	flow, discharge
-scope	skōp	instrument to view
-scopy	skŏ-pē	visual examination
-spasm	spăzm	involuntary contraction, twitching
-stenosis	stĕ-nō-sĭs	stricture, narrowing

PREFIXES

Suffix (Prefix)	Pronunciation	Meaning
ab-	ăb	away from
dys-	dĭs	bad, painful, difficult
epi-	ĕp-ĭ	above, upon
hyper-	hī-pĕr	above, excessive
hypo-	hī-pō	under, below
peri-	pĕr-ĭ	around
sub-	sŭb	under, below

Urinary System

The urinary system includes two kidneys, two ureters, the urinary bladder, and the urethra (Fig. 3–1). These organs are present in both men and women, but the function in each sex differs. In the woman, the only function of the urethra is urination. In the man, the urethra has a dual function: urination and conveying secretions produced by the reproductive glands. In both sexes, the primary purpose of the urinary system is production and elimination of urine to help maintain a constant balance (homeostasis) of water, salts, and acids in the body fluids.

The combining forms related to the urinary system are summarized here. Review this information before you begin to work the frames.

COMBINING FORMS

Combining Form	Meaning	Example	Pronunciation
cyst/o	bladder	cyst/o/scope instrument to view	SĬST-ō-skōp
vesic/o		vesic/o/ureter/al pertaining to	vĕs-ĭ-kō-ū-RĒ-tĕr-ăl
ureter/o	ureter	ureter/o/lith stone, calculus	ū-RĒ-tĕr-ō-lĭth
glomerul/o	glomerulus	glomerul/o/pathy disease	glō-mĕr-ū-LŎP-ă-thē
nephr/o	kidney	nephr/itis inflammation	nĕf-RĪ-tĭs
ren/o		ren/al pertaining to	RĒ-năl

pyel/o	renal pelvis	pyel/o/lith/o/tomy
		   stone incision
		    calculus
			pī-ĕ-lō-lĭth-ŎT-ō-mē

ureter/o	ureter	ureter/o/cele herniation	ū-RĒ-tĕr-ō-sĕl
urethr/o	urethra	urethr/o/dynia pain	ū-RĒ-thrō-dĭn-ē-ă
ur/o	urine	ur/emia blood	ū-RĒ-mē-ă
urin/o		urin/ary pertaining to	Ū-rĭ-nār-ē

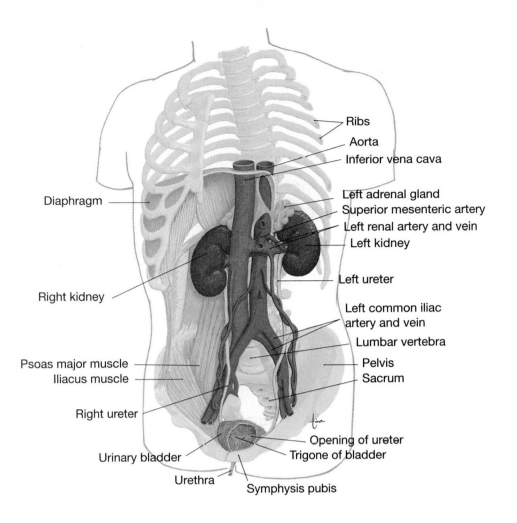

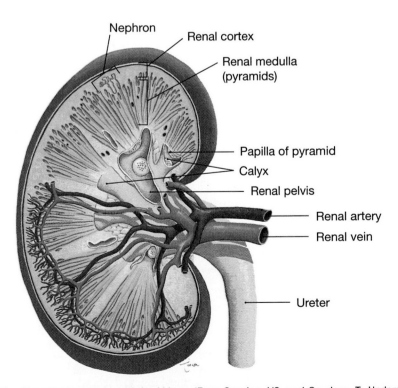

Figure 3–1. The urinary system and the kidney. (From Scanlon, VC, and Sanders, T: Understanding Human Structure and Function. FA Davis, Philadelphia, 1997, pp 325–326, with permission.)

KIDNEYS

3–1 Use the Index of Medical Word Elements in Part A of Appendix A to define the following word elements.

Medical Word Element	Meaning
-osis	_____
-pathy	_____
-pexy	_____
-ptosis	_____
supra-	_____

3–2 Use the Index of Medical Word Elements in Part B of Appendix A to write the medical word elements for the following English terms.

English Term	Medical Word Element
abnormal condition (produced by something specified)	_____
enlargement	_____
hardening	_____ / _____
kidney	_____ / _____ or
	_____ / _____
stone, calculus	_____

3–3 The main function of the **(1) kidneys** is to remove waste products from the blood in the form of urine. Label the kidney in Figure 3–2 as you learn the names of the parts of the urinary system.

---

enlargement

kidney(s)

3–4 **Nephr/o** and **ren/o** are combining forms that refer to the kidney. Nephr/o/megaly and ren/o/megaly both mean an _____ of the _____ .

---

inflammation

excision, removal

3–5 Remember that -itis refers to _____ , and -ectomy means _____ or _____ .

---

nephr/ectomy
(nĕ-FRĔK-tō-mē)
nephr/itis
(nĕf-RĪ-tĭs)

3–6 Use **nephr/o** to form medical words meaning

excision of a kidney: _____ / _____

inflammation of a kidney: _____ / _____

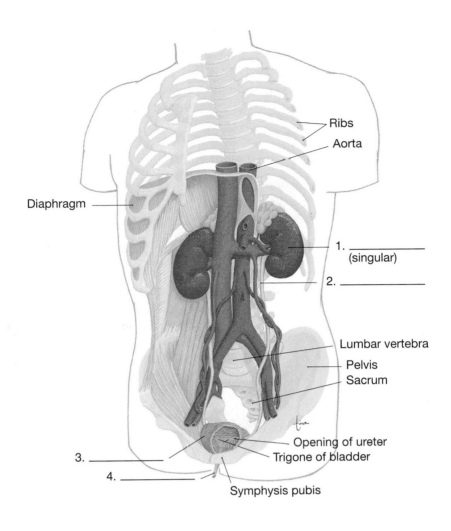

Ribs

Aorta

Diaphragm

1. _____
(singular)

2. _____

Lumbar vertebra

Pelvis

Sacrum

Opening of ureter

Trigone of bladder

3. _____

4. _____

Symphysis pubis

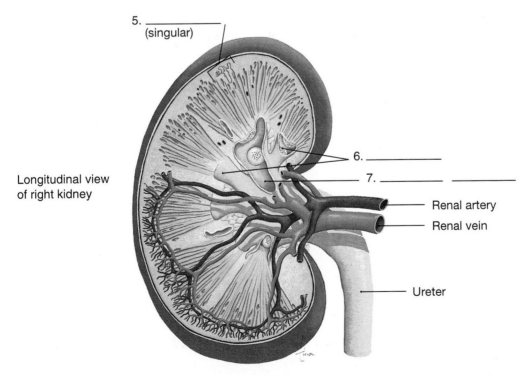

5. _____
(singular)

Longitudinal view
of right kidney

6. _____

7. _____ _____

Renal artery

Renal vein

Ureter

Figure 3–2. The urinary system, including the longitudinal section (*inset*) of a left kidney. (Adapted from Scanlon, VC, and Sanders, T: Understanding Human Structure and Function. FA Davis, Philadelphia, 1997, pp 325–326, with permission.)

kidney stomach pertaining to	**3–7** Analyze ren/o/gastr/ic by defining the elements. **ren/o** refers to _____ . **gastr** refers to _____ . -ic refers to _____ _____ (adjective ending).
kidney(s)	**3–8** Ren/o/intestin/al means pertaining to the _____ and intestine.
lith/iasis (lĭth-Ī-ă-sĭs)	**3–9** Recall the suffix -iasis is used to describe an abnormal condition (produced by something specified). An abnormal condition of stones is called _____ / _____ .
nephr/o/lith (NĔF-rō-lĭth) nephr/o/lith/iasis (nĕf-rō-lĭth-Ī-ă-sĭs)	**3–10** Use **nephr/o** to construct medical words meaning stone (in the) kidney: _____ / ___ / _____ abnormal condition of kidney stone(s): _nephro_ / _o_ / _lith_ / _iasis_
nephr/o/lith/iasis (nĕf-rō-lĭth-Ī-ă-sĭs)	**3–11** Once kidney stones are present, they can be extremely painful. A person with kidney stones suffers from _nephro_ / _o_ / _lith_ / _iasis_ .
	3–12 The surgical suffixes -ectomy , -tomy , and -tome are often confusing to beginning medical terminology students. To reinforce your understanding of their meanings, review them in the following chart. *Surgical Suffix* — *Meaning* -ectomy — excision, removal -tomy — incision, cut into -tome — instrument to cut
incision stone or calculus	**3–13** Stones that are trapped in the kidney or ureter may need to be removed surgically. Nephr/o/lith/o/tomy is an _____ to remove a ren/al _____ .
kidney abnormal condition	**3–14** High blood pressure and diabetes damage the kidneys and cause nephr/osis. Analyze nephr/osis by defining the elements. **nephr/o** means _____ . -osis means _____ _____ .

A combining vowel is not used to link a suffix that begins with a vowel.	**3-15** State the rule for forming nephr/osis. _____ _____
swelling	**3-16** A patient with nephr/osis exhibits edema (swelling) in the body, especially around the ankles, feet, and eyes. The term edema indicates a _____ .
edema (ĕ-DĒ-mă)	**3-17** Although there are various types of edema, they all mean swelling. The medical word for swelling is _____ .
edema (ĕ-DĒ-mă)	**3-18** When body tissues contain an excessive amount of fluid, a swelling or _____ results.
diuretic (dī-ū-RĔT-ĭc)	**3-19** Diuretics are agents or drugs that stimulate the flow of urine; they are used to control edema. A diet that is high in sodium causes a swelling around the ankles and feet. When this occurs, the physician may prescribe a _____ .
diuretic (dī-ū-RĔT-ĭc)	**3-20** Coffee increases the production of urine, which means that it is a _____ .
-pathy ren/o	**3-21** Ren/o/pathy is a disease of the kidney. Determine the element in ren/o/pathy that means disease: _-pathy_ kidney: _reno_ / _o_
nephr/o/pathy (nĕ-FRŎP-ĕ-thē) ren/o/pathy (rē-NŎP-ă-thē)	**3-22** Use **nephr/o** and **ren/o** to develop words meaning disease of the kidney. _nephr._ / _o_ / _pathy_ and _reno_ / _o_ / _pathy_
supra- ren -al	**3-23** Supra/ren/al is a directional term that means above the kidney. The element in supra/ren/al that means above is _supra-_ . The element that means kidney is _ren_ . The element that means pertaining to is _al_ .

scler/o	**3–24** The combining form **scler/o** is used in words to indicate a hardening of a body part. It also refers to the sclera, or white of the eye (covered in Unit 10). To indicate a hardening, use the combining form _____ / _____ .
hardening	**3–25** Scler/osis is an abnormal condition of _____ .
nephr/osis (něf-RŌ-sĭs) nephr/o/scler/osis (něf-rō-sklě-RŌ-sĭs) nephr/o/lith (NĚF-rō-lĭth) nephr/o/lith/iasis (něf-rō-lĭth-Ī-ă-sĭs)	**3–26** Use **nephr/o** to form medical words meaning an abnormal condition of a kidney: _nephr_ / _osis_ an abnormal condition of kidney hardening: _nephr_ / _o_ / _scler_ / _osis_ a stone in a kidney: _nephr_ / _o_ / _lith_ abnormal condition of kidney stone(s): _nephr_ / _o_ / _lith_ / _iasis_
-megaly	**3–27** Recall the suffix for enlargement is _-megaly_ .
nephr/o/megaly (něf-rō-MĚG-ă-lē)	**3–28** When the kidneys become diseased, an enlargement of one or both kidneys may result. Use **nephr/o** to formulate a word meaning enlargement of a kidney: _nephr_ / _o_ / _megaly_
kidney stone or calculus	**3–29** A lith/o/tomy is an incision to remove a stone or calculus. A nephr/o/lith/o/tomy is an incision of the _kidney_ to remove a _stone or calculus_.
nephr/ectomy (ně-FRĚK-tō-mē) nephr/o/rrhaphy (něf-RŌR-ă-fē) nephr/o/tomy (ně-FRŎT-ō-mē) nephr/o/lith/o/tomy (něf-rō-lĭth-ŎT-ō-mē)	**3–30** Use **nephr/o** to construct surgical words meaning excision of a kidney: _nephr_ / _ectomy_ suture of a kidney: _nephr_ / _o_ / _rrhaphy_ incision of the kidney: _nephr_ / _o_ / _tomy_ incision of a kidney stone: _nephr_ / _o_ / _lith_ / _o_ / _tomy_

nephr/o/ptosis (nĕf-rŏp-TŌ-sĭs)	**3–31** A kidney may prolapse or drop from its normal position because of a birth defect or injury. Combine **nephr/o** and **-ptosis** to build a word meaning prolapse of a kidney. _nephr_ / _o_ / _ptosis_
-ptosis nephr/o	**3–32** Determine the element in nephr/o/ptosis that means prolapse, falling, dropping: _ptosis_ kidney: _nephr_ / _o_
nephr/o/ptosis (nĕf-rŏp-TŌ-sĭs)	**3–33** A downward displacement of a kidney, or kidneys, because of a birth defect or injury is also called _nephr_ / _o_ / _ptosis_ .
-pexy -ptosis	**3–34** Nephr/o/pexy is the surgical procedure performed to correct nephr/o/ptosis. Determine the element in this frame that means surgical fixation: _pexy_ prolapse, falling, dropping: _ptosis_
nephr/o/ptosis (nĕf-rŏp-TŌ-sĭs) nephr/o/pexy (NĔF-rō-pĕks-ē) nephr/osis (nĕf-RŌ-sĭs)	**3–35** Use **nephr/o** to build medical words meaning prolapse of a kidney: _nephr_ / _o_ / _ptosis_ fixation or suspension of a kidney: _nephr_ / _o_ / _pexy_ abnormal condition of a kidney: _nephr_ / _osis_

Review

Select the element(s) that match(es) the meaning.

lith/o ✓
nephr/o
ren/o ✓
scler/o ✓

-ectomy
-iasis ✓
-lith ✓
-megaly ✓
-oma
-osis ✓
-pathy
-pexy ✓
-ptosis ✓
-rrhaphy ✓
-tome ✓
-tomy

supra- ✓

a. _____-osis_____ abnormal condition

b. _____-iasis_____ abnormal condition (produced by something specified)

c. _____supra-_____ above

d. _____ disease

e. _____-megaly_____ enlargement

f. _____ excision, removal

g. _____pexy_____ fixation

h. _____scler/o_____ hardening

i. _____-tome_____ instrument to cut

j. _____ incision, cut into

k. _____ren/o_____ kidney

l. _____-ptosis_____ prolapse, falling, dropping

m. _____-lith_____ stone, calculus

n. _____-rrhaphy_____ suture

Check your answers with the Review Answer Key on the following page.

Review Answer Key

a. -osis

b. -iasis

c. supra-

d. -pathy

e. -megaly

f. -ectomy

g. -pexy

h. scler/o

i. -tome

j. -tomy

k. nephr/o, ren/o

l. -ptosis

m. -lith, lith/o

n. -rrhaphy

REINFORCEMENT FRAME: If you are not satisfied with your level of comprehension, go back to Frame 3–1 and rework the frames. You can also make your own flash cards to reinforce your learning of the medical word elements presented in this section.

REMINDER FRAME: Define medical words by first defining the suffix and then the first part(s) of the word. Refer to the Informative Frame on page 27 to review this method.

URETER, BLADDER, URETHRA

3–36 Use the Index of Medical Word Elements in Part B of Appendix A to define the word elements used in this unit.

English Term	Medical Word Element
expansion, dilation	_– ectasis_
bladder	_____ / ____ or
	_____ / ____
crushing	_____
gland	_____ / ____
intestine	_____ / ____
ureter	_____ / ____
urethra	_____ / ____

3–37 Urine is conveyed from each kidney through its **(2) ureter** and stored in the urinary **(3) bladder** until it is expelled from the body through the **(4) urethra**.

Label Figure 3–2 as you learn the names of the structures in the urinary system.

---

ureters
(Ū-rĕ-tĕrs)

3–38 Locate the two pencil-like tubes in Figure 3–2 that transport urine from the kidneys to the urinary bladder. These are the _ureters_ .

---

enlargement, ureter
(Ū-rĕ-tĕr)

3–39 The combining form **ureter/o** refers to the ureter.

Ureter/o/megaly is an _elongemnt_ of the _ureter_ .

---

ureter/o

-ectasis

3–40 Ureter/ectasis is a dilation of the ureter.

The combining form for ureter is _ureter_ / _o_ .

Write the word element that denotes expansion or dilation: _–ectasis_ .

---

ureter/o/lith
(ū-RĒ-tĕr-ō-lĭth)

ureter/o/lith/iasis
(ū-rĕ-tĕr-ō-lĭth-Ī-ăs-ĭs)

3–41 When a patient experiences pain or other difficulties because of calculi, the physician may decide to remove the stones.

Develop medical words that mean

stone in the ureter: _ureter_ / _o_ / _lith_

abnormal condition of a ureter(al) stone:
ureter / _o_ / _lith_ / _iasis_

---

incision, ureter

stone or calculus

3–42 Ureter/o/lith/o/tomy is an _incision_ of the _ureter_ to remove a _stone or calculus_

dilation ureter (Ū-rĕ-tĕr)	**3–43** Ureter/ectasis is an expansion or _____ of the _____ .

ureter/ectasis (ū-rē-tĕr-ĔK-tă-sĭs)	**3–44** When kidney stones get trapped in the ureter, the urine is blocked, causing pressure on the walls of the ureter. This blockage results in an expansion or dilation of the ureter, which is called _____ / _____ .

lith/o/tripsy (LĬTH-ō-trĭp-sē)	**3–45** Stones are formed in the urinary tract by the deposit of various crystalline substances excreted in the urine. In some cases, the stone may be surgically crushed so that it is excreted in the urine. The suffix -tripsy is used in words to mean crushing. Combine **lith/o** and **-tripsy** to form a word that means surgical crushing of a stone: _____ / _____ / _____

-tripsy lith/o	**3–46** List the element in lith/o/tripsy that denotes crushing: _–tripsy_____ a stone or calculus: __lith__ / _o_

cyst/o/lith (SĬS-tō-lĭth) cyst/o/lith/iasis (sĭs-tō-lĭ-THĪ-ă-sĭs) cyst/o/lith/o/tomy (sĭs-tō-lĭth-ŎT-ō-mē)	**3–47** The urinary bladder, which is a muscular sac, stores urine until it is voided. The combining forms **cyst/o** and **vesic/o** are used in words to refer to the bladder. Use **cyst/o** to form words meaning a stone in the bladder: _____ / _____ / _____ an abnormal condition of a bladder stone: _____ / _____ / _____ / _____ an incision into the bladder to remove a stone: _____ / _____ / _____ / _____ / _____

instrument ureter	**3–48** A ureter/o/cyst/o/scope is an _____ used to view the _____ and bladder.

ureter/algia (ū-rē-tĕr-ĂL-jē-ă)	**3–49** When ureter/o/liths get trapped in the ureter, a person may experience ureter/o/dynia or _____ / _____ .

ureter/o/liths
(ū-RĒ-tĕr-ō-lĭths)

ureter/o/cyst/o/scope
(ū-rē-tĕr-ō-SĬS-tō-skōp)

ureter/o/cyst/o/scopy
(ū-rē-tĕr-ō-sĭs-TŎS-kō-pē)

3-50 Form medical words to mean stones

in the ureter:

_____ / ___ / _____

an instrument to view the ureter and bladder:

_____ / ___ / _____ / ___ / _____

visual examination of the ureter and bladder:

_____ / ___ / _____ / ___ / _____

---

suture
(SŪ-chūr)

3-51 Remember that the surgical suffix -rrhaphy is used in words to mean

_____ .

---

ureter/o/rrhaphy
(ū-rē-tĕr-ŎR-ră-fē)

cyst/o/rrhaphy
(sĭs-TŎR-ă-fē)

3-52 Construct surgical words meaning

suture of the ureter: _____ / ___ / _____

suture of the bladder: _____ / ___ / _____

---

dictionary

vesic/o

cyst/o

3-53 When forming medical words, you may have a choice of two or more elements that have the same meaning. For example, **vesic/o** and **cyst/o** both mean bladder. Refer to a medical dictionary when you are in doubt about which combining form to use.

Keep a medical _____ handy as a reference when you need additional information about a word.

The combining forms for bladder are _____ / ___ and

_____ / ___ .

---

medical

3-54 Whenever you are in doubt about a medical word, look it up in your _____ dictionary.

---

bladder

intestine

3-55 Vesic/o/enter/ic means pertaining to the _____ and

_____ .

---

bladder

surgical repair

3-56 After childbirth, some women suffer a prolapse of the bladder into the vagina, which results in an inability to retain urine. Cyst/o/plasty is performed to repair the problem. Analyze cyst/o/plasty by defining the elements:

cyst/o means _____

-plasty means _____ _____

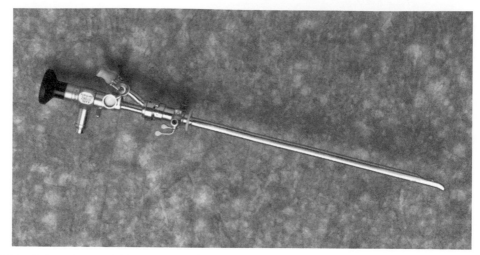

Figure 3–3. As assembled cystoscope. (From Brubaker, LT, and Saclarides, TJ: The Female Pelvic Floor: Disorders of Function and Support. FA Davis, Philadelphia, 1996, p 115, with permission.)

cyst/o/scopy
(sĭs-TŎS-kō-pē)

3–57   A cyst/o/scope (Fig. 3–3) is an instrument that is used to view the bladder.

Form a medical term that means visual examination of the bladder:

_____ / _____ / _____

---

cyst/ectomy
(sĭs-TĔK-tō-mē)
cyst/o/plasty
(SĬS-tō-plăs-tē)
cyst/o/scope
(SĬST-ō-skōp)

3–58   Construct surgical words meaning

excision of the bladder: _____ / _____

surgical repair of the bladder: _____ / _____ / _____

instrument to view the bladder: _____ / _____ / _____

---

urethr/o

3–59   The urethra differs in men and women. In men it serves a dual purpose of conveying sperm and discharging urine from the bladder. The female urethra performs only the latter function. The combining form for urethra is

_____ / _____ .

---

urethr/itis
(ū-rē-THRĪ-tĭs)
urethr/ectomy
(ū-rē-THRĔK-tō-mē)
urethr/o/pexy
(ū-RĒ-thrō-pĕks-ē)
urethr/o/plasty
(ū-RĒ-thrō-plăs-tē)

3–60   Formulate medical words meaning

inflammation of the urethra: _____ / _____

excision of the urethra: _____ / _____

surgical fixation of the urethra: _____ / _____ / _____

surgical repair of the urethra: _____ / _____ / _____

---

pain, urethra
(ū-RĒ-thră)

3–61   Urethr/o/dynia is a _____ in the _____ .

3–62 In addition to the urethr/o/dynia, construct another word meaning pain in the urethra: _____ / _____

urethr/algia
(ū-rē-THRĂL-jē-ă)

3–63 Cyst/itis and urethr/itis are two common lower urinary tract infections (UTIs) that almost always occur in women. Write the terms that mean

inflammation of the bladder: _____ / _____

inflammation of the urethra: _____ / _____

Write the abbreviation for urinary tract infection: _____ .

cyst/itis
(sĭs-TĪ-tĭs)
urethr/itis
(ū-rē-THRĪ-tĭs)

UTI

3–64 Urethr/o/rect/al means pertaining to the _____ and

_____ .

urethra
(ū-RĒ-thră)
rectum
(RĔK-tŭm)

3–65 Construct a medical word meaning inflammation of the urethra and bladder: _____ / ____ / _____ / _____

urethr/o/cyst/itis
(ū-rē-thrō-sĭs-TĪ-tĭs)

3–66 Form medical words to mean

an instrument to view the urethra:

_____ / ____ / _____

visual examination of the urethra:

_____ / ____ / _____

urethr/o/scope
(ū-RĒ-thrō-skōp)

urethr/o/scopy
(ū-rē-THRŎS-kō-pē)

3–66A Cyst/o/urethr/o/scopy (Fig. 3–4) is performed to examine the urethra and bladder. The instrument used to perform a cyst/o/urethr/o/scopy is a

_____ / ____ / _____ / ____ / _____

cyst/o/urethr/o/scope
(sĭs-tō-ū-RĒ-thrō-skōp)

3–67 Identify the element that denotes a noun ending in -algia, -dynia,

-pepsia, and -phagia : _____

-ia

3–68 The element in the suffixes in Frame 3–67 that means condition is

_____ .

-ia

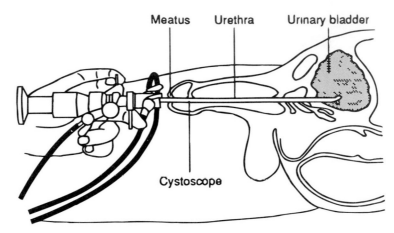

Figure 3–4. Cystourethroscopy. (From Watson, J, and Jaffe, MS: Nurse's Manual of Laboratory and Diagnostic Tests, ed 2. FA Davis, Philadelphia, 1995, p 526, with permission.)

malignant (mă-LĬG-nănt) benign (bĕ-NĪN)	**3–69** Malignant tumors or growths are cancerous, whereas benign tumors are noncancerous. Use the words "malignant" or "benign" to complete this frame. A cancerous tumor is a _____ tumor. A noncancerous tumor is a _____ tumor.
noncancerous	**3–70** Benign tumors are contained within a capsule and do not invade the surrounding tissue. They harm the individual only in that they place pressure on adjacent structures. Benign tumors are (cancerous, noncancerous) _____ growths.
cancerous	**3–71** Malignant tumors spread rather rapidly, are invasive, and are life threatening. Malignant tumors are (cancerous, noncancerous) _____ .
pain, gland	**3–72** The combining form **aden/o** is used in words to denote a gland. An aden/o/dynia is a _____ in a _____ .

gland
 	
cancer
 	
tumor
	3–73 Tumors of the urinary tract may be benign or malignant. An aden/o/carcin/oma is the most common malignant tumor of the kidney.
	
	Analyze aden/o/carcin/oma by defining the elements.
	
	    aden/o refers to _____ .
	
	    carcin/o refers to _____ .
	
	    -oma refers to _____ .

3–74 An aden/oma is a benign glandular tumor composed of the tissue from which it is developing; an aden/o/carcin/oma is a malignant glandular tumor.

Determine the words in this frame that mean

aden/oma
(ăd-ĕ-NŌ-mă)

noncancerous glandular tumor: _____ / _____

cancerous glandular tumor:

_____ / _____ / _____/_____

aden/o/carcin/oma
(ăd-ĕ-nō-kăr-sĭn-Ō-mă)

3–75 Form medical words to mean

aden/itis
(ăd-ĕ-NĪ-tĭs)
aden/oma
(ăd-ĕ-NŌ-mă)
aden/o/pathy
(ăd-ĕ-NŎP-ă-thē)

inflammation of a gland: _____ / _____

tumor of a gland: _____ / _____

disease of a gland: _____ / _____ / _____

3–76 Urinary tract infections (UTIs) account for the majority of office visits by individuals experiencing urinary tract problems.

urinary tract infection(s)

Define UTI(s): _____ _____ _____ .

Review

Select the element(s) that match(es) the meaning.

aden / o	-algia	-oma
carcin / o	-dynia	-pathy
cyst / o	-ectomy	-plasty
enter / o	-ectasis	-rrhaphy
rect / o	-iasis	-scope
ureter / o	-itis	-scopy
urethr / o	-lith	-tomy
vesic / o	-megaly	

a. _____ abnormal condition (produced by something specified)

b. _____ bladder

c. _____ cancer

d. _____ disease

e. _____ enlargement

f. _____ excision, removal

g. _____ expansion, dilation

h. _____ gland

i. _____ incision, cut into

j. _____ inflammation

k. _____ instrument to view

l. _____ intestines

m. _____ pain

n. _____ rectum

o. _____ stone, calculus

p. _____ surgical repair

q. _____ suture

r. _____ tumor

s. _____ ureter

t. _____ urethra

u. _____ visual examination

Check your answers with the Review Answer Key on the following page.

Review Answer Key

a. -iasis

b. cyst/o, vesic/o

c. carcin/o

d. -pathy

e. -megaly

f. -ectomy

g. -ectasis

h. aden/o

i. -tomy

j. -itis

k. -scope

l. enter/o

m. -algia, -dynia

n. rect/o

o. -lith

p. -plasty

q. -rrhaphy

r. -oma

s. ureter/o

t. urethr/o

u. -scopy

REINFORCEMENT FRAME: If you are not satisfied with your level of comprehension, go back to Frame 3–36 to rework the frames. You can also make your own flash cards to reinforce your learning of the medical word elements presented in this section.

NEPHRON

3–77   Use the Index of Medical Word Elements in Part A of Appendix A, to define the word elements used in this unit.

Element	Meaning
cyt/o, -cyte	_____
glomerul/o	_____
-gram	_____
intra-	_____
-pathy	_____
pyel/o	_____
ur/o	_____
ven/o	_____

3–78   The **(5) nephrons** are the microscopic filtering units; they produce urine and are responsible for continually keeping body fluids in balance. Each kidney consists of approximately 1 million nephrons.

Label the nephron in Figure 3–2 and note its location in the kidney.

nephr/o/ptosis
(nĕf-rŏp-TŌ-sĭs)
nephr/o/pexy
(NĔF-rō-pĕks-ē)

3–79   Use **nephr/o** to form medical words meaning

dropping or prolapse of a kidney: _____ / _____ / _____

surgical fixation of kidney: _____ / _____ / _____

3–80   Urine flows from the funnel-shaped extension called the **(6) calyx** (plural, **calyces**), to the **(7) renal pelvis** and into the ureter.

Label Figure 3–2 as you learn about the structures of the kidney.

inflammation

3–81   The combining form **pyel/o** refers to the renal pelvis. Pelvis is a word denoting any bowl-shaped structure. Pyel/itis is an _____ of the renal pelvis.

pyel/o/pathy
(pī-ĕ-LŎP-ă-thē)
pyel/o/tomy
(pī-ĕ-LŎT-ō-mē)

pyel/o/stomy
(pī-ĕ-LŎS-tō-mē)

3–82   Construct medical words meaning

disease of the renal pelvis: _____ / _____ / _____

incision of the renal pelvis: _____ / _____ / _____

forming a new opening or mouth into the renal pelvis:

_____ / _____ / _____

VALIDATION FRAME: Check your labeling of Figure 3–2 in the Answer Key, Appendix B.

3–83   Besides numerous other structures, each nephron contains a tiny ball of very small, coiled and intertwined capillaries called the **(1) glomerulus** (plural, **glomeruli**) and a **(2) collecting tubule** that carries the urine to the renal pelvis. The capsule that surrounds and encloses the glomerulus is **(3) Bowman's capsule**.

Label the structures in Figure 3–5.

---

glomerul/itis
(glō-mĕr-ū-LĪ-tĭs)
glomerul/o/pathy
(glō-mĕr-ū-LŎP-ă-thē)

3–84   Use **glomerul/o** to form medical words meaning

an inflammation of a glomerulus: _____ / _____

disease of a glomerulus: _____ / _____ / _____

---

glomerulus, hardening
(glō-MĔR-ū-lŭs)

3–85   Glomerul/o/scler/osis literally means an abnormal condition of

_____ (singular) _____ .

VALIDATION FRAME: Check your labeling of Figure 3–5 with the Answer Key in Appendix B.

3–86   Define *micturition* using your medical dictionary.

_____

_____

---

pyel/itis
(pī-ĕ-LĪ-tĭs)

pyel/o/plasty
(PĪ-ĕ-lō-plăs-tē)

ureter/o/pyel/o/plasty
(ū-rē-tĕr-ō-PĪ-ĕl-ō-plăs-tē)

3–87   Form medical words to mean

inflammation of the renal pelvis: _____ / _____

surgical repair of the renal pelvis: _____ / _____ / _____

surgical repair of the ureter and renal pelvis:

_____ / _____ / _____ / _____ / _____

---

intra/ven/ous
(ĭn-tră-VĒ-nŭs)
pyel/o/gram
(PĪ-ĕ-lō-grăm)
nephr/o/liths
(NĔF-rō-lĭths)
ureter/o/liths
(ū-RĒ-tĕr-ō-lĭths)

3–88   An intra/ven/ous pyel/o/gram (IVP) permits visualization of the kidneys, ureter, and bladder. It is used to verify kidney function or identify nephr/o/liths and ureter/o/liths.

Determine the words in this frame that mean

within a vein: _____ / _____ / _____

record (x-ray) of the renal pelvis: _____ / _____ / _____

stones in the kidney: _____ / _____ / _____

stones in the ureter: _____ / _____ / _____

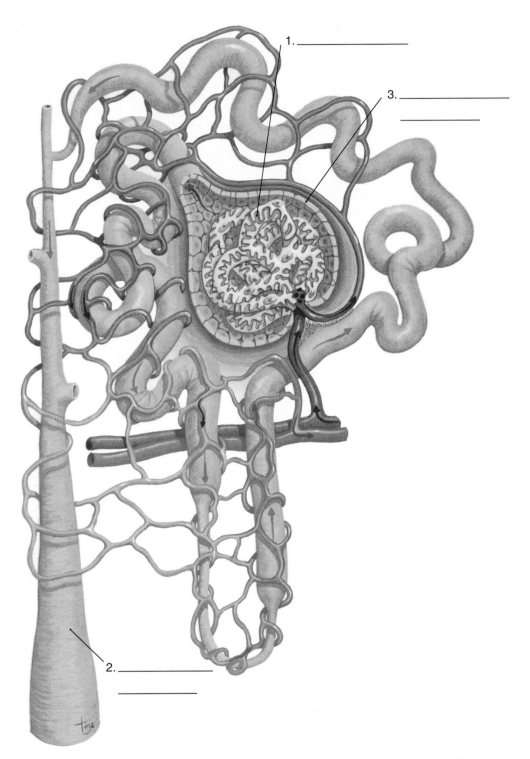

1. _____

3. _____
   _____

2. _____
   _____

Figure 3–5. A nephron. (Adapted from Scanlon, VC, and Sanders, T: Understanding Human Structure and Function. FA Davis, Philadelphia, 1997, p 327, with permission.)

IVP	**3–89** Write the abbreviation for intra/ven/ous pyel/o/gram: _____

3–90 An intra/ven/ous pyel/o/gram is an x-ray film of the kidneys after an injection of dye into a vein.

Identify the elements in this frame that mean

intra- within: _____

ven vein: _____

-ous pertaining to: _____ (adjective ending)

pyel/o renal pelvis: _____ / _____

-gram record: _____

3–91 Use **nephr/o** to construct medical terms meaning

nephr/o/scope
(NĔF-rō-skōp) an instrument to view the kidney: _____ / _____ / _____

nephr/o/scopy
(nĕ-FRŎ-skŏ-pē) visual examination of the kidney: _____ / _____ / _____

3–92 An incision in the renal pelvis is made to insert the nephr/o/scope to view the inside of the kidney. A visual examination of the kidney is called

nephr/o/scopy
(nĕ-FRŎ-skŏ-pē) _____ / _____ / _____ .

3–93 There are various types of nephr/itis. The usual form is glomerul/o/nephr/itis or Bright's disease, in which the glomeruli within the kidneys are inflamed.

Analyze glomerul/o/nephr/itis by defining the elements.

glomerulus
(glō-MĔR-ū-lŭs) **glomerul/o** refers to _____ (singular).

kidney(s) **nephr/o** refers to _____ .

inflammation -itis refers to _____ .

Bright's	**3–94** Another name for glomerul/o/nephr/itis is _____ disease.

3–95 Pyel/o/nephr/itis is a bacterial infection of the renal pelvis caused by bacterial invasion from the middle and lower urinary tract or bloodstream. Bacteria may gain access to the bladder via the urethra and ascend to the kidney.

Form medical words meaning

pyel/itis
(pī-ĕ-LĪ-tĭs) inflammation of the renal pelvis: _____ / _____

  inflammation of the renal pelvis and kidney:

pyel/o/nephr/itis
(pī-ĕ-lō-nĕ-FRĪ-tĭs) _____ / _____ / _____ / _____

3–96 Pyel/o/nephr/itis is very dangerous in pregnant women because it can cause premature labor. A woman who has a bacterial infection of the renal pelvis and kidneys has a condition called

pyel/o/nephr/itis
(pĭ-ĕ-lō-nĕ-FRĪ-tĭs)

_____ / _____ / _____ / _____ .

---

bladder

3–97 A cyst/o/cele is a protrusion or herniation of the _____ .

-cele

cyst/o

3–98 Identify the elements in cyst/o/cele that mean

hernia or swelling: _____

bladder: _____ / _____

-cele

3–99 A hernia is a protrusion or projection of an organ through the wall of the cavity that normally contains it. The suffix for hernia or swelling is _____ .

---

bladder

urethra
(ū-RĒ-thră)
rectum
(RĔK-tŭm)
intestine
(ĭn-TĔS-tĭn)

3–100 Four common types of hernias or protrusions that occur as downward displacements are:

cyst/o/cele, a protrusion or herniation of the _____ .

urethr/o/cele, a protrusion or herniation of the _____ .

rect/o/cele, a protrusion or herniation of the _____ .

enter/o/cele, a protrusion or herniation of the _____ .

---

cyst/o/cele
(SĬS-tō-sēl)
urethr/o/cele
(ū-RĒ-thrō-sēl)
rect/o/cele
(RĔK-tō-sēl)

3–101 Develop medical words meaning

herniation of the bladder: _____ / _____ / _____

herniation of the urethra: _____ / _____ / _____

herniation of the rectum: _____ / _____ / _____

---

white

red

3–102 The combining form **erythr/o** denotes the color red, and **leuk/o** denotes white.

Leuk/o/rrhea is a discharge that is _____ .

Erythr/uria is urine that is _____ .

---

cell

cell

3–103 The combining form for cell is **cyt/o**. The suffix -cyte also means cell. An erythr/o/cyte is a red blood _____ ; a leuk/o/cyte is a white blood _____ .

| pain | 3-104 Ur/o/dynia indicates _____ associated with urination. |
| ur/o | From ur/o/dynia, identify the combining form for urine: _____ / _____ |

| urine (Ū-rĭn) | 3-105 Ur/o/toxin is a poisonous substance in the _____ . |

| toxin (TŎKS-ĭn) | 3-106 From ur/o/toxin, determine the element meaning poisonous: _____ |

| poison | 3-107 A toxic substance in the body is a substance that resembles or is caused by a _____ . |

| ur/o/logy (ū-RŎL-ō-jē) ur/o/logist (ū-RŎL-ō-jĭst) | 3-108 Use **ur/o** to form words meaning

study of urine: _____ / _____ / _____

specialist in the study of urine: _____ / _____ / _____ |

INFORMATIVE FRAME: Two combining forms that sound somewhat alike but have different meanings are **pyel/o** and **py/o**. You will find the following clarification useful.

Combining Form	Meaning	Example
pyel/o	renal pelvis	pyel/o/pathy
py/o	pus	py/o/rrhea

| pyel/o/plasty (PĪ-ĕ-lō-plăs-tē) pyel/o/gram (PĪ-ĕ-lō-grăm) | 3-109 Formulate medical words to mean

surgical repair of the renal pelvis: _____ / _____ / _____

a record (x-ray) of the renal pelvis: _____ / _____ / _____ |

| py/o/rrhea (pī-ō-RĒ-ă)

py/o/nephr/osis (pī-ō-nĕf-RŌ-sĭs) | 3-110 Use **py/o** (pus) to build words meaning

discharge or flow of pus: _____ / _____ / _____

abnormal condition of pus from the kidney (Remember not to use -iasis because the pus is not produced by something specified.):

_____ / _____ / _____ / _____ |

3–111   Use the Index of Medical Word Elements in Part A of Appendix A to define the following elements. Use this information to complete Frame 3–113 through Frame 3–131.

Medical Word Element	*Meaning*
a-, an-	_____
hemat/o	_____
olig/o	_____
poly-	_____
-uria	_____

3–112   Use the Index of Medical Word Elements in Part B of Appendix A to define the medical word elements for the following English terms. Use this information to complete Frame 3–113 through Frame 3–130.

English Term	*Medical Word Element*
fear	_____
night	_____ / _____
pus	_____ / _____

---

py/uria
(pī-Ū-rē-ă)

3–113   The suffix -uria refers to urine or urination. Hemat/uria is a condition of blood in the urine. Form a word meaning pus in the urine: _____ / _____

---

an/uria
(ăn-Ū-rē-ă)

3–114   The prefixes a- and an- are used in words to mean without or not. The a- is usually used before a consonant. The an- is usually used before a vowel.

Construct a medical word meaning without urination:

_____ / _____

---

an/uria
(ăn-Ū-rē-ă)

3–115   Stoppage of urine production by the kidney can be a serious health problem if it persists. This condition is known as _____ / _____ .

---

py/uria
(pī-Ū-rē-ă)

3–116   Pus may be present in the urine if there is a kidney infection. A person with pus in the urine has a condition called _____ / _____ .

---

olig/uria
(ŏl-ĭg-Ū-rē-ă)

3–117   The combining form **olig/o** means scanty, or little. Combine **olig/o** and -uria to form a word meaning scanty urination:

_____ / _____

olig/uria (ŏl-ĭg-Ū-rē-ă)	**3-118** A diminished or scanty amount of urine formation is known as _____ / _____ .
scanty, or little, saliva	**3-119** Recall that **sial/o** refers to saliva. Olig/o/sial/ia is a condition of _____ _____ .
urination	**3-120** The prefix poly- means many, much, or an excess of. Poly/uria is a condition of excessive _____ .
poly/phobia (pŏl-ē-FŌ-bē-ă)	**3-121** The suffix -phobia refers to fear. A condition in which a person experiences many fears is called _____ / _____ .
inflammation, many	**3-122** Poly/aden/itis is an _____ of _____ glands.
night	**3-123** The combining form for night is **noct/o**. Noct/uria refers to urination at _____ .
noct/uria (nŏk-TŪ-rē-ă)	**3-124** Children have a tendency to urinate at night. This condition is called _____ / _____ .
urination	**3-125** Continence indicates self-control, and is the ability to control urination and defecation. A person who has urinary continence is able to control urination. A person with urinary in/continence is not able to control _____ .
in/continence (ĭn-KŎN-tĭ-něns)	**3-126** Many patients in nursing homes experience uncontrolled loss of urine from the bladder. These patients suffer from urinary _____ / _____ .

ur/o/logist or
(ū-RŎL-ō-jĭst)
  nephr/o/logist
  (nĕ-FRŎL-ō-jĭst)
	3-127 Persons with urinary disorders will see the medical specialist called a
	_____ / _____ / _____ .

Review

Select the combining form(s) that match(es) the meaning.

cyst/o
cyt/o
enter/o
erythr/o
glomerul/o
hemat/o
leuk/o
nephr/o

olig/o
pyel/o
py/o
ren/o
scler/o
ureter/o
urethr/o
ur/o

-uria

a. _____ bladder

b. _____ blood

c. _____ cell

d. _____ glomerulus

e. _____ hardening

f. _____ intestines

g. _____ kidney

h. _____ pus

i. _____ red

j. _____ renal pelvis

k. _____ scanty, little

l. _____ ureter

m. _____ urethra

n. _____ urine

o. _____ white

Check your answers with the Review Answer Key on the following page.

Review Answer Key

a. cyst/o

b. hemat/o

c. cyt/o

d. glomerul/o

e. scler/o

f. enter/o

g. nephr/o, ren/o

h. py/o

i. erythr/o

j. pyel/o

k. olig/o

l. ureter/o

m. urethr/o

n. ur/o

o. leuk/o

REINFORCEMENT FRAME: If you are not satisfied with your level of comprehension, go back to Frame 3–77 to rework the frames.

3-128 Cyst/itis is frequently caused by bacteria that originates in the fecal matter of the colon. The bacteria enters the urethra and ascends to the bladder.

cyst/itis
(sĭs-TĪ-tĭs)

An inflammation of the bladder is called _____ / _____ .

3-129 Cyst/itis is more common in women, owing to their shorter urethra and the closeness of the urethr/al orifice to the anus. Symptoms of cyst/itis include dys/uria (painful urination), bacteri/uria (bacteria in the urine), and py/uria (pus in the urine).

Identify the words in this frame that mean

dys/uria
(dĭs-Ū-rē-ă)
bacteri/uria
(băk-tē-rē-Ū-rē-ă)
py/uria
(pī-Ū-rē-ă)
cyst/itis
(sĭs-TĪ-tĭs)

    painful urination: _____ / _____

    bacteria in the urine: _____ / _____

    pus in the urine: _____ / _____

    inflammation of the bladder: _____ / _____

3-130 Pyel/o/nephr/itis, an inflammation of the renal pelvis and the kidney, is a common type of kidney disease and a frequent complication of cystitis.

Build a medical term that means

nephr/itis
(nĕf-RĪ-tĭs)

pyel/o/nephr/itis
pī-ĕ-lō-nĕ-FRĪ-tĭs)

    an inflammation of the kidney: _____ / _____

    an inflammation of the renal pelvis and kidney:

    _____ / _____ / _____ / _____

3-131 Glomerul/o/nephr/itis, a form of nephr/itis in which the lesions involve primarily the glomeruli, may result in protein/uria and hemat/uria.

Determine the medical words in this frame that mean

hemat/uria
(hĕm-ă-TŪ-rē-ă)
protein/uria
(prō-tē-ĭn-Ū-rē-ă)
nephr/itis
(nĕf-RĪ-tĭs)

    blood in the urine: _____ / _____

    protein in the urine: _____ / _____

    inflammation of the kidney: _____ / _____

3-132 A form of nephr/itis that involves the glomeruli is called

glomerul/o/nephr/itis
glō-mĕr-ū-lō-nĕ-FRĪ-tĭs)

_____ / _____ / _____ / _____ .

3-133 Any condition that impairs the flow of blood to the kidneys, such as shock, injury, or exposure to toxins, may result in acute renal failure (ARF).

acute renal

failure

The abbreviation ARF refers to _____ _____

_____ .

lith/ectomy
(lĭ-THĔK-tō-mē)

lith/o/tripsy
(LĬTH-ō-trĭp-sē)

nephr/o/lith/iasis
(nĕf-rō-lĭth-Ī-ă-sĭs)

3–134 Nephr/o/lith/iasis occurs when salts in the urine precipitate (settle out of solution and grow in size). Elimination of the stone(s) may occur spontaneously, but lith/o/tripsy or lith/ectomy may be performed to remove the stone(s).

Build medical terms that mean

excision of a stone: _____ / _____

crushing a stone: _____ / _____ / _____

abnormal condition (produced by something specified) of kidney stone(s):

_____ / _____ / _____ / _____

Review

Select the element(s) that match(es) the meaning.

-al   -plasty   a-
-cele   -ptosis   an-
-cyte   -rrhea   intra-
-dynia   -scope   poly-
-gram   -scopy
-itis
-lith
-ous
-pathy

a. _____ cell

b. _____ disease

c. _____ flow, discharge

d. _____ hernia, swelling

e. _____ inflammation

f. _____ instrument to view

g. _____ many, much

h. _____ pain

i. _____ pertaining to

j. _____ prolapse, falling, dropping

k. _____ record

l. _____ stone, calculus

m. _____ surgical repair

n. _____ visual examination

o. _____ within

p. _____ without, not

Check your answers with the Review Answer Key on the following page.

Review Answer Key

a. -cyte

b. -pathy

c. -rrhea

d. -cele

e. -itis

f. -scope

g. poly-

h. -dynia

i. -al, -ous

j. -ptosis

k. -gram

l. -lith

m. -plasty

n. -scopy

o. intra-

p. a-, an-

REINFORCEMENT FRAME: If you are not satisfied with your level of comprehension, go back to Frame 3–77 and rework the frames.

Other Pathological Conditions Related to the Urinary System

azoturea (ăz-ō-TŪ-rē-ă): an increase in nitrogenous compounds, especially urea, in urine.

bladder neck obstruction (BNO): blockage of the bladder outlet.

diuresis (dī-ū-RĒ-sĭs): abnormal secretion of large amounts of urine.

dysuria (dĭs-Ū-rē-ă): painful or difficult urination, symptomatic of numerous conditions.

end-stage renal disease: the final phase of a kidney disease process; kidney disease has advanced to the point that the kidneys can no longer adequately filter the blood.

enuresis (ĕn-ū-RĒ-sĭs): involuntary discharge of urine after the age by which bladder control should have been established. In children, voluntary control of urination is usually present by the age of 5. Also called *bed-wetting* at night.

hypospadias (hī-pō-SPĀ-dē-ăs): abnormal congenital opening of the male urethra upon the undersurface of the penis.

interstitial nephritis (ĭn-tĕr-STĪSH-ăl nĕf-RĪ-tĭs): nephritis associated with pathological changes in the renal interstitial tissue that in turn may be primary or due to a toxic agent such as a drug or chemical. The end result is that the nephrons are destroyed and renal function is seriously impaired.

phimosis (fī-MŌ-sĭs): stenosis or narrowness of the foreskin opening over the glans penis in men.

renal hypertension (RĒ-năl hī-pĕr-TĔN-shŭn): high blood pressure that results from a kidney disease.

uremia (ū-RĒ-mē-ă): elevated level of urea or other protein waste products in the blood.

Wilms' tumor (VĬLMZ TŪ-mŏr): rapidly developing kidney tumor that usually occurs in children. The cause of this tumor is unknown.

Medical Record

The reports that follow are related to the medical specialty called nephrology and urology. Nephrologists and urologists specialize in diagnosing and treating diseases and disorders of the urinary system of women and the genitourinary system of men.

MEDICAL RECORD 3–1. Cystitis

Dictionary Exercise

This exercise will help you master the terminology in the medical record. Underline the following terms in the reading exercise and use a medical dictionary to define the words. The pronunciations of medical terms in this report are included in the Audiocassette Exercise on pages 127–130.

appendectomy _____

cholecystectomy _____

cholecystitis _____

choledocholithiasis _____

choledocholithotomy _____

cholelithiasis _____

cystitis _____

cystoscopy _____

epigastric _____

hematuria _____

nocturia _____

pelvic _____

polyuria _____

spasm _____

urinary incontinence _____

urinary frequency _____

Word Element Exercise

Break down the following words into their basic elements. The first one is completed for you.

pelv/ic
cystoscopy
cystitis
nocturia
epigastric
polyuria

hematuria
cholelithiasis
choledocholithiasis
cholecystectomy
choledocholithotomy
appendectomy

VALIDATION FRAME: Check your answers in Appendix B, Answer Key.

Reading Exercise

Read the case study out loud.

This 50-year-old white woman has been complaining of diffuse pelvic pain with urinary bladder spasm since cystoscopy 10 days ago, at which time marked cystitis was noted. She reports nocturia three to four times, urinary frequency, urgency, and epigastric discomfort. The patient has had a history of polyuria, hematuria, and urinary incontinence. There is a history of numerous stones, large and small, in the gallbladder. In 19XX she was admitted to the hospital with cholecystitis, chronic and acute; cholelithiasis; and choledocholithiasis. Subsequently, cholecystectomy, choledocholithotomy, and incidental appendectomy were performed. My impression is that the urinary incontinence is due to cystitis and is temporary in nature.

MEDICAL RECORD EVALUATION 3–1. Cystitis

1. What was found when the patient had a cystoscopy?

2. What are the symptoms of cystitis?

3. What is the patient's past surgical history?

4. What is the treatment for cystitis?

5. What are the dangers of untreated cystitis?

6. What instrument is used to perform a cystoscopy?

MEDICAL RECORD 3–2. Benign Prostatic Hypertrophy

Dictionary Exercise

This exercise will help you master the terminology in the medical record. Underline the following terms in the reading exercise and use a medical dictionary to define the words. The pronunciations of medical terms in this report are included in the Audiocassette Exercise on pages 127–130.

asymptomatic _____

auscultation _____

benign _____

bilateral _____

carcinoma _____

catheterization _____

colectomy _____

hemorrhoid _____

hernia _____

hydrocele _____

hypertrophy _____

impotence _____

normocephalic _____

percussion _____

pneumothorax _____

preoperative _____

prostatic _____

rectal _____

retinal _____

transurethral _____

urological _____

venereal _____

voiding _____

Word Element Exercise

Break down the following words into their basic elements. The first one is completed for you.

pneum/o/thorax   carcinoma
colectomy   hydrocele
transurethral   hypertrophy
retinal

VALIDATION FRAME: Check your answers in Appendix B, Answer Key.

Reading Exercise

Read the case study out loud.

The patient is a 72-year-old white man with no significant voiding symptoms before this admission and recently was found to have colon cancer and is being admitted for colectomy.

History of Present Illness: Preoperative catheterization was not possible and consultation with Dr. Moriarty was obtained.

Past History: Negative for transurethral resection of the prostate or any urological trauma or venereal disease. The past history is positive for hemorrhoid symptoms and history of bilateral inguinal hernia repair, history of high cholesterol, history of retinal surgery, spontaneous pneumothorax times two and had chest tubes in the past. He also had a basal cell carcinoma.

Physical Examination: Head: Normocephalic. Eyes, Ears, Nose, and Throat: Within normal limits. Neck: No nodes. No bruits over carotids. Chest: Clear to auscultation and percussion. Heart: Normal heart sounds. No murmur. Abdomen: Soft and nontender. No masses are palpable. It is very distended. Penis: Normal. There is a right hydrocele. Rectal: Examination reveals 35 to 40 grams of benign prostatic hypertrophy.

Assessment

1. Mild to moderate benign prostatic hypertrophy
2. Status post colon resection for carcinoma of the colon
3. Right hydrocele, asymptomatic
4. Impotence

MEDICAL RECORD EVALUATION 3–2. Benign Prostatic Hypertrophy

1. What was wrong with the patient's prostate?

2. Did it cause him any urinary difficulty?

3. Why did the surgeon call in Dr. Moriarty?

4. Did the patient have any previous surgery on his prostate?

5. Where was the patient's hernia?

6. Was the patient's past medical history contributory for his present urological problem?

ABBREVIATIONS

Abbreviation	Meaning	Abbreviation	Meaning
cysto	cystoscopic examination	TURP	transurethral resection of the prostate
IVP	intravenous pyelogram	UA	urinalysis
KUB	kidney, ureter, bladder	UTI	urinary tract infection
RP	retrograde pyelogram		

Audiocassette Exercise

The audiocassette tape helps you master the pronunciation of medical words. Listen to the tape for instructions to complete this exercise. You may also use this list without the audiotape to practice correct pronunciation and spelling of the terms.

Frame	Word	Pronunciation	Spelling Exercise
3–75	[] adenitis	(ăd-ĕ-NĪ-tĭs)	_____
3–74	[] adenocarcinoma	(ăd-ĕ-nō-kăr-sĭn-Ō-mă)	_____
3–72	[] adenodynia	(ăd-ĕ-nō-DĬN-ē-ă)	_____
3–74	[] adenoma	(ăd-ĕ-NŌ-mă)	_____
3–75	[] adenopathy	(ăd-ĕ-NŎP-ă-thē)	_____
3–114	[] anuria	(ăn-Ū-rē-ă)	_____
Reading Exercise	[] appendectomy	(ăp-ĕn-DĔK-tō-mē)	_____
Reading Exercise	[] asymptomatic	(ā-sĭmp-tō-MĂT-ĭk)	_____
Reading Exercise	[] auscultation	(ăws-kŭl-TĀ-shŭn)	_____
3–129	[] bacteriuria	(băk-tē-rē-Ū-rē-ă)	_____
3–69	[] benign	(bē-NĪN)	_____
Reading Exercise	[] bilateral	(bī-LĂT-ĕr-ăl)	_____
3–93	[] Bright's disease	(BRĪTZ dĭ-ZĒZ)	_____
Reading Exercise	[] bruits	(BROOTZ)	_____
Reading Exercise	[] carcinoma	(kăr-sĭ-NŌ-mă)	_____
Reading Exercise	[] carotids	(kă-RŎT-ĭdz)	_____
Reading Exercise	[] catheterization	(kăth-ĕ-tĕr-ĭ-ZĀ-shŭn)	_____
Reading Exercise	[] cholecystectomy	(kō-lē-sĭs-TĔK-tō-mē)	_____
Reading Exercise	[] cholecystitis	(kō-lē-sĭs-TĪ-tĭs)	_____
Reading Exercise	[] choledocholithiasis	(kō-lĕd-ō-kō-lĭ-THĪ-ă-sĭs)	_____
Reading Exercise	[] choledocholithotomy	(kō-lĕd-ō-kō-lĭth-ŎT-ō-mē)	_____
Reading Exercise	[] cholelithiasis	(kō-lē-lĭ-THĪ-ă-sĭs)	_____
Reading Exercise	[] colectomy	(kō-LĔK-tō-mē)	_____
3–125	[] continence	(KŎN-tĭ-nĕns)	_____
3–58	[] cystectomy	(sĭs-TĔK-tō-mē)	_____
3–63	[] cystitis	(sĭs-TĪ-tĭs)	_____
3–101	[] cystocele	(SĬS-tō-sēl)	_____
3–47	[] cystolith	(SĬS-tō-lĭth)	_____
3–47	[] cystolithiasis	(sĭs-tō-lĭ-THĪ-ă-sĭs)	_____
3–47	[] cystolithotomy	(sĭs-tō-lĭth-ŎT-ō-mē)	_____
3–58	[] cystoplasty	(SĬS-tō-plăs-tē)	_____
3–52	[] cystorrhaphy	(sĭst-ŎR-ă-fē)	_____
3–57	[] cystoscopy	(sĭs-TŎS-kō-pē)	_____
3–19	[] diuretic	(dī-ū-RĔT-ĭk)	_____
3–129	[] dysuria	(dĭs-Ū-rē-ă)	_____
3–17	[] edema	(ĕ-DĒ-mă)	_____
3–100	[] enterocele	(ĔN-tĕr-ō-sēl)	_____
Reading Exercise	[] epigastric	(ĕp-ĭ-GĂS-trĭk)	_____

Frame	Word	Pronunciation	Spelling Exercise
3–103	[] erythrocyte	(ĕ-RĬTH-rō-sīt)	_____
3–102	[] erythruria	(ĕr-ĭ-THRŪ-rē-ă)	_____
3–84	[] glomerulitis	(glō-mĕr-ū-LĪ-tĭs)	_____
3–132	[] glomerulonephritis	(glō-mĕr-ū-lō-nĕ-FRĪ-tĭs)	_____
3–84	[] glomerulopathy	(glō-mĕr-ū-LŎP-ă-thē)	_____
3–85	[] glomerulosclerosis	(glō-mĕr-ū-lō-sklē-RŌ-sĭs)	_____
3–85	[] glomerulus	(glō-MĔR-ū-lŭs)	_____
3–131	[] hematuria	(hĕm-ă-TŪ-rē-ă)	_____
Reading Exercise	[] hemorrhoid	(HĔM-ō-royd)	_____
3–99	[] hernia	(HĔR-nē-ă)	_____
Reading Exercise	[] hydrocele	(HĪ-drō-sēl)	_____
Reading Exercise	[] hypertrophy	(hī-PĔR-trŏ-fē)	_____
Reading Exercise	[] impotence	(ĬM-pō-tĕns)	_____
3–126	[] incontinence	(ĭn-KŎN-tĭ-nĕns)	_____
3–88	[] intravenous	(ĭn-tră-VĒ-nŭs)	_____
3–103	[] leukocyte	(LOO-kō-sīt)	_____
3–102	[] leukorrhea	(loo-kō-RĒ-ă)	_____
3–134	[] lithectomy	(lĭ-THĔK-tō-mē)	_____
3–9	[] lithiasis	(lĭth-Ī-ă-sĭs)	_____
3–45	[] lithotripsy	(LĬTH-ō-trĭp-sē)	_____
3–69	[] malignant	(mă-LĬG-nănt)	_____
3–86	[] micturition	(mĭk-tū-RĬ-shŭn)	_____
3–6	[] nephrectomy	(nĕ-FRĔK-tō-mē)	_____
3–6	[] nephritis	(nĕf-RĪ-tĭs)	_____
3–10	[] nephrolith	(NĔF-rō-lĭth)	_____
3–10	[] nephrolithiasis	(nĕf-rō-lĭth-Ī-ă-sĭs)	_____
3–30	[] nephrolithotomy	(nĕf-rō-lĭth-ŎT-ō-mē)	_____
3–28	[] nephromegaly	(nĕf-rō-MĔG-ă-lē)	_____
3–78	[] nephron	(NĔF-rŏn)	_____
3–22	[] nephropathy	(nĕ-FRŎP-ă-thē)	_____
3–35	[] nephropexy	(NĔF-rō-pĕks-ē)	_____
3–31	[] nephroptosis	(nĕf-rŏp-TŌ-sĭs)	_____
3–30	[] nephrorrhaphy	(nĕf-RŎR-ă-fē)	_____
3–26	[] nephrosclerosis	(nĕf-rō-sklĕ-RŌ-sĭs)	_____
3–91	[] nephroscope	(NĔF-rō-skōp)	_____
3–91	[] nephroscopy	(nĕf-RŎS-kō-pē)	_____
3–26	[] nephrosis	(nĕf-RŌ-sĭs)	_____
3–30	[] nephrotomy	(nĕ-FRŎT-ō-mē)	_____
3–124	[] nocturia	(nŏk-TŪ-rē-ă)	_____
Reading Exercise	[] normocephalic	(nŏr-mō-SĔF-ă-lĭk)	_____
3–119	[] oligosialia	(ŏl-ĭ-gō-sī-ĂL-ē-ă)	_____
3–117	[] oliguria	(ŏl-ĭg-Ū-rē-ă)	_____
Reading Exercise	[] pelvic	(PĔL-vĭk)	_____

Frame	Word	Pronunciation	Spelling Exercise
3–81	[] pelvis	(PĔL-vĭs)	——————
Reading Exercise	[] percussion	(pĕr-KŬSH-ŭn)	——————
Reading Exercise	[] pneumothorax	(nū-mō-THŌ-răks)	——————
3–122	[] polyadenitis	(pŏl-ē-ăd-ĕ-NĪ-tĭs)	——————
3–121	[] polyphobia	(pŏl-ē-FŌ-bē-ă)	——————
3–120	[] polyuria	(pŏl-ē-Ū-rē-ă)	——————
Reading Exercise	[] preoperative	(prē-ŎP-ĕr-ă-tĭv)	——————
Reading Exercise	[] prostatic	(prŏs-TĂT-ĭk)	——————
3–131	[] proteinuria	(prō-tē-ĭn-Ū-rē-ă)	——————
3–87	[] pyelitis	(pī-ĕ-LĪ-tĭs)	——————
3–88	[] pyelogram	(PĪ-ĕ-lō-grăm)	——————
3–95	[] pyelonephritis	(pī-ĕ-lō-nĕ-FRĪ-tĭs)	——————
3–82	[] pyelopathy	(pī-ĕ-LŎP-ăth-ē)	——————
3–87	[] pyeloplasty	(PĪ-ĕ-lō-plăs-tē)	——————
3–110	[] pyonephrosis	(pī-ō-nĕf-RŌ-sĭs)	——————
3–110	[] pyorrhea	(pī-ō-RĒ-ă)	——————
3–113	[] pyuria	(pī-Ū-rē-ă)	——————
Reading Exercise	[] rectal	(RĔK-tăl)	——————
3–101	[] rectocele	(RĔK-tō-sēl)	——————
3–7	[] renogastric	(rē-nō-GĂS-trĭk)	——————
3–8	[] renointestinal	(rē-nō-ĭn-TĔS-tĭn-ăl)	——————
3–4	[] renomegaly	(rē-nō-MĔG-ă-lē)	——————
3–22	[] renopathy	(rē-NŎP-ă-thē)	——————
Reading Exercise	[] retinal	(RĔT-ĭ-năl)	——————
3–25	[] sclerosis	(sklĕ-RŌ-sĭs)	——————
Reading Exercise	[] spasm	(SPĂZM)	——————
3–23	[] suprarenal	(soo-pră-RĒ-năl)	——————
3–107	[] toxic	(TŎKS-ĭk)	——————
Reading Exercise	[] transurethral	(trăns-ū-RĒ-thrăl)	——————
Reading Exercise	[] trauma	(TRAW-mă)	——————
3–49	[] ureteralgia	(ū-rē-tĕr-ĂL-jē-ă)	——————
3–44	[] ureterectasis	(ū-rē-tĕr-ĔK-tă-sĭs)	——————
3–50	[] ureterocystoscope	(ū-rē-tĕr-ō-SĬS-tō-skōp)	——————
3–49	[] ureterodynia	(ū-rē-tĕr-ō-DĬN-ē-ă)	——————
3–41	[] ureterolith	(ū-RĒ-tĕr-ō-lĭth)	——————
3–41	[] ureterolithiasis	(ū-rē-tĕr-ō-lĭth-Ī-ă-sĭs)	——————
3–42	[] ureterolithotomy	(ū-rē-tĕr-ō-lĭth-ŎT-ō-mē)	——————
3–39	[] ureteromegaly	(ū-rē-tĕr-ō-MĔG-ă-lē)	——————
3–87	[] ureteropyeloplasty	(ū-rē-tĕr-ō-PĪ-ĕl-ō-plăs-tē)	——————
3–52	[] ureterorrhaphy	(ū-rē-tĕr-ŎR-ră-fē)	——————
3–61	[] urethra	(ū-RĒ-thră)	——————
3–62	[] urethralgia	(ū-rē-THRĂL-jē-ă)	——————
3–60	[] urethrectomy	(ū-rē-THRĔK-tō-mē)	——————

Frame	Word	Pronunciation	Spelling Exercise
3–60	[] urethritis	(ū-rē-THRĪ-tĭs)	_____
3–101	[] urethrocele	(ū-RĒ-thrō-sēl)	_____
3–65	[] urethrocystitis	(ū-rē-thrō-sĭs-TĪ-tĭs)	_____
3–61	[] urethrodynia	(ū-rē-thrō-DĬN-ē-ă)	_____
3–60	[] urethropexy	(ū-RĒ-thrō-pĕks-ē)	_____
3–60	[] urethroplasty	(ū-RĒ-thrō-plăs-tē)	_____
3–64	[] urethrorectal	(ū-rē-thrō-RĔK-tăl)	_____
3–66	[] urethroscope	(ū-RĒ-thrō-skōp)	_____
3–66	[] urethroscopy	(ū-rē-THRŎS-kō-pē)	_____
Reading Exercise	[] urinary incontinence	(Ū-rĭ-nār-ē ĭn-KŎN-tĭ-nĕns)	_____
3–104	[] urodynia	(ū-rō-DĬN-ē-ă)	_____
3–108	[] urologist	(ū-RŎL-ō-jĭst)	_____
3–108	[] urology	(ū-RŎL-ō-jē)	_____
3–105	[] urotoxin	(ū-rō-TŎK-sĭn)	_____
Reading Exercise	[] venereal	(vĕ-NĒ-rē-ăl)	_____
Reading Exercise	[] voiding	(VOYD-ĭng)	_____
3–55	[] vesicoenteric	(vĕs-ĭ-kō-ĕn-TĔR-ĭk)	_____

Unit Exercises

DEFINITIONS

Review the Unit Summary (pages 137–139) before completing this exercise.
Write the meaning for each word part.

SUFFIXES, PREFIXES, AND ABBREVIATIONS

Element	Meaning

SURGICAL SUFFIXES

1. -ectomy _____
2. -pexy _____
3. -plasty _____
4. -rrhaphy _____
5. -tome _____
6. -tomy _____

OTHER SUFFIXES

7. -algia _____
8. -cele _____
9. -cyte _____
10. -dynia _____
11. -ectasis _____
12. -gram _____
13. -iasis _____
14. -ic _____
15. -itis _____
16. -lith _____
17. -logist _____
18. -logy _____
19. -megaly _____
20. -oma _____
21. -osis _____
22. -ous _____
23. -pathy _____
24. -phagia _____
25. -ptosis _____
26. -rrhea _____
27. -scope _____
28. -scopy _____

PREFIXES AND ABBREVIATIONS

29. a- _____
30. an- _____
31. poly- _____

Element	Meaning
32. supra-	_____
33. UTI	_____
34. IVP	_____

COMBINING FORMS RELATED TO THE URINARY SYSTEM

35. cyst/o   _____

36. glomerul/o   _____

37. nephr/o   _____

38. pyel/o   _____

39. ren/o   _____

40. ureter/o   _____

41. ur/o   _____

42. vesic/o   _____

OTHER COMBINING FORMS IN UNIT 3

43. aden/o   _____

44. carcin/o   _____

45. enter/o   _____

46. erythr/o   _____

47. gastr/o   _____

48. hemat/o   _____

49. lith/o   _____

50. rect/o   _____

51. scler/o   _____

VALIDATION FRAME: Check your answers in the Index of Medical Word Elements, Appendix A. If you scored less than _____ %,* review Unit Summary (pages 137–139) and retake this exercise.

   To obtain a percentage score, multiply the number of correct answers times 2.

Number of Correct Answers: _____   **Percentage Score:** _____

*Enter the percentage required by your instructor to complete this course.

Vocabulary

Match the medical word(s) below the definitions in the numbered list.

acute renal failure	hematuria	nocturia
anuria	IVP	oliguria
benign	lithotripsy	polyuria
Bright's disease	malignant	renal pelvis
cystocele	nephrolithotomy	spasm
diuretics	nephrons	ureteropyeloplasty
edema	nephropexy	urinary incontinence
	nephroptosis	

1. _____ Tending or threatening to produce death; harmful. Refers to cancerous growths.

2. _____ The microscopic filtering units in the kidney that are responsible for keeping body fluids in balance.

3. _____ A form of glomerulonephritis.

4. _____ The funnel-shaped reservoir that is the basin of the kidney.

5. _____ X-ray film of the kidneys after an injection of dye.

6. _____ Drugs that stimulate the flow of urine.

7. _____ Swelling of body tissue.

8. _____ Not cancerous.

9. _____ An incision into a kidney to remove a stone.

10. _____ Condition that results from a lack of blood flow to the kidneys.

11. _____ Downward displacement of a kidney.

12. _____ Surgical repair of a ureter and renal pelvis.

13. _____ Twitching, involuntary contraction.

14. _____ Excessive urination at night.

15. _____ Inability to hold urine.

16. _____ Presence of blood cells in the urine.

17. _____ Excessive discharge of urine.

18. _____ Diminished amount of urine formation.

19. _____ Absence of urine formation.

20. _____ A urinary bladder hernia.

VALIDATION FRAME: Check your answers in Appendix B, Answer Key. If you scored less than

_____ %, review the vocabulary and retake the exercise.

To obtain a percentage score, multiply the number of correct answers times 5.

Number of Correct Answers: _____   **Percentage Score:** _____

Pathological Conditions

Match the medical word(s) below with the definitions in the numbered list.

azoturea
diuresis
dysuria
end-stage renal disease
enuresis

hypospadias
interstitial nephritis
phimosis
uremia
Wilms' tumor

1. _____ Stenosis of the foreskin opening over the glans penis in men.

2. _____ Kidney tumor that occurs in children.

3. _____ An increase in nitrogenous compounds, especially urea, in urine.

4. _____ Painful or difficult urination, symptomatic of numerous conditions.

5. _____ Abnormal secretion of large amounts of urine.

6. _____ The final phase of a kidney disease process; kidney disease has advanced to the point that the kidneys can no longer adequately filter the blood.

7. _____ Abnormal congenital opening of the male urethra upon the undersurface of the penis.

8. _____ Nephritis associated with pathological changes in the renal interstitial tissue that in turn may be primary or due to a toxic agent such as a drug or chemical.

9. _____ Elevated urea level or other protein waste products in the blood.

10. _____ Urinary incontinence, including bed-wetting.

VALIDATION FRAME: Check your answers in Appendix B, Answer Key. If you scored less than _____ %, review the vocabulary and retake the exercise.

To obtain a percentage score, multiply the number of correct answers times 10.

Number of Correct Answers: _____   **Percentage Score:** _____

Unit Summary

COMBINING FORMS RELATED TO THE URINARY SYSTEM

Form	Pronunciation	Meaning
cyst/o vcsic/o	sĭs-tō ⎫ vĕs-ĭ-kō ⎭	bladder
glomerul/o	glō-mĕr-ū-lō	glomerulus
nephr/o ren/o	nĕf-rō ⎫ rē-nō ⎭	kidney
pyel/o	pī-ĕ-lō	renal pelvis
ureter/o	ū-rē-tĕr-ō	ureter
urethr/o	ū-rē-thrō	urethra
ur/o	ū-rō	urine

OTHER COMBINING FORMS IN UNIT 3

Form	Pronunciation	Meaning
aden/o	ăd-ĕ-nō	gland
carcin/o	kăr-sĭn-ō	cancer
enter/o	ĕn-tĕr-ō	intestines (usually small)
erythr/o	ĕ-rĭth-rō	red
gastr/o	găs-trō	stomach
hemat/o	hĕm-ă-tō	blood
hepat/o	hĕp-ă-tō	liver
lith/o	lĭth-ō	stone, calculus
noct/o	nŏk-tō	night
olig/o	ō-lĭ-gō	scanty
py/o	pī-ō	pus
rect/o	rĕk-tō	rectum
scler/o	sklē-rō	hardening
sial/o	sī-ă-lō	saliva, salivary glands
ven/o	vē-nō	vein

SUFFIXES AND PREFIXES

Suffix (Prefix)	Pronunciation	Meaning
ADJECTIVE-ENDING SUFFIXES		
-al -ic -ous	ăl ⎫ ĭk ⎬ ŭs ⎭	pertaining to

Suffix (Prefix)	Pronunciation	Meaning
NOUN-ENDING SUFFIXES		
-ia	ē-ă	condition
-ist	ĭst	specialist
SURGICAL SUFFIXES		
-ectomy	ĕk-tō-mē	excision, removal
-pexy	pĕks-ē	fixation
-plasty	plăs-tē	surgical repair
-rrhaphy	ră-fē	suture
-stomy	stō-mē	forming a new opening or mouth
-tome	tōm	instrument to cut
-tomy	tō-mē	incision, cut into
-tripsy	trĭp-sē	crushing
OTHER SUFFIXES		
-algia -dynia	ăl-jē-ă dĭn-ē-ă	pain
-cele	sēl	hernia, swelling
-cyte	sīt	cell
-ectasis	ĕk-tă-sĭs	dilation, expansion
-edema	ĕ-dē-mă	swelling
-emesis	ĕm-ĕ-sĭs	vomiting
-gram	grăm	record
-graphy	gră-fē	process of recording
-iasis	ī-ă-sĭs	abnormal condition (produced by something specified)
-itis	ī-tĭs	inflammation
-lith	lĭth	stone, calculus
-logist	lō-jĭst	specialist in the study of
-logy	lō-jē	study of
-megaly	mĕg-ă-lē	enlargement
-oma	ō-mă	tumor
-osis	ō-sĭs	abnormal condition
-pathy	pă-thē	disease
-pepsia	pĕp-sē-ă	digestion
-phagia	fā-jē-ă	swallow, eat
-phobia	fō-bē-ă	fear

Suffix (Prefix)	Pronunciation	Meaning
-ptosis	tō-sĭs	prolapse, falling, dropping
-rrhea	rē-ă	flow, discharge
-scope	skōp	instrument to view
-scopy	skŏ-pē	visual examination
-uria	ū-rē-ă	urine, urination

PREFIXES

Suffix (Prefix)	Pronunciation	Meaning
a-	ă	without, not
an-	ăn	without, not
dys-	dĭs	bad, painful, difficult
in-	ĭn	not, in
intra-	ĭn-tră	within
poly-	pŏl-ē	many, much
supra-	soo-pră	above

Integumentary System

The integumentary system consists of tissues structurally joined together to perform specific activities. It includes the skin and its accessory organs, which are the hair, nails, sebaceous glands, and sweat glands. The skin covers the entire body and provides protection against injuries, infection, and toxic compounds. It also contains many nerve endings and serves as a sensory receptor for pain, temperature, pressure, and touch (Fig. 4–1).

The combining forms related to the integumentary system are summarized here. Review this information before you begin to work the frames.

COMBINING FORMS

Combining Form	Meaning	Example	Pronunciation
adip/o	fat	adip/osis abnormal condition	ăd-ĭ-PŌ-sĭs
lip/o		lip/oid resembling	LĬP-oyd
steat/o		steat/oma tumor	stē-ă-TŌ-mă
cutane/o	skin	sub/cutane/ous under pertaining to	sŭb-kū-TĀ-nē-ŭs
dermat/o		dermat/o/logy study of	dĕr-mă-TŎL-ō-jē
derm/o		hypo/derm/ic under, pertaining to below	hī-pō-DĔR-mĭk
hidr/o*	sweat	an/hidr/osis abnormal condition (of)	ăn-hī-DRŌ-sĭs
kerat/o	horny tissue	kerat/osis hard abnormal condition (of)	kĕr-ă-TŌ-sĭs
myc/o	fungus	onych/o/myc/osis nail abnormal condition (of)	ŏn-ĭ-kō-mī-KŌ-sĭs
onych/o	nail	onych/o/malacia softening	ŏn-ĭ-kō-mă-LĀ-sē-ă
pil/o	hair	pil/o/nid/al nest pertaining to	pī-lō-NĪ-dăl
trich/o		trich/o/pathy disease	trĭk-ŎP-ă-thē
scler/o	hardening	scler/osis abnormal condition (of)	sklĕ-RŌ-sĭs
xer/o	dry	xer/o/derma skin	zē-rō-DĔR-mă

*Do not confuse **hidr/o** (sweat) with **hydr/o** (water).

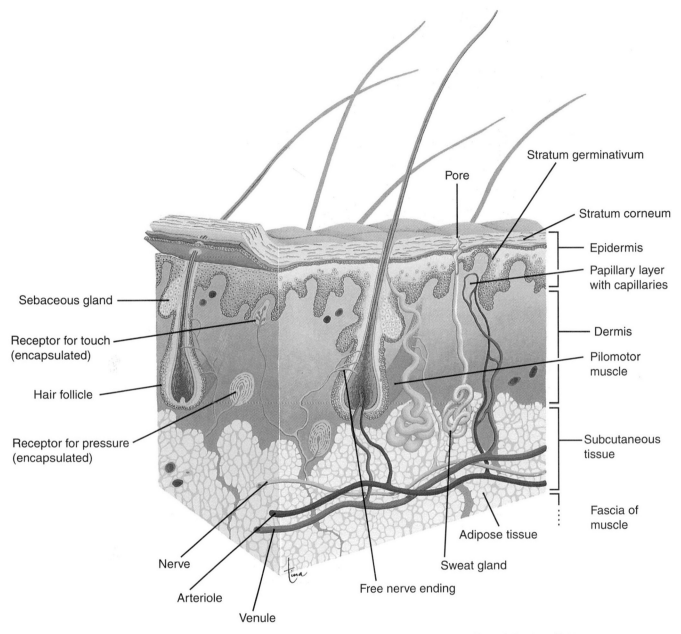

Figure 4–1. Structure of the skin and subcutaneous tissue. (From Scanlon, VC, and Sanders, T: Understanding Human Structure and Function. FA Davis, Philadelphia, 1997, p 75, with permission.)

SKIN

4–1 Use the Index of Medical Word Elements, Part A of Appendix A, to define the following word elements.

Medical Word Element	Meaning
-cyte	_____
hidr/o	_____
hydr/o	_____
myc/o	_____
-phagia	_____
sub-	_____

4–2 Use the Index of Medical Word Elements, Part B of Appendix A, to write the medical word elements for the following English terms.

English Term	Medical Word Element
above, upon	_____
fat	_____ / _____ or
	_____ / _____
flow, discharge	_____
hardening	_____ / _____

4–3 The skin is composed of two layers of tissue. The outer, thinner layer that is visible to the naked eye is the **(1) epidermis**. The second layer of skin is the **(2) dermis**.

Label the two layers of skin in Figure 4–2.

---

epi-

4–4 The element in epi / derm / is that means above or upon is _____ .

---

skin

4–5 The combining form **derm / o** refers to the skin. Derm / o / pathy is a disease of the _____ .

-pathy

derm / o

4–6 Identify the elements in derm / o / pathy that mean

disease: _____

skin: _____ / _____

---

epi / derm / is
(ĕp-ĭ-DĔR-mĭs)

4–7 The epi / derm / is forms the protective covering of the body, and does not have a blood or nerve supply. When you talk about the outer layer of skin, you are referring to the _____ / _____ / _____ .

---

skin

4–8 Two other combining forms for skin are **dermat / o** and **cutane / o**. Cutane / ous means pertaining to the _____ .

---

skin

4–9 A dermat / o / tome is an instrument to cut or incise the _____ .

---

dermat / itis
dĕr-mă-TĪ-tĭs)

4–10 Use **dermat** to build a word meaning inflammation of the skin.

_____ / _____

---

skin

4–11 The prefixes sub- and hypo- mean below or under. A hypo / derm / ic needle is inserted under the _____ .

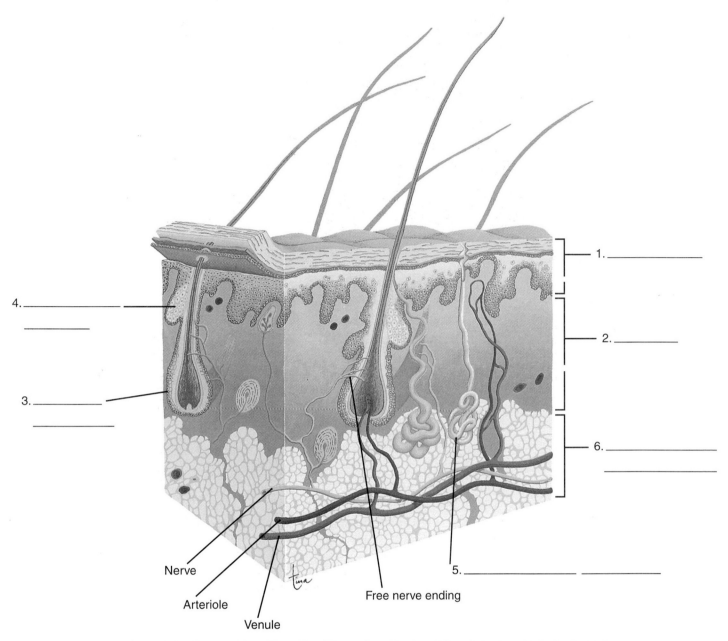

Figure 4–2. Cross-section of the skin. (Adapted from Scanlon, VC, and Sanders, T: Understanding Human Structure and Function. FA Davis, Philadelphia, 1997, p 75, with permission.)

skin	**4–12** Sub / cutane / ous literally means pertaining to under the _____ .
skin	**4–13** When you see the words derm / a, derm / is, derm / ic, you will know they refer to the _____ .
skin	**4–14** Each of the terminal endings or suffixes -a , -is , and -ic in Frame 4–13 designates a part of speech. The important thing for you to remember is that derm / a, derm / is, and derm / ic all refer to the _____ .

adjective	**4-15** Derm/a and derm/is both have noun endings. Derm/ic has an _____ ending.

4-16 The second layer of skin, the derm/is, contains the **(3) hair follicle, (4) sebaceous glands** (oil glands), and **(5) sudoriferous glands** (sweat glands). Label Figure 4-2 as you learn about the parts of the dermis.

inflammation, skin	**4-17** Dermat/itis is an _____ of the _____ .

disease, skin	**4-18** Derm/o/pathy is a disease of the skin. Dermat/o/pathy is also a _____ of the _____ .

epi/derm/is, derm/is (ĕp-ĭ-DĔR-mĭs) (DĔR-mĭs)	**4-19** The two layers of the skin are the _____ / _____ / _____ and _____ / _____

hidr/osis (hī-DRŌ-sĭs)	**4-20** The combining form for sweat is **hidr/o**. Use -osis to form a word meaning an abnormal condition of sweat _____ / _____ .

sweat flow, discharge sweat, abnormal condition excessive, sweat abnormal condition	**4-21** The term "diaphoresis" is usually used to denote profuse or excessive sweating. Define the elements of three other words listed here that mean sweating. hidr/o/rrhea means: hidr/o _____ ; -rrhea _____ , or _____ . hidr/osis means: hidr/o _____ ; -osis _____ _____ hyper/hidr/osis means: hyper- _____ ; hidr/o _____ ; -osis _____ _____

sweat, water	**4-22** Even though **hidr/o** and **hydr/o** both sound alike they have different meanings. **Hidr/o** refers to _____ ; **hydr/o** refers to _____ .

hidr/osis (hī-DRŌ-sĭs)	**4-23** Hidr/osis is a condition that can cause blistering and peeling of the palms and soles. Build a word that means an abnormal condition of sweating: _____ / _____

sweating or sweat	**4-24** An/hidr/osis is an abnormal condition of diminished or absence of _____ .

aden
 	
-oma
	4-25 Remember that an aden/oma is a glandular tumor composed of glandular tissue.
	
	Identify the elements in the word aden/oma that mean:
	
	    gland: _____
	
	    tumor: _____

sweat gland	**4-26** Hidr/aden/oma is a tumor of the _____ _____ .
adip/ectomy (ăd-ĭ-PĔK-tō-mē)	**4-27** **Lip/o** and **adip/o** are combining forms meaning fat. A lip/ectomy is the excision of fat or adipose tissue. Use **adip/o** to form another surgical term meaning excision of fat. _____ / _____
adip/o, lip/o steat/o	**4-28** Adip/oma, lip/oma, and steat/oma refer to a fatty tumor. The three combining forms for fat are _____ / _____ , _____ / _____ , and _____ / _____ .
	4-29 The dermis is attached to the underlying structures of the skin by **(6) subcutaneous tissue**. Label the section of subcutaneous tissue in Figure 4-2.

sub/cutane/ous
(sŭb-kū-TĀ-nē-ŭs)
lip/o/cytes
(LĬP-ō-sītz)
	4-30 Sub/cutane/ous tissue forms lip/o/cytes, or fat cells.
	
	Determine the words in this frame that mean
	
	    pertaining to under the skin: _____ / _____ / _____
	
	    fat cells: _____ / _____ / _____

cell	**4-31** A lip/o/cyte is a fat _____ .

VALIDATION FRAME: Check your labeling of Figure 4-2 in Appendix B, Answer Key.

sub/cutane/ous
(sŭb-kū-TĀ-nē-ŭs)
lip/ectomy
(lĭ-PĔK-tō-mē)
	4-32 Suction lip/ectomy is the removal of sub/cutane/ous fat tissue (see Fig. 4-2) using a blunt-tipped cannula (tube) introduced into the fatty area through a small incision. Suction is then applied and fat tissue is removed.
	
	Identify the terms in this frame that mean
	
	    under the skin: _____ / _____ / _____
	
	    excision of fat: _____ / _____

excision or removal, fat	**4–33** Suction lip/ectomy is performed for cosmetic reasons. Lip/ectomy literally means _____ of _____ .

derm/o, dermat/o, cutane/o	**4–34** List the three combining forms that refer to the skin: _____ / _____ , _____ / _____ , and _____ / _____ .

dermat/o/plasty (DĔR-mă-tō-plăs-tē)	**4–35** Use **dermat/o** to form a word meaning plastic surgery (of the) skin: _____ / _____ / _____

log -ist	**4–36** The following noun suffixes include the same root and are easier to define if you analyze their components. The -y and -ist denote a noun ending. -logy means study of -logist means specialist in the study of The root in each suffix that means study of is _____ . The element in the suffix -logist that means specialist is: _____

dermat/o/logy (dĕr-mă-TŎL-ō-jē) dermat/o/logist (dĕr-mă-TŎL-ō-jĭst)	**4–37** Refer to Frame 4–36 and use **dermat/o** to develop words meaning study of the skin: _____ / _____ / _____ specialist in the study of the skin: _____ / _____ / _____

dermat/oma (dĕr-mă-TŌ-mă) dermat/o/pathy (DĔR-mă-tō-pă-thē) dermat/o/logy (dĕr-mă-TŎL-ō-jē)	**4–38** Use **dermat/o** to practice forming words meaning tumor of the skin: _____ / _____ disease of the skin: _____ / _____ / _____ study of the skin: _____ / _____ / _____

dermat/o/logist (dĕr-mă-TŎL-ō-jĭst)	**4–39** A physician specializing in treating diseases of the stomach is a gastr/o/logist. A physician specializing in treating diseases of the skin is a _____ / _____ / _____ .

dermat/o/logy (dĕr-mă-TŎL-ō-jē)	**4–40** The medical specialty concerned with the treatment of stomach diseases is gastr/o/logy. The medical specialty concerned with the treatment of skin diseases is _____ / _____ / _____ .

hardening	**4–41** Scler/osis is an abnormal condition of _____ .
scler/o dermat, derm	**4–42** Dermat/o/scler/osis or scler/o/derm/a is a rare, devastating disease of unknown cause that results in scarring or hardening of vital organs and eventually death. The combining form for hardening is _____ / _____ . The roots in this frame meaning skin are _____ and _____ .
skin	**4–43** The combining form **kerat/o** means hard or horny tissue. It also refers to the cornea of the eye (see Unit 10). Kerat/osis is a condition of the skin characterized by the formation of horny growths or an excessive development of the horny growth. A person with kerat/osis has horny growths on the _____ .
kerat/o	**4–44** The combining form for horny tissue is _____ / _____ .
sub/cutane/ous (sŭb-kū-TĀ-nē-ŭs)	**4–45** A sub/cutane/ous surgery is performed through a small opening in the skin. The word that means pertaining to under the skin is _____ / _____ / _____ (adjective ending).
sebaceous (sē-BĀ-shŭs)	**4–46** Refer to Figure 4–2 to complete this frame. The oil-secreting glands of the skin are the _____ glands.
sudoriferous (sū-dŏr-ĬF-ĕr-ŭs)	**4–47** The sweat glands of the skin are known as the _____ glands.

Hair and Nails

derm cutane	**4–48** We associate the epi/derm/is, derm/is, and sub/cutane/ous tissues with the skin, but we do not think of the hair and nails as skin. However, these structures are modified forms of skin cells. The elements in this frame that refer to the skin are _____ and _____ .
cutane/ous (kū-TĀ-nē-ŭs)	**4–49** Combine **cutane** + **-ous** to build a medical word meaning pertaining to the skin: _____ / _____ .

derm/o/pathy (dĕr-MŎP-ă-thē)	**4–50** Use **derm/o** to form a medical term that means disease of the skin: _____ / ____ / _____ .
myc/osis (mī-KŌ-sĭs)	**4–51** The combining form **myc/o** refers to a fungus, (fungi: plural). Combine **myc/o** + -osis to form a word meaning an abnormal condition or disease caused by fungi: _____ / _____ .
skin	**4–52** Dermat/o/myc/osis is a term meaning a fungal infection of the _____ .
dermat/itis dĕr-mă-TĪ-tĭs)	**4–53** Form a medical word that means an inflammation of the skin: _____ / _____ .
fungus	**4–54** Myc/o/dermat/itis, an inflammation of the skin, is caused by a _____ .
trich/o/pathy (trĭk-ŎP-ă-thē) trich/osis (trī-KŌ-sĭs)	**4–55** The combining form **trich/o** refers to the hair. Construct medical terms meaning disease of the hair: _____ / ____ / _____ abnormal condition of the hair: _____ / _____
trich/o/myc/osis (trĭk-ō-mī-KŌ-sĭs)	**4–56** Combine **trich/o** + **myc** + -osis to form a medical term that means any disease of the hair caused by a fungus: _____ / ____ / _____ / _____ .
hair	**4–57** Another combining form for the hair is **pil/o**. Whenever you see **pil/o** or **trich/o** in a word, you will know it refers to the _____ .
pil/o	**4–58** Pil/o/cyst/ic means pertaining to a derm/oid cyst containing hair. The element in this frame that refers to hair is _____ / ____ .
onych/oma (ŏn-ĭ-KŌ-mă) onych/o/pathy ŏn-ĭ-KŎP-ăth-ē)	**4–59** The combining form **onych/o** refers to the nail. Form medical words meaning tumor of the nail: _____ / _____ disease of the nails: _____ / ____ / _____

onych/oma (ŏn-ĭ-KŌ-mă)	**4-60** A tumor of the nail (or nailbed) is known as _____ / _____ .

onych/o/malacia (ŏn-ĭ-kō-mă-LĀ-sē-ă)	**4-61** Malacia is an abnormal softening of tissue; this word can also be used as a suffix. Use -malacia to form a medical word meaning softening of the nail: _____ / _____ / _____ .

onych/o myc -osis	**4-62** The nails become white, opaque, thickened, and brittle when a person suffers from the disease called onych/o/myc/osis. Identify the word elements in onych/o/myc/osis that mean nail: _____ / _____ fungus: _____ abnormal condition or disease: _____

xer/o	**4-63** The noun suffix -derma is also used to denote skin. A person with excessive dryness of skin has a condition called xer/o/derm/a. From xer/o/derm/a; identify the combining form that means dry: _____ / _____ .

dry eat(ing), swallow(ing)	**4-64** Xer/o/phagia is a condition of eating dry food only. Analyze xer/o/phagia by defining the elements: **xer/o** means _____ . -phagia means _____ or _____ .

-cele	**4-65** Recall that a cyst/o/cele is a hernia of the bladder. The word element meaning hernia or swelling is _____ .

lip/o/cele (LĬP-ō-sēl)	**4-66** A hernia containing fat or fatty tissue is called an adip/o/cele or _____ / _____ / _____ .

Review

Select the element(s) that match(es) the meaning.

adip/o
cutane/o
dcrm/o
dermat/o
hidr/o
lip/o
onych/o
scler/o
trich/o
xer/o

-cele
-derma
-logist
-logy
-malacia
-oma
-pathy
-phagia
-rrhea

epi-
hypo-
sub-

a. _____ disease

b. _____ dry

c. _____ fat

d. _____ flow, discharge

e. _____ hair

f. _____ hardening

g. _____ hernia, swelling

h. _____ nail

i. _____ skin

j. _____ softening

k. _____ specialist in the study of

l. _____ study of

m. _____ swallow, eat

n. _____ sweat

o. _____ tumor

p. _____ under, below

q. _____ upon

Check your answers with the Review Answer Key on the following page.

Review Answer Key

a. -pathy

b. xer/o

c. lip/o, adip/o

d. -rrhea

e. trich/o

f. scler/o

g. -cele

h. onych/o

i. derm/o, dermat/o, cutane/o

j. -malacia

k. -logist

l. -logy

m. -phagia

n. hidr/o

o. -oma

p. sub-, hypo-

q. epi-

REINFORCEMENT FRAME: If you are not satisfied with your level of comprehension, go back to Frame 4–1 to rework the frames.

COMBINING FORMS DENOTING COLORS

4-67 Examine the combining forms that denote color, and use a slash to break each word down into its basic elements. The first word is completed for you.

Combining Form	Meaning	Example
leuk/o	white	l e u k/o/d e r m a
cyan/o	blue	c y a n o d e r m a
erythr/o	red	e r y t h r o d e r m a
melan/o	black	m e l a n o d e r m a
xanth/o	yellow	x a n t h o m a

leuk/o/derma
cyan/o/derma
erythr/o/derma
melan/o/derma
xanth/oma

---

nouns

4-68 The -a ending in cyanoderma, erythroderma, leukoderma, and melanoderma specifies that these words are (adjectives, nouns) _____ .

---

erythr/o/derma
(ĕ-rĭth-rō-DĔR-mă)
melan/o/derma
(mĕl-ăn-ō-DĔR-mă)
xanth/o/derma
(zăn-thō-DĔR-mă)
xer/o/derma
(zē-rō-DĔR-mă)

4-69 Use **-derma** to build medical words meaning

skin that is red: _____ / _____ / _____

skin that is black: _____ / _____ / _____

skin that is yellow: _____ / _____ / _____

skin that is dry: _____ / _____ / _____

CELLS

4-70 Cells are the smallest basic units of the human organism. Every tissue and organ in your body is made up of cells (Figs. 4–3 and 4–4). Look under the main heading of "cell" in your medical dictionary and define the following terms:

adipose cell: _____

red cell: _____

blood cell: _____

---

cell

4-71 Remember that **cyt/o** and -cyte are used to build words that designate a _____ .

---

cells

4-72 Cyt/o/logy is the study of _____ .

---

erythr/o/cyte
(ĕ-RĬTH-rō-sīt)
leuk/o/cyte
(LOO-kō-sīt)
melan/o/cyte
(MĔL-ăn-ō-sīt)
xanth/o/cyte
(ZĂN-thō-sīt)

4-73 Use -cyte to form words meaning a

cell that is red: _____ / _____ / _____

cell that is white: _____ / _____ / _____

cell that is black: _____ / _____ / _____

cell that is yellow: _____ / _____ / _____

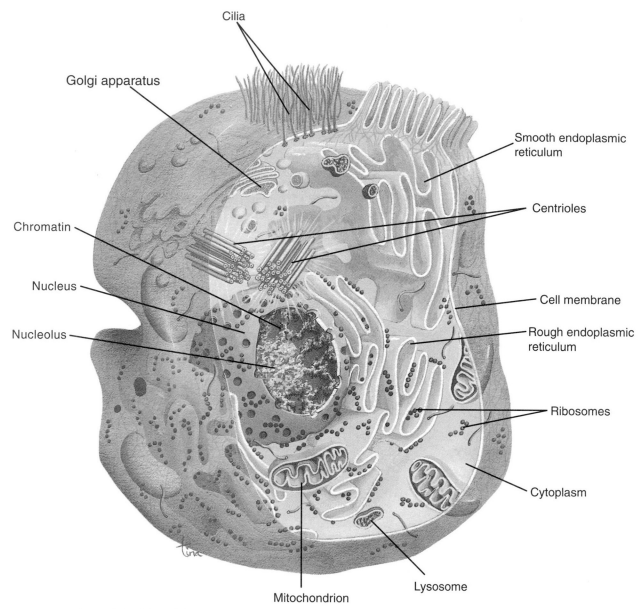

Figure 4–3. The cell. (Adapted from Scanlon, VC, and Sanders, T: Understanding Human Structure and Function. FA Davis, Philadelphia, 1997, p 42, with permission.)

	4–74 Leuk/o/cyt/o/penia is a decrease in white blood cells. The word leuk/o/cyt/o/penia is formed from the following word elements:
-penia	The suffix meaning decrease is _____ .
leuk/o	The combining form for white is _____ / _____ .
cyt/o	The combining form for cell is _____ / _____ .
leuk/o/cyt/o/penia (loo-kō-sī-tō-PĒ-nē-ă)	**4–75** When a person does not produce an adequate amount of white blood cells, his or her white blood cell (count) (WBC) decreases. This person has a condition called _____ / _____ / _____ / _____ / _____ .
WBC	**4–76** The abbreviation for white blood cell (count) is _____ .

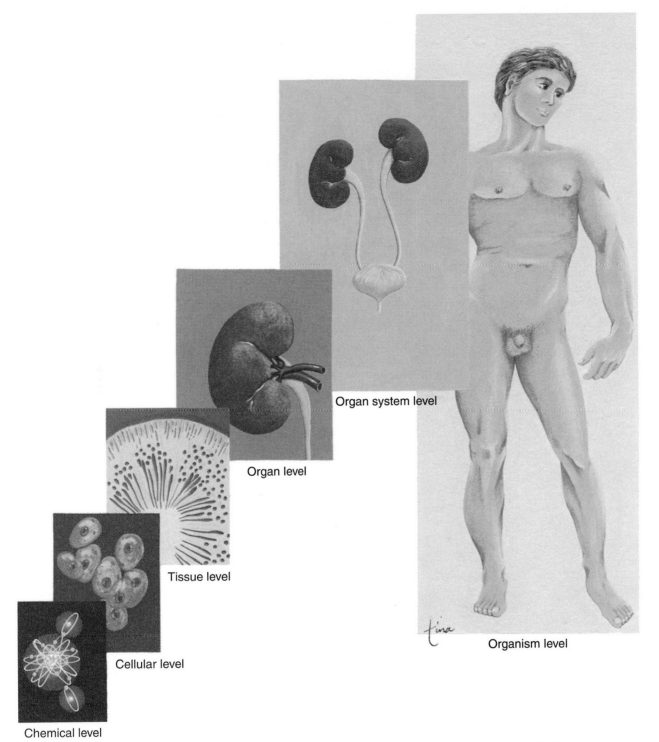

Figure 4–4. Levels of organization of the body. (Adapted from Scanlon, VC, and Sanders, T: Understanding Human Structure and Function. FA Davis, Philadelphia, 1997, p 3, with permission.)

Organ system level

Organ level

Tissue level

Cellular level

Chemical level

Organism level

4-77 Leuk/emia is a progressive malignant disease of the blood-forming organs, marked by proliferation and development of leuk/o/cytes in the blood and bone marrow.

blood

white

Leuk/emia literally means white _____ .

Leuk/o/cytes are _____ blood cells.

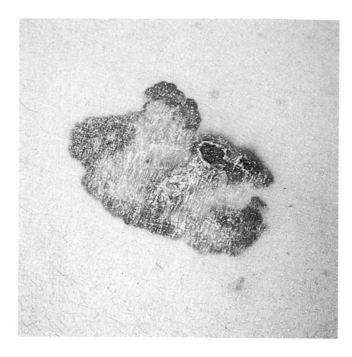

Figure 4–5. Superficial spreading melanoma. Healed areas in center are devoid of malignant cells. (From Reeves, JT, and Maibach, H: Clinical Dermatology Illustrated, A Regional Approach, ed 3. FA Davis, Philadelphia, 1998, p 340, with permission.)

leuk/emia (loo-KĒ-mē-ă)	**4–78** A disease of unrestrained growth of white blood cells is called _____ / _____ .
melan/oma (měl-ă-NŌ-mă)	**4–79** Melan/oma (Fig. 4–5) is a dark or black malignant skin tumor. If it is not detected early, it is fatal. Form a word meaning a tumor that is black: _____ / _____ .
abnormal condition black	**4–80** A dark pigment normally found in the hair and skin is melanin. Melan/osis literally means an _____ _____ of _____ .
melan/oma (měl-ă-NŌ-mă)	**4–81** A person with a black tumor could be diagnosed with a _____ / _____ .
blue	**4–82** Lack of oxygen causes cyan/o/derma or cyan/osis. Both words mean a condition in which the color of the skin is _____ .
cyan/o/derma (sī-ă-nō-DĔR-mă)	**4–83** A person with a bluish discoloration of skin exhibits cyan/osis or _____ / ____ / _____ .

4-84 Use -osis to develop medical words meaning

cyan/osis
(sī-ă-NŌ-sĭs)
erythr/osis
(ĕr-ĭ-THRŌ-sĭs)
melan/osis
(mĕl-ăn-Ō-sĭs)
xanth/osis
(zăn-THŌ-sĭs)

abnormal condition of blue (skin): _____ / _____

abnormal condition of red (skin): _____ / _____

abnormal condition of black (pigmentation): _____ / _____

abnormal condition of yellow (skin): _____ / _____

4-85 Skin cancer is the most common type of cancer. Recently there has been an increase in the rate of skin cancer, mainly caused by exposure to ultraviolet rays in sunlight.

Sun exposure, especially excessive tanning of the skin, can cause the lethal black

melan/oma
(mĕl-ă-NŌ-mă)

tumor called _____ / _____ .

4-86 Basal cell carcin/oma is a type of skin cancer that affects the basal cell layer of the epidermis.

Form a medical word that means a tumor that is cancerous:

carcin/oma
(kăr-sĭ-NŌ-mă)

_____ / _____ .

4-87 The lesion of melan/oma (see Fig. 4-5) is characterized by its asymmetry, irregular border, and lack of uniform color. Malignant melan/oma is the most dangerous form of skin cancer because of its tendency to metastasize rapidly.

melan/oma
(mĕl-ă-NŌ-mă)

The medical term for a black tumor is _____ / _____ .

4-88 A decubitus ulcer, or bedsore, is an example of a skin lesion that penetrates the epidermis and dermis layers of the skin. These ulcers are caused by prolonged pressure against an area of the skin from a bed or chair. The

decubitus ulcer
(dĕ KŪ-bĭ-tŭs ŬL-sĕr)

medical term for a bedsore is _____ _____ .

4-89 Psoriasis (Fig. 4-6) is a common chronic dermatitis characterized by red lesions covered by silvery scales. The appearance of silvery scales on the skin is

psoriasis
(sō-RĪ-ă-sĭs)

typical of the dermat/itis called _____ .

4-90 Kaposi's sarcoma, a malignant skin tumor frequently associated with patients who have acquired immunodeficiency syndrome (AIDS), is often fatal. Initially the tumor appears as a purplish-brown lesion.

AIDS

Kaposi's sarcoma
(KĂH-pō-sēz- săr-KŌ-mă)

The abbreviation for acquired immunodeficiency syndrome is _____ .

A type of skin cancer associated with the AIDS virus is _____

_____ .

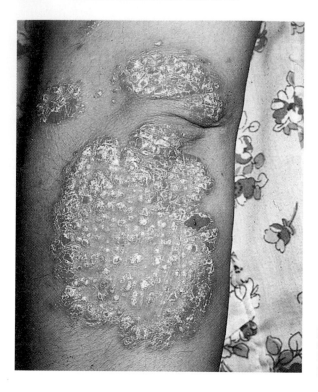

Figure 4–6. Psoriasis. Typical bright red scaly plaque of psoriasis with silvery scale, over a joint. (From Reeves, JT, and Maibach, H: Clinical Dermatology Illustrated, A Regional Approach, ed 3. FA Davis, Philadelphia, 1998, p 189, with permission.)

blood	**4–91** The suffix -emia is used in words to mean blood. Xanth/emia, an occurrence of yellow pigment in the blood, literally means yellow _____ .
xanth/omas (zăn-THŌ-măs)	**4–92** High cholesterol levels may cause small yellow tumors called _____ / _____ .
death or dead	**4–93** The combining form **necr/o** is used in words to denote death or dead. Necr/o/tic is a word that means pertaining to _____ .
dead	**4–94** Necr/osis is a word that is used to denote the death of areas of tissue or bone surrounded by healthy tissue. Cellular necr/osis means that the cells are _____ .
dead	**4–95** Necr/o/cyt/osis means that the cells are _____ .
necr/osis (nĕ-KRŌ-sĭs)	**4–96** Bony necr/osis occurs when dead bone tissue results from the loss of blood supply (e.g., after a fracture). The term that means abnormal condition of death is _____ / _____ .

4–97 Gangrene is a form of necr/osis associated with loss of blood supply. Before healing can take place, the dead matter must be removed. When there is an injury to blood flow, a form of necr/osis may develop that is known as

gangrene
(GĂNG-grēn)

_____ .

4–98 In the English language an auto/graph is a signature written by oneself. In medical words, auto- is used as a prefix and means self.

self

Auto/hypnosis is hypnosis of one's _____ .

self

Auto/examination is an examination of one's _____ .

self

An auto/graft is skin transplanted from one's _____ .

4–99 A graft is tissue that is transplanted or implanted in a part of the body to repair a defect. Grafts done with tissue transplanted from the patient's own skin

auto/grafts
(AW-tō-grăfts)

are called _____ / _____ .

4–100 A dermat/o/tome is an instrument used to incise or cut. When the physician wants to graft a thin slice of skin, the physician asks for an instrument

dermat/o/tome
(DĔR-mă-tō-tōm)

called a _____ / _____ / _____ .

4–101 Skin transplanted from another person will not survive very long, so a graft is performed using tissue transplanted from the patient's own skin. This

auto/graft
(AW-tō-grăft)

surgical procedure is called an _____ / _____ .

Review

Select the element(s) that match the meaning.

cyt/o   -cyte   auto-
cyan/o   -derma
erythr/o   -emia
leuk/o   -oma
melan/o   -pathy
necr/o   -penia
xanth/o   -rrhea

a. _____ black

b. _____ blue

c. _____ blood

d. _____ cell

e. _____ decrease

f. _____ disease

g. _____ flow, discharge

h. _____ red

i. _____ self

j. _____ skin

k. _____ tumor

l. _____ white

m. _____ yellow

n. _____ dead, death

Check your answers with the Review Answer Key on the following page.

Review Answer Key

a. melan/o

b. cyan/o

c. -emia

d. cyt/o, -cyte

e. -penia

f. -pathy

g. -rrhea

h. erythr/o

i. auto-

j. -derma

k. -oma

l. leuk/o

m. xanth/o

n. necr/o

REINFORCEMENT FRAME: If you are not satisfied with your level of comprehension, go back to Frame 4–67 and rework the frames.

Additional Pathological Conditions

Skin lesions are not always a sign of disease but may be a variation from the normal surface of the skin. Several common skin lesions are described here and illustrated in Figure 4–7.

abrasion (ă-BRĀ-zhŭn): scraping away of a portion of skin or of a mucous membrane as a result of injury or by mechanical means, as in dermabrasion for cosmetic purposes.

alopecia (ăl-ō-PĒ-shē-ă): absence or loss of hair, especially of the head; baldness.

comedo (KŎM-ē-dō): blackhead; discolored dried sebum plugging an excretory duct of the skin.

contusion (kŏn-TOO-zhŭn): injury in which the skin is not broken; a bruise.

cyst (SĬST): closed sac or pouch in or under the skin, with a definite wall, that contains fluid, semifluid, or solid material.

ecchymosis (ĕk-ĭ-MŌ-sĭs): discoloration on the skin consisting of large, irregularly formed hemorrhagic areas. The color is blue-black, changing in time to greenish-brown or yellow; commonly called a bruise.

eczema (ĔK-zĕ-mă): inflammatory skin disease characterized by redness, itching, and blisters.

fissure (FĬSH-ŭr): small cracklike sore or break exposing the dermis; usually red.

hirsutism (HŬR-sūt-ĭzm): condition characterized by excessive growth of hair or presence of hair in unusual places, especially in women.

impetigo (ĭm-pĕ-TĪ-gō): inflammatory skin disease characterized by isolated pustules that become crusted and rupture (Fig. 4–8).

laceration (lăs-ĕr-Ā-shŭn): wound or irregular tear of the flesh.

macule (MĂK-ūl): flat, discolored circumscribed lesion of any size.

nodule (NŎD-ūl): palpable circumscribed lesion, larger than a papule, 1 to 2 cm in diameter.

papule (PĂP-ūl): solid elevated lesion, <1 cm in diameter.

petechia (pē-TĒ-kē-ă): minute or small hemorrhagic spot on the skin. (A petechia is a smaller version of an ecchymosis.)

pustule (PŬS-tūl): small elevation of skin filled with lymph or pus.

scabies (SKĀ-bēz): contagious skin disease transmitted by the itch mite.

scales (SKĀLZ): excessive dry exfoliations shed from upper layers of the skin.

tinea (TĬN-ē-ă): any fungal skin disease, frequently caused by ringworm, whose name indicates the body part affected (e.g., tinea barbae (beard), tinea corporis (body), tinea pedis (athlete's foot).

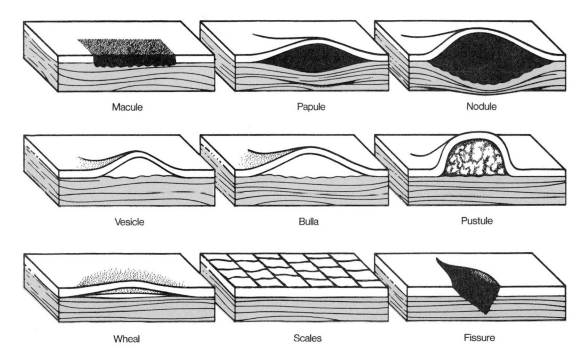

Macule   Papule   Nodule

Vesicle   Bulla   Pustule

Wheal   Scales   Fissure

Figure 4–7. Skin lesions. (From Gylys, BA, and Wedding, ME: Medical Terminology: A Systems Approach, ed 3. FA Davis, Philadelphia, 1995, p 70, with permission.)

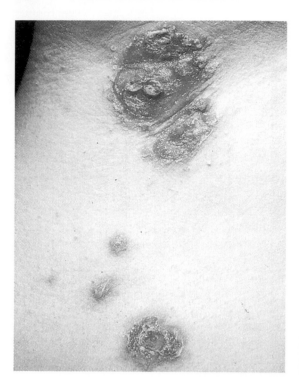

Figure 4–8. Typical impetigo contageosa: honey-colored crusts on red erosions in a fold area of the axilla (armpit). (From Reeves, JT, and Maibach, H: Clinical Dermatology Illustrated, A Regional Approach, ed 3. FA Davis, Philadelphla, 1998, p 250, with permission.)

urticaria (ŭr-tĭ-KĀ-rē-ă): allergic reaction of the skin characterized by eruption of pale-red elevated patches called wheals (hives).

vesicle (VĔS-ĭ-kl) and bulla (BŬL-lă): elevated lesion that contains fluid; a bulla is a vesicle >0.5 cm.

vitiligo (vĭt-ĭl-Ī-gō): localized loss of skin pigmentation characterized by milk-white patches.

wart (WORT): rounded epidermal growths caused by a virus, which include plantar warts, juvenile warts, and venereal warts; removable by cryosurgery, electrocautery, or acids; able to regrow if virus remains in the skin.

wheal (HWĒL): dome-shaped or flat-topped elevated lesion, slightly reddened and often changing in size and shape, usually accompanied by intense itching.

Medical Record

The reports that follow are related to the medical specialty called dermatology. Dermatologists treat diseases of the skin; plastic surgeons also perform procedures to enhance the integumentary system.

MEDICAL RECORD 4–1. Compound Nevus

Dictionary Exercise

This exercise will help you master the terminology in the medical record. Underline the following terms in the reading exercise and use a medical dictionary to define the words. The pronunciations of medical terms in this report are included in the Audiocassette Exercise on pages 169–172.

nevus _____

cm _____

crusting _____

circumscribed _____

diameter _____

melanoma _____

vermilion border _____

Check your answers in Appendix B, Answer Key.

Word Element Exercise

Break down the following words into their basic elements.

chronic
sinusitis
abdominal

histiocytoma
colitis
enteritis

Check your answers in Appendix B, Answer Key.

Reading Exercise

Read the medical report out loud.

A 29-year-old married white woman was referred for surgical treatment of a nevus of the right lower lip. The patient has had a small nevus located at the vermilion border of her lower lip all of her life, but recently it has enlarged somewhat and has become irritated with crusting and bleeding, through local trauma.

The lesion was evaluated initially about 1 month ago during a period of trauma, but it could not be removed at that time because the patient had a prominent upper respiratory infection. Subsequently, there has been healing of the local inflammatory component and the nevus is clear at this time.

Examination reveals a brownish lesion with a flat, somewhat irregular, border that is fairly circumscribed, measuring 0.5 cm in the greatest diameter and located just at the edge of the vermilion border on the right side of the lower lip.

IMPRESSION: Compound nevus, lower lip, rule out melanoma.

MEDICAL RECORD EVALUATION 4–1. Compound Nevus

1. What is a nevus?

2. Locate the vermilion border on your lip and tell where it is located?

3. Was the lesion limited to a certain area?

4. In the impression, the pathologist has ruled out melanoma. What does this mean?

5. What is unusual about a melanoma?

6. Is a melanoma a dangerous condition? If so, explain why.

MEDICAL RECORD 4–2. Psoriasis

Dictionary Exercise

This exercise will help you master the terminology in the medical record. Underline the following terms in the reading exercise and use a medical dictionary to define the words. The pronunciations of medical terms in this report are included in the Audiocassette Exercise on pages 169–172.

abdominal regions _____

Bartholin's gland _____

chronic _____

colitis _____

diabetes mellitus _____

_____

diaphoresis _____

Dx _____

enteritis _____

erythematous _____

FH _____

histiocytoma _____

intermittent _____

macule _____

multiple _____

papule _____

PE _____

pruritis _____

psoriasis _____

scales _____

sclerosed _____

sinusitis _____

syncope _____

vulgaris _____

Reading Exercise

Read the medical report out loud.

Patient is a 24-year-old white woman who has experienced intermittent psoriasis since her early teens in various stages of severity. Her condition has become more troublesome over the past year since May because of an increase of symptoms after being exposed to the sun. Her past history indicates she had chronic sinusitis of 3 years' duration. Her Bartholin's gland was excised in 19XX. She has had pruritus of the scalp and abdominal regions. There is no FH of psoriasis (see Fig. 4–6). An uncle has had diabetes mellitus since the age of 43. Patient has occasional abdominal pains accompanied by diaphoresis and/or syncope. PE showed the patient to have psoriatic involvement of the scalp, external ears, trunk, and, to a lesser degree, legs. There are many scattered erythematous (light ruby) thickened plaques covered by thick yellowish-white scales. A few areas on the legs and arms show multiple, sclerosed, brown macules and papules.

Dx:

1. psoriasis vulgaris

2. multiple histiocytomas

3. abdominal pain, by history; rule out colitis, regional enteritis

MEDICAL RECORD EVALUATION 4–2. Psoriasis

1. What causes psoriasis?

2. On what parts of the body does psoriasis typically occur?

3. How is psoriasis treated?

4. What is a histiocytoma?

Abbreviations

Abbreviation	Meaning	Abbreviation	Meaning
AIDS	acquired immunodeficiency syndrome	ID	intradermal
Bx	biopsy	I&D	incision and drainage
decub.	decubitus	PE	physical examination
derm.	dermatology	SC	subcutaneous
Dx	diagnoses	ung	ointment
FH	family history	WBC	white blood cell (count); white blood cell
FS	frozen section		

Audiocassette Exercise

The audiocassette tape helps you master the pronunciation of medical words. Listen to the tape for instructions to complete this exercise. You may also use this exercise without the audiotape to practice correct pronunciation and spelling of the terms.

Frame	Word	Pronunciation	Spelling Exercise
4–25	[] adenoma	(ăd-ĕ-NŌ-mă)	_____
4–27	[] adipectomy	(ăd-ĭ-PĔK-tō-mē)	_____
4–66	[] adipocele	(ĂD-ĭ-pō-sēl)	_____
4–27	[] adipose tissue	(ĂD-ĭ-pōs TĬSH-ū)	_____
Combining Forms	[] adiposis	(ăd-ĭ-PŌ-sĭs)	_____
Additional Pathological Conditions	[] alopecia	(ăl-ō-PĒ-shē-ă)	_____
4–24	[] anhidrosis	(ăn-hī-DRŌ-sĭs)	_____
4–98	[] autograft	(ĂW-tō-grăft)	_____
Reading Exercise	[] Bartholin's gland	(BĂR-tō-lĭnz GLĂND)	_____
4–86	[] basal cell carcinoma	(BĀ-săl SĔL kăr-sĭ-NŌ-mă)	_____
Reading Exercise	[] colitis	(kō-LĪ-tĭs)	_____
Additional Pathological Conditions	[] comedo	(KŎM-ē-dō)	_____
Additional Pathological Conditions	[] contusion	(kŏn-TOO-zhŭn)	_____
4–67	[] cyanoderma	(sī-ă-nō-DĔR-mă)	_____
4–82	[] cyanosis	(sī-ă-NŌ-sĭs)	_____
Additional Pathological Conditions	[] cyst	(SĬST)	_____
4–65	[] cystocele	(sĭs-tō-sēl)	_____
4–88	[] decubitus ulcer	(dē-KŪ-bĭ-tŭs ŬL-sĕr)	_____
4–10	[] dermatitis	(dĕr-mă-TĪ-tĭs)	_____
4–37	[] dermatologist	(dĕr-mă-TŎL-ōl-jĭst)	_____
4–37	[] dermatology	(dĕr-mă-TŎL-ō-jē)	_____
4–9	[] dermatotome	(DĔR-mă-tōm)	_____
4–52	[] dermatomycosis	(dĕr-mă-tō-mī-KŌ-sĭs)	_____
4–5	[] dermatopathy	(DĔR-mă-tŏ-păth-ē)	_____
4–35	[] dermatoplasty	(DĔR-mă-tō-plăs-tē)	_____
4 42	[] dermatosclerosis	(dĕr-mă-tō-sklĕ-RŌ-sĭs)	_____
4–3	[] dermis	(DĔR-mĭs)	_____
4–18	[] dermopathy	(dĕr-MŎP-ă-thē)	_____
Reading Exercise	[] diabetes mellitus	(dī-ă-BĒ-tēz mĕ-LĪ-tŭs)	_____
4–22	[] diaphoresis	(dī-ă-fō-RĒ-sĭs)	_____
Additional Pathological Conditions	[] ecchymosis	(ĕk-ĭ-MŌ-sĭs)	_____
Additional Pathological Conditions	[] eczema	(ĔK-zĕ-mă)	_____
Reading Exercise	[] enteritis	(ĕn-tĕr-Ī-tĭs)	_____
4–7	[] epidermis	(ĕp-ĭ-DĔR-mĭs)	_____

Frame	Word	Pronunciation	Spelling Exercise
Reading Exercise	[] erythematous	(ĕr-ĭ-THĔM-ă-tŭs)	_____
4–73	[] erythrocyte	(ĕ-RĬTH-rō-sīt)	_____
4–67	[] erythroderma	(ĕ-rĭth-rō-DĔR-mă)	_____
4–84	[] erythrosis	(ĕr-ĭ-THRŌ-sĭs)	_____
Additional Pathological Conditions	[] fissure	(FĬSH-ŭr)	_____
4–97	[] gangrene	(GĂNG-grēn)	_____
4–39	[] gastrologist	(găs-TRŎL-ō-jĭst)	_____
4–40	[] gastrology	(găs-TRŎL-ō-jē)	_____
4–26	[] hidradenoma	(hī-drăd-ĕ-NŌ-mă)	_____
4–22	[] hidrorrhea	(hī-drō-RĒ-ă)	_____
4–21	[] hidrosis	(hī-DRŌ-sĭs)	_____
Additional Pathological Conditions	[] hirsutism	(HŬR-sūt-ĭzm)	_____
Reading Exercise	[] histiocytoma	(hĭs-tē-ō-sī-TŌ-mă)	_____
4–22	[] hyperhidrosis	(hī-pĕr-hī-DRŌ-sĭs)	_____
4–11	[] hypodermic	(hī-pō-DĔR-mĭk)	_____
Additional Pathological Conditions	[] impetigo	(ĭm-pĕ-TĪ-gō)	_____
4–90	[] Kaposi's sarcoma	(KĂH-pō-sēz săr-KŌ-mă)	_____
4–43	[] keratosis	(kĕr-ă-TŌ-sĭs)	_____
Additional Pathological Conditions	[] laceration	(lăs-ĕr-Ā-shŭn)	_____
4–87	[] lesion	(LĒ-zhŭn)	_____
4–77	[] leukemia	(loo-KĒ-mē-ă)	_____
4–73	[] leukocyte	(LOO-kō-sīt)	_____
4–74	[] leukocytopenia	(loo-kō-sī-tō-PĒ-nē-ă)	_____
4–27	[] lipectomy	(lĭ-PĔK-tō-mē)	_____
4–66	[] lipocele	(LĬP-ō-sēl)	_____
4–31	[] lipocyte	(LĬP-ō-sīt)	_____
4–28	[] lipoma	(lĭ-PŌ-mă)	_____
Additional Pathological Conditions	[] macule	(MĂK-ūl)	_____
4–87	[] malignant melanoma	(mă-LĬG-nănt mĕl-ă-NŌ-mă)	_____
4–73	[] melanocyte	(MĔL-ăn-ō-sīt)	_____
4–67	[] melanoderma	(mĕl-ăn-ō-DĔR-mă)	_____
4–79	[] melanoma	(mĕl-ă-NŌ-mă)	_____
4–80	[] melanosis	(mĕl-ăn-Ō-sĭs)	_____
4–95	[] necrocytosis	(nĕk-rō-sī-TŌ-sĭs)	_____
4–94	[] necrosis	(nĕ-KRŌ-sĭs)	_____
4–93	[] necrotic	(nĕ-KRŎT-ĭk)	_____
Reading Exercise	[] nevus	(NĒ-vŭs)	_____
Additional Pathological Conditions	[] nodule	(NŎD-ūl)	_____
4–59	[] onychoma	(ŏn-ĭ-KŌ-mă)	_____

Frame	Word	Pronunciation	Spelling Exercise
4–61	[] onychomalacia	(ŏn-ĭ-kō-mă-LĀ-sē-ă)	_____
4–62	[] onychomycosis	(ŏn-ĭ-kō-mī-KŌ-sĭs)	_____
4–59	[] onychopathy	(ŏn-ĭ-KŎP-ăth-ē)	_____
Additional Pathological Conditions	[] papule	(PĂP-ūl)	_____
Additional Pathological Conditions	[] petechia	(pē-TĒ-kē-ă)	_____
4–58	[] pilocystic	(pī-lō-SĬS-tĭk)	_____
Combining Forms	[] pilonidal	(pī-lō-NĪ-dăl)	_____
Reading Exercise	[] pruritus	(proo-RĪ-tŭs)	_____
4–89	[] psoriasis	(sō-RĪ-ă-sĭs)	_____
Reading Exercise	[] psoriasis vulgaris	(sō-RĪ-ă-sĭs vŭl-GĂ-rĭs)	_____
Reading Exercise	[] psoriatic	(sō-RĪ-ă-tĭc)	_____
Additional Pathological Conditions	[] pustule	(PŬS-tūl)	_____
Additional Pathological Conditions	[] scabies	(SKĀ-bēz)	_____
Additional Pathological Conditions	[] scales	(SKĀLZ)	_____
4–42	[] scleroderma	(sklĕr-ō-DĔR-mă)	_____
4–41	[] sclerosis	(sklĕ-RŌ-sĭs)	_____
4–16	[] sebaceous gland	(sē-BĀ-shŭs GLĂND)	_____
Reading Exercise	[] sinusitis	(sī-nŭs-Ī-tĭs)	_____
4–28	[] steatoma	(stē-ă-TŌ-mă)	_____
4–12	[] subcutaneous	(sŭb-kū-TĀ-nē-ŭs)	_____
4–33	[] suction lipectomy	(SŬK-shŭn lĭ-PĔK-tō-mē)	_____
4–16	[] sudoriferous gland	(soo-dŏr-ĬF-ĕr-ŭs GLĂND)	_____
Reading Exercise	[] syncope	(SĬN-kŭ-pē)	_____
Additional Pathological Conditions	[] tinea	(TĬN-ē-ă)	_____
4–56	[] trichomycosis	(trĭk-ō-mī-KŌ-sĭs)	_____
4–55	[] trichopathy	(trĭk-ŎP-ă-thē)	_____
4–55	[] trichosis	(trī-KŌ-sĭs)	_____
Additional Pathological Conditions	[] urticaria	(ŭr-tĭ-KĀ-rē-ă)	_____
Reading Exercise	[] vermilion border	(vĕr-MĬL-ē-ŏn BŎRD-ĕr)	_____
Additional Pathological Conditions	[] vesicle	(VĔS-ĭ-kl)	_____
Additional Pathological Conditions	[] vitiligo	(vĭt-ĭ-LĪ-gō)	_____
Reading Exercise	[] vulgaris	(vŭl-GĀ-rĭs)	_____
Additional Pathological Conditions	[] wart	(WŎRT)	_____
Additional Pathological Conditions	[] wheal	(HWĒL)	_____
4–91	[] xanthemia	(zăn-THĒ-mē-ă)	_____

Frame	Word	Pronunciation	Spelling Exercise
4–73	[] xanthocyte	(ZĂN-thō-sīt)	_____
4–67	[] xanthoderma	(zăn-thō-DĔR-mă)	_____
4–84	[] xanthosis	(zăn-THŌ-sĭs)	_____
4–63	[] xeroderma	(zē-rō-DĔR-mă)	_____
4–64	[] xerophagia	(zē-rō-FĀ-jē-ă)	_____

Unit Exercises

DEFINITIONS

Review Unit Summary (pages 179–180) before completing this exercise. Write the definition for each word part.

SUFFIXES, PREFIXES, AND ABBREVIATIONS

Element	Meaning
SUFFIXES	
1. -cele	_____
2. -cyte	_____
3. -emia	_____
4. -logist	_____
5. -logy	_____
6. -malacia	_____
7. -oma	_____
8. -osis	_____
9. -pathy	_____
10. -penia	_____
11. -phagia	_____
12. -rrhea	_____
PREFIXES AND ABBREVIATIONS	
13. auto-	_____
14. epi-	_____
15. sub-	_____
16. Dx	_____
17. FH	_____
18. PE	_____
19. WBC	_____
COMBINING FORMS	
20. adip/o	_____
21. cutane/o	_____
22. cyt/o	_____
23. derm/o, dermat/o	_____
24. hidr/o	_____
25. hydr/o	_____
26. lip/o	_____
27. onych/o	_____
28. scler/o	_____
29. trich/o	_____
30. xer/o	_____

Element	Meaning

COMBINING FORMS OF COLORS

31. cyan / o _____

32. erythr / o _____

33. leuk / o _____

34. melan / o _____

35. xanth / o _____

VALIDATION FRAME: Check your answers with the Index of Medical Word Elements, Appendix A. If you scored less than _____ %,* review Unit Summary (pages 179–180). To obtain a percentage score, multiply the number of correct answers times 2.9.

Number of Correct Answers: _____   **Percentage Score:** _____

*Enter the percentage required by your instructor to complete this course.

Vocabulary

Match the medical term(s) below with the definitions in the numbered list.

autograft
decubitus ulcer
diabetes mellitus
diaphoresis
ecchymosis
hidrorrhea
hirsutism
leukemia

lipocele
lipoma
Kaposi's sarcoma
macules
melanoma
onychomalacia
papules

psoriasis
pustule
subcutaneous
suction lipectomy
trichopathy
vulgaris
xeroderma

1. _____ Beneath the layers of the skin.

2. _____ A condition in which a person sweats excessively; profuse perspiration.

3. _____ Any disease of the hair.

4. _____ A graft transferred from one part to another part of a patient's body.

5. _____ A type of skin tumor associated with AIDS.

6. _____ Excision of subcutaneous fat tissue by use of a blunt-tipped cannula (tube), done for cosmetic reasons.

7. _____ Medical term for discolored patches on the skin, such as flat moles, freckles, or measles rash.

8. _____ Caused by prolonged pressure against an area of skin from a bed or chair.

9. _____ Excessive production of white blood cells; literally white blood.

10. _____ Black-and-blue mark on the skin; a bruise.

11. _____ Usually a chronic skin disease marked by itchy, scaly, red patches covered by silvery gray scales.

12. _____ Excessive body hair, especially in women.

13. _____ An elevated lesion containing pus.

14. _____ The medical term for warts, moles, and pimples.

15. _____ A disease resulting from a breakdown in the body's ability to produce or utilize insulin.

16. _____ Excessive dryness of skin.

17. _____ Black or dark tumor.

18. _____ A hernia that contains fat or fatty cells.

19. _____ Ordinary, common.

20. _____ Softening of the nail or nailbed.

VALIDATION FRAME: Check your answers in Appendix B, Answer Key. If you scored less than _____ %, review the vocabulary and retake the exercise.

To obtain a percentage score, multiply the number of correct answers times 5.

Number of Correct Answers: _____   **Percentage Score:** _____

Additional Pathological Conditions

Match the medical term(s) below with the definitions in the numbered list.

alopecia	laceration	tinea
comedo	nodule	urticaria
contusion	papule	vesicle
cyst	petechia	vitiligo
fissure	pustule	wart
eczema	scabies	wheal
impetigo	scales	

1. _____ Rounded epidermal growth caused by a virus.

2. _____ Localized loss of skin pigmentation characterized by eruption of pale red elevated patches.

3. _____ Any fungal skin disease, frequently caused by ringworm, whose name indicates the body part affected.

4. _____ Small elevation of skin filled with lymph or pus.

5. _____ Small cracklike break that exposes the dermis; usually red.

6. _____ Inflammatory skin disease characterized by redness, itching, and blisters.

7. _____ Inflammatory skin disease characterized by isolated pustules that become crusted and rupture.

8. _____ Allergic reaction of the skin characterized by eruption of pale-red elevated patches called hives.

9. _____ Slightly elevated dome-shaped lesion that is slightly redder or paler than the surrounding skin accompanied by itching.

10. _____ A large fluid-filled blister.

11. _____ Excessive dry exfoliations shed from upper layers of the skin.

12. _____ Contagious skin disease transmitted by the itch mite.

13. _____ Palpable circumscribed lesion, larger than a papule, 1 to 2 cm in diameter.

14. _____ Absence or loss of hair, especially of the head; baldness.

15. _____ A blackhead.

16. _____ A cut.

17. _____ A fluid-filled or solid sac in or under the skin.

18. _____ An injury in which the skin is not broken.

19. _____ A solid elevated lesion, <1 cm in diameter.

20. _____ Minute hemorrhagic spots on the skin that are smaller versions of ecchymosis.

VALIDATION FRAME: Check your answers in Appendix B, Answer Key. If you scored less than _____ %, review the vocabulary and retake the exercise.

To obtain a percentage score, multiply the number of correct answers times 5.

Number of Correct Answers: _____   **Percentage Score:** _____

UNIT SUMMARY

COMBINING FORMS RELATED TO THE INTEGUMENTARY SYSTEM

Combining Form	Pronunciation	Meaning
adip / o lip / o steat / o	ăd-ĭ-pō lĭ-pō stē-ă-tō	fat
cyt / o	sī-tō	cell
cutane / o derm / o dermat / o	kū-tā-nē-ō dĕr-mō dĕr-mă-tō	skin
hidr / o	hī-drō	sweat
hydr / o	hī-drō	water
kerat / o	kĕr-ă-tō	horny
myc / o	mī-kō	fungus
necr / o	nĕk-rō	dead, death
onych / o	ŏn-ĭ-kō	nail
scler / o	sklĕ-rō	hardening
pil / o trich / o	pī-lō trĭ-kō	hair
xer / o	zē-rō	dry

COMBINING FORMS DENOTING COLOR

Combining Form	Pronunciation	Meaning
cyan / o	sī-ăn-ō	blue
erythr / o	ē-rĭth-rō	red
leuk / o	loo-kō	white
melan / o	mĕl-ă-nō	black
xanth / o	zăn-thō	yellow

SUFFIXES AND PREFIXES

Suffix (Prefix)	Pronunciation	Meaning
SURGICAL SUFFIXES		
-ectomy	ĕk-tō-mē	excision, removal
-plasty	plăs-tē	surgical repair
-tome	tōm	instrument to cut

Suffix (Prefix)	Pronunciation	Meaning
OTHER SUFFIXES		
-cele	sēl	hernia, swelling
-cyte	sīt	cell
-derma	dĕr-mă	skin
-emia	ē-mē-ă	blood
-logist	lō-jĭst	specialist in the study of
-logy	lō-jē	study of
-malacia	mă-lā-shē-ă	softening
-oma	ō-mă	tumor
-osis	ō-sĭs	abnormal condition
-pathy	pă-thē	disease
-penia	pē-nē-ă	decrease
-phagia	fā-jē-ă	swallow, eat
-rrhea	rē-ă	flow, discharge
PREFIXES		
auto-	aw-tō	self
epi-	ĕp-ĭ	above, upon
sub-	sŭb	under, below

5

Reproductive System

Even though the structures of the female and male reproductive systems (Fig. 5–1) are different, both have a common purpose, which is to produce offspring.

Female Reproductive System

In the woman, reproduction is accomplished when the egg (ovum; plural: ova) produced by the ovaries is fertilized by male sperm.

The combining forms related to the female reproductive system are summarized here. Review this information before you begin to work the frames.

COMBINING FORMS

Form	Meaning	Example	Pronunciation
cervic/o	neck, cervix uteri (neck of uterus)	cervic/itis inflammation	sĕr-vĭ-SĪ-tĭs
colp/o	vagina	colp/o/rrhaphy suture	kŏl-PŎR-ă-fē
vagin/o		vagin/itis inflammation	văj-ĭn-Ī-tĭs
episi/o	vulva	episi/o/tomy incision, cut into	ĕ-pĭs-ē-ŌT-ō-mē
vulv/o		vulv/ectomy excision	vŭl-VĔK-tō-mē
gynec/o	woman, female	gynec/o/logist specialist in the study (of)	gī-nĕ-KŎL-ō-jĭst
hyster/o	uterus	hyster/ectomy excision, removal	hĭs-tĕr-ĔK-tō-mē
metr/o		metr/o/rrhagia bursting forth (of)	mē-trŏ-RĀ-jē-ă
uter/o		uter/al pertaining to	Ū-tĕr-ăl
lapar/o	abdomen	lapar/o/scopy visual examination	lăp-ăr-ŎS-kō-pē
mamm/o	breast	mamm/o/gram record (x-ray)	MĂM-ō-grăm
mast/o		mast/o/dynia pain	măst-ō-DĬN-ē-ă
men/o	menses, menstruation	men/o/rrhea flow, discharge	mĕn-ō-RĒ-ă

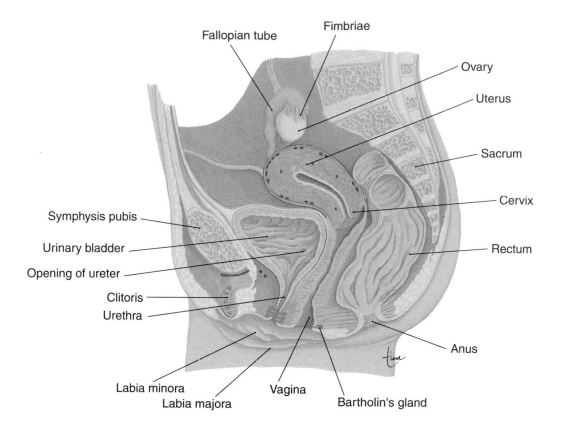

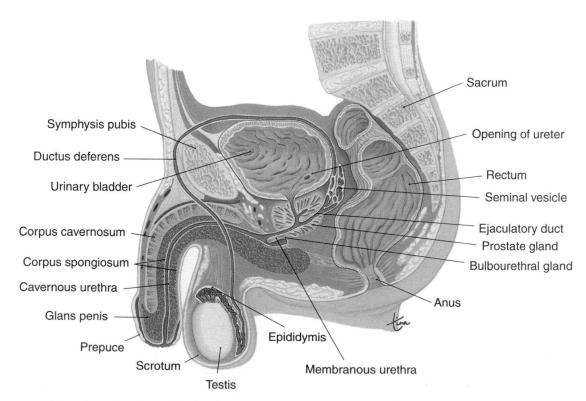

Figure 5–1. Structures of the female and male reproductive systems. (From Scanlon, VC, and Sanders, T: Understanding Human Structure and Function. FA Davis, Philadelphia, 1997, pp 357, 361, with permission.)

Form	Meaning	Example	Pronunciation
oophor/o	ovary	oophor/itis inflammation	ō-ŏf-ō-RĪ-tĭs
ovari/o		ovari/o/cele hernia, swelling	ō-VĀ-rē-ō-sēl
salping/o	fallopian (uterine) tube, eustachian (auditory) tube	salping/o/scopy visual examination	săl-pĭng-GŎS-kō-pē

Internal Structures

5–1 Use the Index of Medical Word Elements, Part A of Appendix A, to define the following elements.

Medical Word Element	*Meaning*
hemat/o	_____
hem/o	_____
hyster/o	_____
metr/o	_____
oophor/o	_____
salping/o	_____

5–2 Use the Index of Medical Word Elements, Part B of Appendix A, to write the medical word elements for the following English terms.

English Term	*Medical Word Element*
bursting forth (of)	_____
fat	_____ / _____ or _____ / _____
hernia, swelling	_____
vomit	_____
woman	_____ / _____

5–3 The female reproductive system is composed of internal and external organs of reproduction. The internal reproductive organs are the **(1) ovaries, (2) fallopian tubes, (3) uterus**, and **(4) vagina**.

Label Figures 5–2 and 5–3 as you learn the names of the internal reproductive organs.

tumor (TOO-mŏr)	**5–4** An oophor/oma is an ovarian _____ . Pronounce both initial o's in words with **oophor/o**.

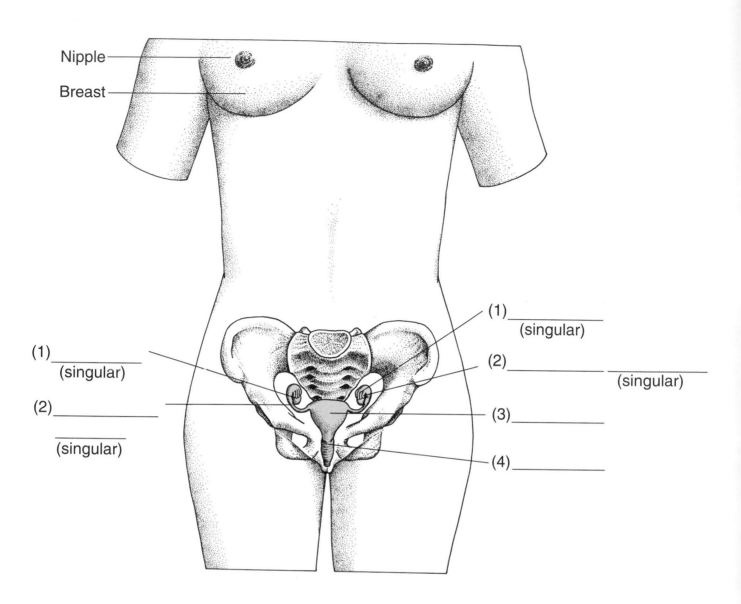

Nipple

Breast

(1)_____ (singular)

(1)_____ (singular)

(2)_____ (singular)

(2)_____ (singular)

(3)_____

(4)_____

Figure 5–2. Female reproductive system, frontal view. (Adapted from Gylys, BA, and Wedding, ME: Medical Terminology: A Systems Approach, ed 3. FA Davis, Philadelphia, 1995, p 265.)

oophor/o (ō-ŎF-ŏr-ŏ)	**5–5** The main purpose of the ovaries is to produce ovum, the female reproductive cell. This process is called ovulation. Another important function of the ovaries is to produce the hormones estrogen and progesterone. From oophor/oma, construct the combining form for ovary: _____ / _____ .
oophor/o/pathy (ō-ŏf-ŏr-ŎP-ă-thē) oophor/o/plasty (ō-ŎF-ŏr-ō-plăs-tē) oophor/o/pexy (ō-ŏf-ō-rō-PĔK-sē)	**5–6** Form medical words meaning disease of the ovaries: _____ / _____ / _____ surgical repair of an ovary: _____ / _____ / _____ fixation of a displaced ovary: _____ / _____ / _____

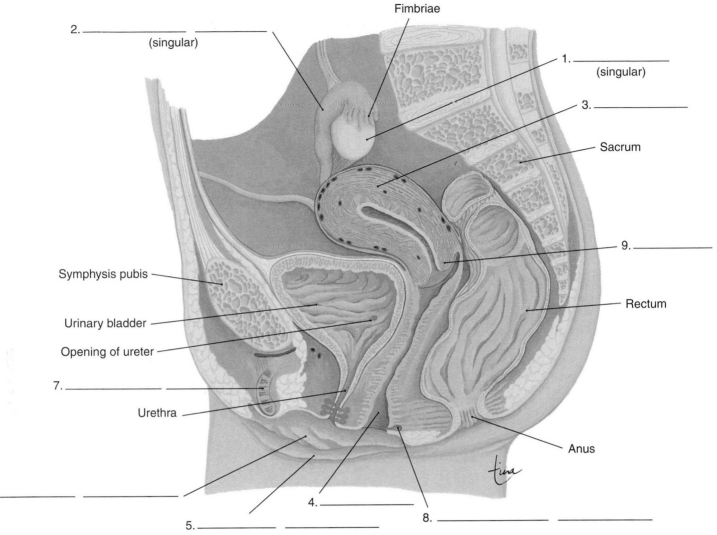

Fimbriae

2. _____ _____
(singular)

1. _____
(singular)

3. _____

Sacrum

9. _____

Symphysis pubis

Urinary bladder

Opening of ureter

Rectum

7. _____ _____

Urethra

Anus

6. _____ _____

4. _____

5. _____ _____

8. _____ _____

Figure 5–3. The female reproductive system, lateral view. (Adapted from Scanlon, VC, and Sanders, T: Understanding Human Structure and Function. FA Davis, Philadelphia, 1997, p 361, with permission.)

5-7 The combining form **salping/o** is used to build words that refer to the fallopian (uterine) tube(s), also called oviduct(s). (**Salping/o** also refers to the eustachian (auditory) tube, covered in Unit 10.)

The surgical repair of a fallopian tube is called

_____ / ___ / _____ .

salping/o/plasty
(săl-PĬNG-gō-plăs-tē)

5-8 About once a month, one of the two fallopian tubes (Fig. 5–2) transports the egg from an ovary to the uterus, a process called ovulation. Union of the ovum with sperm results in fertilization, or pregnancy.

To form words for the fallopian tube(s), uterine tube(s), or oviduct(s), use the combining form _____ / ___ .

salping/o
(săl-PĬNG-gō)

salping/ectomy (săl-pĭn-JĔK-tō-mē)	**5–9** If the fertilized egg attaches to the wall of the fallopian tube (instead of the uterus), the tube must be removed to prevent serious bleeding in or even death of the mother. When a fallopian tube(s) is removed, the surgical procedure is called _____ / _____ .
instrument	**5–10** A salping/o/scope is an _____ to view the fallopian tube(s).
salping/o/scopy (săl-pĭng-GŎS-kō-pē)	**5–11** A visual examination of the fallopian tube(s) is called _____ / _____ / _____ .
salping/o/cele (săl-PĬNG-ō-sēl)	**5–12** A hernia (hernial protrusion) of a fallopian tube(s) is known as _____ / _____ / _____ .
oviducts (Ŏ-vĭ-dŭkts)	**5–13** Locate the two small tubes leading to an ovary (see Fig. 5–2). They are called fallopian tubes, uterine tubes, or _____ .
excision or removal (ĕk-SĬ-zhŭn) **uterus** (Ū-tĕr-ŭs)	**5–14** The uterus, also called the womb, is the organ that contains and nourishes the embryo and fetus from the time the fertilized egg is implanted to the time of birth. The combining form **hyster/o** is used to form words about the uterus as an organ. A hyster/ectomy is an _____ of the _____ .
hyster/o/pathy (hĭs-tĕr-ŎP-ă-thē) **hyster/algia** (hĭs-tĕr-ĂL-jē-ă) **hyster/o/dynia** (hĭs-tĕr-ō-DĬ-nē-ă) **hyster/o/spasm** (HĬS-tĕr-ō-spăzm)	**5–15** Use **hyster/o** to construct medical words meaning disease of the uterus: _____ / _____ / _____ pain in the uterus: _____ / _____ or _____ / _____ / _____ spasm of the uterus: _____ / _____ / _____
hyster/ectomy (hĭs-tĕr-ĔK-tō-mē) **hyster/o/tomy** (hĭs-tĕr-ŎT-ō-mē)	**5–16** The most frequent reason to remove the uterus is the presence of one or more benign or malignant tumors. Use **hyster/o** to form surgical terms meaning excision of the uterus: _____ / _____ incision of the uterus: _____ / _____ / _____

5–17 The combining forms **metr/o** and **uter/o** also denote the uterus.

Metr/o/cele, uter/o/cele, and hyster/o/cele all refer to a hernia of the

_____ .

uterus
(Ū-tĕr-ŭs)

5–18 When you are in doubt about forming medical words with either

hyster/o, uter/o, or **metr/o,** refer to your medical _____ .

dictionary

5–19 The uterus is a muscular, hollow, pear-shaped structure located in the pelvic area between the bladder and rectum (see Fig. 5–2).

Use **hyster/o** and **metr/o** to form two words that both mean an inflammation of the uterus:

_____ / _____

_____ / _____

hyster/itis
(hĭs-tĕr-Ī-tĭs)
metr/itis
(mĕ-TRĪ-tĭs)

5–20 Use **metr/o** to formulate words meaning

incision of the uterus: _____ / ____ / _____

instrument to cut or incise the uterus:
_____ / ____ / _____

metr/o/tomy
(mĕ-TRŎT-ō-mē)

metr/o/tome
(MĔ-trō-tōm)

5–21 Hyster/o/pathy and metr/o/pathy both mean _____ of

the _____ .

disease

uterus
(Ū-tĕr-ŭs)

5–22 A uterine hernia is known as a metr/o/cele or

_____ / ____ / _____ .

hyster/o/cele
(HĬS-tĕr-ō-sēl)

5–23 Birth control pills contain estrogen and progesterone. Recall that the ovaries secrete two hormones called _____ and

_____ .

estrogen
(ĔS-trō-jĕn)
progesterone
(prō-JĔS-tĕr-ōn)

5–24 The suffixes -rrhage and -rrhagia are used in words to mean bursting forth (of). Hem/o/rrhage denotes a _____ _____ (of) blood.

bursting forth

5–25 The combining form in hem/o/rrhage that denotes blood is
_____ / ____ .

hem/o

blood	**5–26** The elements **hemat/o, hem/o**, and -emia refer to _____ .

blood	**5–27** Hemat/o/logy is the study of _____ .

5–28 A hemat/oma is a localized collection or swelling of blood, usually clotted, in an organ, space, or tissue, caused by a break in the wall of a blood vessel.

Analyze hemat/oma by defining the elements.

blood   **hemat/o** refers to _____ .

tumor   -oma refers to a _____ .
(TOO-mor)

5–29 Use **hemat/o** to build medical words meaning

hemat/o/logist   specialist in the study of blood: _____ / _____ / _____
(hē-mă-TŎL-ō-jĭst)

hemat/o/pathy   disease of the blood: _____ / _____ / _____
(hē-mă-TŎP-ăth-ē)

hemat/emesis   vomiting blood: _____ / _____
(hēm-ăt-ĔM-ĕ-sĭs)

5–30 The vagina (Fig. 5–2) is a muscular tube that extends from the cervix (neck of the uterus) to the exterior of the body. As well as serving as the organ of sexual intercourse and the receptor of semen, the vagina discharges the menstrual flow and acts as a passageway for the delivery of the fetus.

The combining forms **colp/o** and **vagin/o** refer to the vagina. Colp/itis is an

inflammation, vagina   _____ of the _____ .
(vă-JĪ-nă)

5–31 Form another word besides colp/itis that means inflammation of the

vagin/itis   vagina: _____ / _____ .
(văj-ĭn-Ī-tĭs)

5–32 Colp/o/dynia is pain in the vagina. Use **colp/o** to build another term for

colp/algia   pain in the vagina: _____ / _____ .
(kŏl-PĂL-jē-ă)

5–33 Use **colp/o** to construct medical words meaning

colp/o/spasm   spasm or twitching of the vagina: _____ / _____ / _____
(KŎL-pō-spăzm)

colp/o/ptosis   prolapse or dropping of the vagina: _____ / _____ / _____
(kŏl-pŏp-TŌ-sĭs)

colp/o/pexy   fixation or suspension of the vagina: _____ / _____ / _____
(KŎL-pō-pĕk-sē)

vagin/o/plasty (vă-JĬ-nō-plăs-tē) **vagin/o/scope** (VĂJ-ĭn-ō-skōp) **vagin/o/tomy** (văj-ĭ-NŎT-ō-mē)	**5-34** Use **vagin/o** to formulate medical words meaning surgical repair of the vagina: _____ / _____ / _____ instrument to view the vagina: _____ / _____ / _____ incision of the vagina: _____ / _____ / _____
suture, vagina (SOO-chŭr) (vă-JĬ-nă)	**5-35** A prolapsed vagina is usually sutured to the abdominal wall. Colp/o/rrhaphy is a _____ of the _____ .
-rrhagia, -rrhage	**5-36** Colp/o/rrhagia is an excessive vaginal discharge or a vaginal hem/o/rrhage. The elements in these words that mean bursting forth (of) are _____ and _____ .
hem/o/rrhage HĔM-ĕ-rĭj)	**5-37** Form a word meaning bursting forth (of) blood: _____ / _____ / _____
hernia, swelling (HĔR-nē-ă)	**5-38** Recall that -cele designates a _____ or _____ .
vagina (vă-JĬ-nă)	**5-39** A colp/o/cyst/o/cele is a protrusion or herniation of the bladder into the _____ .
vagina (vă-JĬ-nă) **bladder** **hernia, swelling** (HĔR-nē-ă)	**5-40** Many women who have had a vagin/al childbirth suffer from herniation of the bladder or colp/o/cyst/o/cele. Identify the elements in colp/o/cyst/o/cele. **colp/o** refers to the _____ . **cyst/o** refers to the _____ . -cele refers to a _____ or _____ .
vagin/al (VĂJ-ĭn-ăl) **hyster/ectomy** (hĭs-tĕr-ĔK-tō-mē)	**5-41** When the uterus is removed by way of the vagina, the surgical procedure is known as a vagin/al hyster/ectomy or a colp/o/hyster/ectomy. Identify the words in this frame that mean pertaining to the vagina: _____ / _____ excision of the uterus: _____ / _____

muc/ous (MŪ-kŭs)	**5–42** The vagina is lubricated by mucus. **Muc/o** is the combining form for mucus. Use the adjective ending -ous to form a word that means pertaining to mucus: _____ / _____ .
-oid	**5–43** Muc/oid means resembling mucus. The adjective ending element meaning resembling is _____ .
resembling fat	**5–44** Lip/oid means _____ _____ .
adip/oid (ĂD-ĭ-poyd)	**5–45** Use **adip/o** to form another term meaning resembling fat: _____ / _____

Review

Select the element(s) that matches the meaning.

adip/o	-algia	-pathy
colp/o	-cele	-pexy
cyst/o	-dynia	-plasty
hemat/o	-ectomy	-ptosis
hem/o	-emia	-rrhage
hyster/o	-itis	-rrhagia
lip/o	-logist	-rrhaphy
metr/o	-logy	-scope
muc/o	-oid	-scopy
oophor/o	-oma	-spasm
salping/o	-ous	-tome
uter/o		-tomy
vagin/o		

a. _____ bladder

b. _____ blood

c. _____ bursting forth (of)

d. _____ fat

e. _____ hernia, swelling

f. _____ incision, cut into

g. _____ instrument to cut

h. _____ instrument to view

i. _____ fallopian (uterine) tube, oviduct

j. _____ fixation

k. _____ mucus

l. _____ ovary

m. _____ pain

n. _____ pertaining to

o. _____ prolapse, falling, dropping

p. _____ resembling

q. _____ specialist in the study of

r. _____ study of

s. _____ surgical repair

t. _____ tumor

u. _____ twitching, involuntary contraction

v. _____ uterus, womb

w. _____ vagina

x. _____ visual examination

Check your answers with the Review Answer Key on the following page.

Review Answer Key

a. cyst / o

b. hemat / o, hem / o, -emia

c. -rrhage, -rrhagia

d. adip / o, lip / o

e. -cele

f. -tomy

g. -tome

h. -scope

i. salping / o

j. -pexy

k. muc / o

l. oophor / o

m. -algia, -dynia

n. -ous

o. -ptosis

p. -oid

q. -logist

r. -logy

s. -plasty

t. -oma

u. -spasm

v. hyster / o, metr / o, uter / o

w. colp / o, vagin / o

x. -scopy

REINFORCEMENT FRAME: If you are not satisfied with your level of comprehension, go back to Frame 5–1 and rework the frames.

External Structures

5–46 The external structures, or genitalia, include the **(5) labia majora** (the outer lips of the vagina), **(6) labia minora** (the smaller, inner lips of the vagina), **(7) clitoris**, and **(8) Bartholin's glands**.

Label Figure 5–3 as you learn the names of the genitalia.

---

vulva

5–47 The combining form **vulv/o** refers to the vulva, the combined external structures of the female reproductive system. Vulv/o/uterine refers to the uterus and _____ .

---

clitoris

Bartholin's glands

5–48 The external structures, or genitalia, also known as the vulva, include labia majora, labia minora, the _____ , and _____ _____ .

---

muc/ous

5–49 The mucus secretions from Bartholin's gland lubricate the vagina. Use -ous to build a word meaning pertaining to mucus: _____ / _____ (adjective ending).

---

vulv/itis
(vŭl-VĪ-tĭs)
vulv/o/pathy
(vŭl-VŎP-ă-thē)
vulv/ectomy
(vŭl-VĔK-tō-mē)

5–50 Use **vulv/o** to construct words meaning

inflammation of the vulva: _____ / _____

disease of the vulva: _____ / ____ / _____

excision of the vulva: _____ / _____

5–51 The **(9) cervix** is a term denoting the neck of the uterus and extends into the top portion of the vagina.

Examine the position of the cervix as you label Figure 5–3.

---

cervic/itis
(sĕr-vĭ-SĪ-tĭs)

5–52 The combining form **cervic/o** denotes either the cervix uteri or the neck. An inflammation of the cervix uteri is called

_____ / _____ .

---

vagina
(vă-JĪ-nă)
uteri
(Ū-tĕ-rē)

5–53 When **cervic/o** is used in a word, you can determine whether it refers to the neck or the cervix uteri by reviewing the other parts of the word. For example, colp/o/cervic/al refers to the _____ and cervix _____ .

colp/o/scopy
(kŏl-PŎS-kō-pē)

5–54 A colp/o/scope, an instrument with a magnifying lens, is used to examine vagin/al and cervic/al tissue. Visual examination of vagin/al and cervic/al tissue using a colposcope is called _____ / _____ / _____ .

colp/o/scope
(KŎL-pō-skōp)

colp/o/scopy
(kŏl-PŎS-kō-pē)
vagin/al
(VĂJ-ĭn-ăl)
cervic/al
(SĔR-vĭ-kăl)

5–55 Determine the words in Frame 5–54 that mean instrument used for examining the vagina and cervix uteri:

_____ / _____ / _____

visual examination of the vagina and cervix uteri using a colp/o/scope:

_____ / _____ / _____

pertaining to the vagina: _____ / _____

pertaining to the cervix uteri: _____ / _____

uterus
(Ū-tĕr-ŭs)

5–56 Cervix uteri refers to the neck of the _____ .

VALIDATION FRAME: Check your labeling of Figures 5–2 and 5–3 with the Answer Key, Appendix B.

gynec/o/logist
(gī-nĕ-KŎL-ō-jĭst)

5–57 Gynec/o/logy literally means study of females or women, and is the medical specialty for treating female disorders or diseases. A specialist in the study of female disorders is called a _____ / _____ / _____ .

gynec/o

5–58 The combining form in the word gynec/o/logy that means woman or female is _____ / _____ .

gynec/o/pathy
(gī-nĕ-KŎP-ă-thē)

5–59 Use -pathy to form a word that means disease of a female: _____ / _____ / _____

gynec/o/logy
(gī-nĕ-KŎL-ō-jē)

5–60 GYN is the abbreviation for gynec/o/logy. OB-GYN refers to obstetrics and _____ / _____ / _____ .

5–61 Use your medical dictionary to define *obstetrics*.

_____

_____

5–62 The combining form **men/o** denotes the menses, also called menstruation, which is the monthly flow of blood and tissue from the uterus.

Men/o/rrhea is a flow of the _____ or _____ .

menses, menstruation
(MĔN-sēz)
(mĕn-stroo-Ā-shŭn)

5–63 Use dys- and men/o/rrhea to develop a word meaning painful or difficult menstrual flow: _____ / _____ / ___ / _____ .

dys/men/o/rrhea
(dĭs-mĕn-ō-RĒ-ă)

5–64 Dys/men/o/rrhea causes pain and tension.

The combining form for menses, or menstruation, is _____ / ___ .

The word element denoting bad, painful, difficult is _____ .

The word element meaning flow or discharge is _____ .

men/o
dys-
-rrhea

5–65 Men/o/rrhagia is excessive bleeding at the time of a menstrual period.

Literally it means _____ _____ (of the)

_____ .

bursting forth

menses or **menstruation**
(MĔN-sēz)
(mĕn-stroo-Ā-shŭn)

5–66 Men/o/pause terminates the reproductive period of life and is a permanent cessation of menses or _____ .

menstruation
(mĕn-stroo-Ā-shun)

5–67 A/men/o/rrhea is the absence or abnormal stoppage of menstruation. Men/o/rrhea is a flow of the menses or _____ .

menstruation
(mĕn-stroo-Ā-shun)

5–68 Identify the element in meno/pause meaning cessation: _____ .

-pause

5–69 Post/men/o/paus/al and pre/men/o/paus/al bleeding is bleeding that occurs at times other than during the normal menstrual flow.

Post- means _____ ; pre- means _____ .

after, before

5–70 Mast/ectomy is an _____ of a breast.

In mast/ectomy, the root for breast is _____ .

excision or **removal**
(ĭk-SĬ-zhŭn)
mast

5–71 To prevent the spread of cancer, a malignant breast may be treated with a partial or complete excision. When a breast has to be removed, the patient will have a _____ / _____ .

mast/ectomy
(măs-TĔK-tō-mē)

mamm / ary (MĂM-ă-rē)	**5–72** The female breast is also referred to as a mamm / ary gland because it produces milk for the newborn. Another combining form for the breast is **mamm / o**. Identify the word in this frame that means pertaining to a breast. _____ / _____
-graphy mamm or mamm / o	**5–73** Mamm / o / graphy, an x-ray examination of the breast, is used in the diagnosis of cancer. Determine the element in this frame that means process of recording: _____ . breast: _____ / _____
mamm / o / plasty (MĂM-ō-plăs-tē)	**5–74** Use **mamm / o** to construct a word meaning surgical reconstruction or surgical repair of a breast: _____ / _____ / _____
mast / o / plasty (MĂS-tō-plăs-tē) mast / o / pexy (MĂS-to-pĕk-sē)	**5–75** Correction of a pendulous breast can be performed by surgical fixation and plastic surgery. Use **mast / o** to develop words meaning surgical repair of the breast: _____ / _____ / _____ fixation of the breast:_____ / _____ / _____
mast / o, mamm / o	**5–76** Two combining forms used to designate the breast are _____ / _____ and _____ / _____ .
inflammation, breast(s)	**5–77** Breast-feeding often causes a blockage of the milk ducts and mast / itis, which is an _____ of the _____ .
mast / o / dynia (măst-ō-DĬN-ē-ă) mast / algia (măst-ĂL-jē-ă)	**5–78** Use **mast / o** to form a word meaning pain in the breast: _____ / _____ / _____ or _____ / _____ .
before after	**5–79** The term nat / al means pertaining to birth. Pre / nat / al means _____ birth; post / nat / al means _____ birth.

neo- nat/o -logy	**5-80** Identify the elements in neo/nat/o/logy that mean new: _____ birth: _____ / _____ study of: _____

neo/nat/o/logist (nē-ō-nā-TŎL-ō-jĭst)	**5-81** Neo/nat/o/logy is the study and treatment of the newborn infant. A specialist in the study and treatment of the newborn infant is called a _____ / _____ / _____ / _____ .

a	**5-82** The word gravida is used to describe a pregnant woman, as is the suffix -gravida . The suffix ending in -gravida that makes the word a noun is _____ .

fourth second	**5-83** The word "gravida" may be followed by numbers to denote the number of pregnancies, as in gravida 1, 2, 3, 4 (or I, II, III, and IV). A gravida 4 is a woman in her _____ pregnancy. A gravida 2 is a woman in her _____ pregnancy.

gravida 3 (GRĂV-ĭ-dă) gravida 5 (GRĂV-ĭ-dă)	**5-84** A woman in her third pregnancy is known as a _____ _____ . A woman in her fifth pregnancy is known as a _____ _____ .

two, five	**5-85** The word **para** refers to a woman who has given birth to an infant, regardless of whether or not the offspring was alive at birth. It may also be followed by numbers to indicate the number of deliveries, as in para 1, 2, 3, 4 (or I, II, III, or IV). Para 2 means _____ deliveries. Para 5 means _____ deliveries.

para 6	**5-86** A woman who has delivered three infants would be described as para 3. A woman who has delivered six infants would be described as _____ _____ .

PID	**5-87** Pelvic inflammatory disease (PID) is a collective term for any extensive bacterial infection of the pelvic organs, especially in the uterus, uterine tubes, or ovaries. The abbreviation for pelvic inflammatory disease is _____ .

pelvic inflammatory disease	**5–88** PID often causes infertility in women, owing to scarring of the fallopian tubes. PID is the abbreviation that means _____ _____ _____ .
salping/ectomy (săl-pĭn-JĔK-tō-mē)	**5–89** A pelvic infection that involves the uterine tubes is known as salping/itis. Form a word that means excision of the uterine tubes: _____ / _____ .
ovary or ovaries (Ō-vă-rē) (Ō-vă-rēz)	**5–90** A pelvic infection that involves the ovaries is known as oophor/itis. **Oophor/o** refers to the _____ .
uterus (Ū-tĕr-ŭs)	**5–91** A hyster/o/tome is an instrument for incising the _____ .
cesarean (sē-SĂR-ē-ăn)	**5–92** The surgical procedure hyster/o/tomy is used to perform a cesarean section. **CS** and **C-section** are abbreviations for _____ section.

5–93 Use your medical dictionary to define *cesarean section*.

_____

_____

Review

Select the element(s) that match the meaning.

cervic / o
colp / o
gynec / o
mamm / o
mast / o
men / o
salping / o
vagin / o
vulv / o

-algia
-ary
-dynia
-ectomy
-itis
-logist
-pathy
-rrhea
-scope
-scopy
-tome

dys-
post-
pre-

a. _____ after

b. _____ bad, painful, difficult

c. _____ before

d. _____ breast

e. _____ disease

f. _____ excision, removal

g. _____ flow, discharge

h. _____ inflammation

i. _____ instrument to cut

j. _____ instrument to view

k. _____ visual examination

l. _____ menses, menstruation

m. _____ neck, cervix uteri

n. _____ pain

o. _____ pertaining to

p. _____ specialist in the study of

q. _____ uterine (fallopian) tube, oviduct

r. _____ vagina

s. _____ vulva

t. _____ woman, female

Check your answers with the Review Answer Key on the following page.

Review Answer Key

a. post-

b. dys-

c. pre-

d. mamm/o, mast/o

e. -pathy

f. -ectomy

g. -rrhea

h. -itis

i. -tome

j. -scope

k. -scopy

l. men/o

m. cervic/o

n. -algia, -dynia

o. -ary

p. -logist

q. salping/o

r. colp/o, vagin/o

s. vulv/o

t. gynec/o

REINFORCEMENT FRAME: If you are not satisfied with your level of comprehension, go back to Frame 5–46 and rework the frames.

Audiocassette Exercise

The audiocassette tape helps you master the pronunciation of medical words. Listen to the tape for instructions to complete this exercise. You may also use this list without the audiotape to practice correct pronunciation and spelling of the terms.

Frame	Word	Pronunciation	Spelling Exercise
5–45	[] adipoid	(ĂD-ĭ-poyd)	_____
5–67	[] amenorrhea	(ă-měn-ō-RĒ-ă)	_____
5–54	[] cervical	(SĚR-vĭ-kăl)	_____
5–52	[] cervicitis	(sěr-vĭ-SĪ-tis)	_____
5–30	[] cervix	(SĚR-vĭks)	_____
5–52	[] cervix uteri	(SĚR-vĭks Ū-těr-ē)	_____
5–46	[] clitoris	(KLĬT-ō-rĭs)	_____
5–30	[] colpitis	(kŏl-PĪ-tĭs)	_____
5–53	[] colpocervical	(kŏl-pō-SĚR-vĭ-kăl)	_____
5–39	[] colpocystocele	(kŏl-pō-SĬS-tō-sēl)	_____
5–32	[] colpodynia	(kŏl-pō-DĪN-ē-ă)	_____
5–41	[] colpohysterectomy	(kŏl-pō-hĭs-těr-ĔK-tō-mē)	_____
5–33	[] colpopexy	(KŌL-pō-pěk-sē)	_____
5–33	[] colpoptosis	(kŏl-pŏp-TŌ-sĭs)	_____
5–36	[] colporrhagia	(kŏl-pō-RĂ-jē-ă)	_____
5–35	[] colporrhaphy	(kŏl-PŌR-ă-fē)	_____
5–54	[] colposcope	(KŎL-pō-skōp)	_____
5–54	[] colposcopy	(kŏl-PŎS-kō-pē)	_____
5–33	[] colpospasm	(KŎL-pō-spăzm)	_____
5–63	[] dysmenorrhea	(dĭs-měn-ō-Rē-ă)	_____
5–5	[] estrogen	(ĔS-trō-jěn)	_____
5–7	[] fallopian tube	(fă-LŌ-pē-ăn toob)	_____
5–82	[] gravida	(GRĂV-ĭ-dă)	_____
5–57	[] gynecologist	(gī-ně-KŎL-ō-jĭst)	_____
5–57	[] gynecology	(gī-ně-KŎL-ō-jē)	_____
5–59	[] gynecopathy	(gī-ně-KŎP-ă-thē)	_____
5–29	[] hematologist	(hēm-ă-TŎL-ō-jĭst)	_____
5–27	[] hematology	(hēm ă TŎL ō jē)	_____
5–24	[] hemorrhage	(HĚM-ě-rĭj)	_____
5–28	[] hematoma	(hē-mă-TŌ-mă)	_____
5–15	[] hysteralgia	(hĭs-těr-ĂL-jē-ă)	_____
5–15	[] hysterodynia	(hĭs-těr-ō-DĪ-nē-ă)	_____
5–14	[] hysterectomy	(hĭs-těr-ĔK-tō-mē)	_____
5–19	[] hysteritis	(hĭs-těr-Ī-tĭs)	_____
5–17	[] hysterocele	(HĬS-těr-ō-sēl)	_____
5–15	[] hysteropathy	(hĭs-těr-ŎP-ă-thē)	_____
5–15	[] hysterospasm	(HĬS-těr-ō-spăzm)	_____
5–91	[] hysterotome	(HĬS-těr-ō-tōm)	_____

Frame	Word	Pronunciation	Spelling Exercise
5–16	[] hysterotomy	(hĭs-tĕr-ŎT-ō-mē)	_____
5–46	[] labia majora	(LĀ-bē-ă mă-JŌR-ă)	_____
5–46	[] labia minora	(LĀ-bē-ă mĭn-ŌR-ă)	_____
5–44	[] lipoid	(LĬ-poyd)	_____
5–72	[] mammary	(MĂM-ă-rē)	_____
5–73	[] mammography	(măm-ŎG-ră-fē)	_____
5–74	[] mammoplasty	(MĂM-ō-plăs-tē)	_____
5–78	[] mastalgia	(măst-ĂL-jē-ă)	_____
5–70	[] mastectomy	(măs-TĔK-tō-mē)	_____
5–77	[] mastitis	(măs-TĪ-tĭs)	_____
5–78	[] mastodynia	(măst-ō-DĬN-ē-ă)	_____
5–75	[] mastopexy	(MĂS-tō-pĕk-sē)	_____
5–75	[] mastoplasty	(MĂS-tō-plăs-tē)	_____
5–66	[] menopause	(mĕn-ō-pawz)	_____
5–65	[] menorrhagia	(mĕn-ō-RĂ-jē-ă)	_____
5–62	[] menorrhea	(mĕn-ō-RĒ-ă)	_____
5–62	[] menses	(mĕn-sēz)	_____
5–62	[] menstruation	(mĕn-stroo-Ā-shŭn)	_____
5–19	[] metritis	(mĕ-TRĪ-tĭs)	_____
5–21	[] metropathy	(mĕ-TRŎP-ă-thē)	_____
5–20	[] metrotome	(MĔ-trō-tōm)	_____
5–20	[] metrotomy	(mĕ-TRŎT-ō-mē)	_____
5–43	[] mucoid	(MŪ-koyd)	_____
5–42	[] mucous	(MŪ-kŭs)	_____
5–81	[] neonatologist	(nē-ō-nā-TŎL-ō-jĭst)	_____
5–80	[] neonatology	(nē-ō-nā-TŎL-ō-jē)	_____
5–60	[] obstetrics	(ŏb-STĔT-rĭks)	_____
5–90	[] oophoritis	(ō-ŏf-ō-RĪ-tĭs)	_____
5–4	[] oophoroma	(ō-ŏf-ō-RŌ-mă)	_____
5–6	[] oophoropathy	(ō-ŏf–ōr-ŎP-ă-thē)	_____
5–6	[] oophoropexy	(ō-ŏf-ō-rō-PĔK-sē)	_____
5–6	[] oophoroplasty	(ō-ŎF-ō-rō-plăs-tē)	_____
5–5	[] ovulation	(ŏv-ū-LĀ-shŭn)	_____
5–85	[] para	(PĂR-ă)	_____
5–87	[] pelvic inflammatory disease	(PĔL-vĭk ĭn-FLĂ-mă-tōr-ē dĭ-ZĒZ)	_____
5–69	[] postmenopausal	(pōst-mĕn-ō-PAW-zăl)	_____
5–79	[] postnatal	(pōst-NĀ-tăl)	_____
5–69	[] premenopausal	(prē-mĕn-ō-PAW-zăl)	_____
5–79	[] prenatal	(prē-NĀ-tăl)	_____
5–5	[] progesterone	(prō-JĔS-tĕr-ōn)	_____
5–9	[] salpingectomy	(săl-pĭn-JĔK-tō-mē)	_____
5–89	[] salpingitis	(săl-pĭn-JĪ-tĭs)	_____

Frame	Word	Pronunciation	Spelling Exercise
5–12	[] salpingocele	(săl-PĬNG-gō-sēl)	_____
5–7	[] salpingoplasty	(săl-PĬNG-gō-plăs-tē)	_____
5–10	[] salpingoscope	(săl-PĬNG-gō-skōp)	_____
5–11	[] salpingoscopy	(săl-pĭng-GŎS-kō-pē)	_____
5–87	[] uterine	(Ū-tĕr-ĭn)	_____
5–40	[] vaginal	(VĂJ-ĭn-ăl)	_____
5–31	[] vaginitis	(văj-ĭn-Ī-tĭs)	_____
5–34	[] vaginoplasty	(vă-JĪ-nō-plăs-tē)	_____
5–34	[] vaginoscope	(VĂJ-ĭn-ō-skōp)	_____
5–34	[] vaginotomy	(văj-ĭ-NŎT-ō-mē)	_____
5–50	[] vulvectomy	(vŭl-VĔK-tō-me)	_____
5–50	[] vulvitis	(vŭl-VĪ-tĭs)	_____
5–50	[] vulvopathy	(vŭl-VŎP-ă-thē)	_____

Male Reproductive System

The organs of the male reproductive system consist of the testes and a number of ducts and glands. Sperm are produced in the testes and transported through the reproductive ducts: epididymis, ductus deferens, ejaculatory duct, and urethra (Fig. 5–4). The reproductive glands produce secretions that become part of semen, the fluid that is ejaculated from the urethra. These glands are the seminal vesicles, prostate gland, and bulbourethral glands.

In the man, the reproductive role is to produce and deliver sperm to the female reproductive organs.

The combining forms related to the male reproductive system are summarized here. Review this information before you begin to work the frames.

COMBINING FORMS

Combining Form	Meaning	Example	Pronunciation
balan/o	glans penis	balan/o/plasty surgical repair	BĂL-ă-nō-plăs-tē
orch/o	testes	orch/itis inflammation	ŏr-KĪ-tĭs
orchi/o		orchi/o/pexy surgical fixation	ŏr-kē-ō-PĔK-sē
orchid/o		orchid/ectomy excision	ŏr-kĭ-DĔK-tō-mē
test/o		test/icle adjective ending	TĔS-tĭ-kl
prostat/o	prostate gland	prostat/o/dynia pain	prŏs-tă-tō-DĬN-ē-ă
spermat/o	sperm	spermat/o/lysis destruction	spĕr-măt-ŎL-ĭ-sĭs
vas/o	vas deferens, vessel	vas/ectomy excision	văs-ĔK-tō-mē

5–94 Use the Index of Medical Word Elements, Part A of Appendix A, to define the following elements.

Medical Word Element	Meaning
-genesis	_____
hydr/o	_____
neo-	_____
-plasia, -plasm	_____
spermat/o	_____
vas/o	_____

5–95 The **(1) testes** (singular, **testis**), also called testicles (singular, testicle), are paired oval glands that descend into the **(2) scrotum**. At the onset of puberty the testes produce the hormone testosterone.

Label Figure 5–5 as you learn about the organs of reproduction.

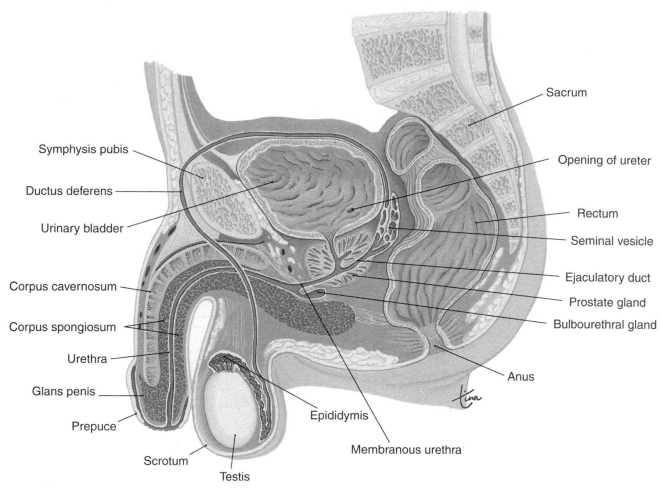

Figure 5–4. The male reproductive systems. (From Scanlon, VC, and Sanders, T: Understanding Human Structure and Function. FA Davis, Philadelphia, 1997, p 357, with permission.)

disease, testes or testicles	**5–96** The combining form **test/o** refers to the testis (singular). Test/o/pathy is a _____ of the _____ (plural).
testis (TĔS-tĭs) **testicle** (TĔS-tĭ-kl)	**5–97** The male hormone, testosterone, stimulates and promotes the growth of secondary sex characteristics in the man. This hormone is produced by the testes (plural). The singular form of testes is _____ . The singular form of testicles is _____ .
test/itis (tĕs-TĪ-tĭs) **test/ectomy** (tĕs-TĔK-tō-mē) **test/o/pathy** (tĕs-TŎP-ă-thē)	**5–98** Use **test/o** to form medical words meaning inflammation of a testis: _____ / _____ excision of a testis: _____ / _____ disease of a testis: _____ / _____ / _____

sperm (SPĔRM)	**5–99** **Spermat/o** is the combining form for sperm, which is the male sex cell produced by the testes. A spermat/o/cyte is a cell that originates from _____ .
calculus, stone (KĂL-kū-lŭs)	**5–100** A spermat/o/lith is a _____ or _____ in the spermatic duct.
spermat/o/genesis (spĕr-măt-ō-JĔN-ĕ-sĭs)	**5–101** The suffix -genesis is used in words to mean producing or forming. Construct a word meaning producing or forming sperm: _____ / ____ / _____ .
spermat/o/cyte (spĕr-MĂT-ō-sīt)	**5–102** Use **spermat/o** to form a word meaning a sperm cell: _____ / ____ / _____ .
spermat/oid (SPĔR-mă-toyd)	**5–103** Build a word that means resembling sperm: _____ / _____ .
spermat/uria (spĕr-mă-TŪ-rē-ă)	**5–104** Spermat/uria is a condition in which there is sperm in the urine. A discharge of semen with urine is also called _____ / _____ .
without	**5–105** A/spermat/ism is a condition in which there is a lack of male sperm. A/spermat/ism literally means _____ sperm.
scanty or little	**5–106** A man who produces a scanty amount of sperm in the semen has a condition known as olig/o/sperm/ia. **Olig/o** refers to _____ .
	5–107 A comma-shaped organ, the **(3) epididymis** stores and propels the sperm toward the urethra during ejaculation. The **(4) vas deferens**, also called **ductus deferens**, is a duct that transports sperm from the testes to the urethra. The sperm is then excreted in the semen. Semen, or seminal fluid, is a mixture of secretions from the **(5) seminal vesicles**, the **(6) prostate gland**, and **(7) Cowper's glands**, also known as the **bulbourethral glands**. Label Figure 5–5 as you learn about the organs related to the male reproductive system.
muc/o	**5–108** The ducts of Cowper's glands open into the urethra and secrete a thick mucus that acts as a lubricant during sexual excitement. Write the combining form that refers to mucus: _____ / ____ .

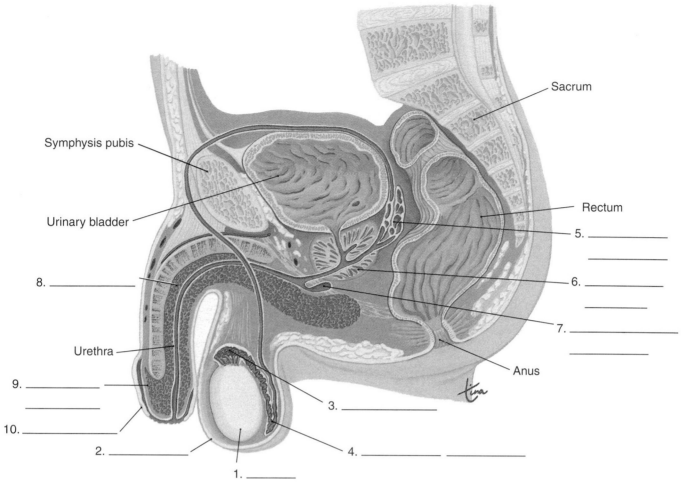

Figure 5–5. The male reproductive system, lateral view. (Adapted from Scanlon, VC, and Sanders, T: Understanding Human Structure and Function. FA Davis, Philadelphia, 1997, p 357, with permission.)

adjective	**5–109** Muc / us is a noun. Muc / ous is a(n) (noun, adjective) _____ .

muc / oid (MŪ-koyd)	**5–110** Use -oid to construct a medical term meaning resembling mucus: _____ / _____ .

orchi / o / plasty (ŌR-kē-ō-plăs-tē) **orchi / o / rrhaphy** (ōr-kē-ŌR-ă-fē) **orchi / o / pexy** (ōr-kē-ō-PĔK-sē)	**5–111** Besides **test / o**, two other combining forms that refer to the testes are **orchi / o** and **orchid / o**. Use **orchi / o** to develop medical words meaning surgical repair of the testicle: _____ / ____ / _____ suture of a testicle: _____ / ____ / _____ fixation of a testicle: _____ / ____ / _____

testicle or testis (TĔS-tĭ-kl) (TĔS-tĭs)	**5-112** Orchid / o / rrhaphy also means suture of a _____ .
testicle or testis (TĔS-tĭ-kl) (TĔS-tĭs)	**5-113** Orchid / o / pexy also means fixation of a _____ .
enlargement	**5-114** The combining form for prostate gland is **prostat / o**. The prostate gland secretes a thick fluid that, as part of the semen, helps the sperm to move spontaneously. Prostat / o / megaly is a(n) _____ of the prostate gland.

prostate gland (PRŎS-tāt) enlargement	**5-115** Almost all men get prostat / o / megaly as they get older. In some cases it causes difficult urination and requires surgery. Analyze prostat / o / megaly by defining the elements.
	
	    prostat / o means _____ _____ .
	
	    -megaly means _____ .

prostate, bladder (PRŎS-tāt)	**5-116** Prostat / o / cyst / o / tomy is an incision of the _____ and _____ .
prostat / o / cyst / itis (prŏs-tă-tō-sĭs-TĪ-tĭs)	**5-117** Form a word meaning inflammation of the prostate and bladder: _____ / _____ / _____ / _____ .

prostat / o / megaly (prŏs-tă-tō-MĔG-ă-lē) prostat / itis (prŏs-tă-TĪ-tis)	**5-118** Construct medical words to mean
	
	    enlargement of the prostate gland:
	
	    _____ / _____ / _____
	
	inflammation of the prostate gland: _____ / _____

	5-119 The **(8) penis** is the male sex organ that transports the sperm into the female vagina. A slightly enlarged region at the tip of the penis is the **(9) glans penis**. The tip of the penis is covered by a fold of skin called the **(10) foreskin** or **prepuce**. Label Figure 5–5 as you learn the names of organs of reproduction.

water
 	
hernia or swelling (HĔR-nē-ă)
	5-120 **Hydro / cele** is a collection of fluid in a saclike cavity, specifically the testis.
	
	Analyze hydr / o / cele by defining the elements.
	
	    hydr / o _____ .
	    -cele means _____ .

VALIDATION FRAME: Check your labeling of Figure 5–5 with the answers in Appendix B, Answer Key.

prostat/ectomy (prŏs-tă-TĔK-tō-mē)	**5–121** Prostat/ic cancer is the third leading cause, after lung and colon cancer, of cancer deaths in men. Surgery may be performed to remove the prostate and adjacent affected tissues. Develop a surgical term meaning excision of the prostate gland: _____ / _____ .
-oma	**5–122** Tumors are growths that arise from normal tissue. The suffix that refers to a tumor is _____ .
threatening	**5–123** Tumors may be either benign or malignant. Benign tumors are not malignant and not life-threatening. A malignant tumor, however, is cancerous and life-_____ .
new formation, growth	**5–124** Use the Index of Medical Terms, Part A of Appendix A, to analyze neo/plasm. neo- means _____ . -plasm means _____ or _____ .
benign (bē-NĪN)	**5–125** Tumors are also called neo/plasms (new growths or formations). Like tumors, neo/plasms can be either malignant or _____ .
liver cancer tumor	**5–126** Hepat/o/carcin/oma is a malignant neo/plasm. Analyze hepat/o/carcin/oma by defining the elements. **hepat/o** means _____ . **carcin/o** means _____ . -oma means _____ .
malignant (mă-LĬG-nănt)	**5–127** The opposite of benign is _____ .
cancer/ous (KĂN-sĕr-ŭs)	**5–128** A benign tumor is non/cancer/ous. A malignant tumor is _____ / _____ .
neo/plasm (NĒ-ō-plăzm)	**5–129** All carcin/omas are also known as malignant neo/plasms. Form a word meaning formation or growth (that is) new _____ / _____ .

neo/plasm (NĒ-ō-plăzm)	**5–130** A new growth in any body system or organ is called a _____ / _____ .
neo/plasm (NĒ-ō-plăzm)	**5–131** Prostat/ic cancer is also known as a malignant _____ / _____ .
growth	**5–132** The suffixes -plasm and -plasia both refer to formation or _____ .
dys- -plasia	**5–133** Dys/plasia is an abnormal development of tissue. Identify the element in dys/plasia that means bad, painful, or difficult: _____ formation or growth: _____
-plasm, -plasia	**5–134** Two suffixes that you have used that mean formation or growth are _____ and _____ .
without formation, growth	**5–135** A/plasia means without formation, and it is a condition that is due to failure of an organ to develop or form normally. Analyze a/plasia by defining the elements. a- means _____ . -plasia means _____ or _____ .
hyper- -plasia	**5–136** Hyper/plasia is an excessive increase in the number of cells in a tissue or organ. Determine the element in hyper/plasia that means excessive: _____ formation or growth: _____
vas/o	**5–137** A vas/ectomy (Fig. 5–6) sterilizes the man and prevents the release of sperm in the semen. With this surgical procedure, a section of the vas deferens duct is cut and closed. From vas/ectomy, construct the combining form for vas deferens, or for any vessel: _____ / ___ .
pain	**5–138** Vas/algia is a _____ in a vessel.

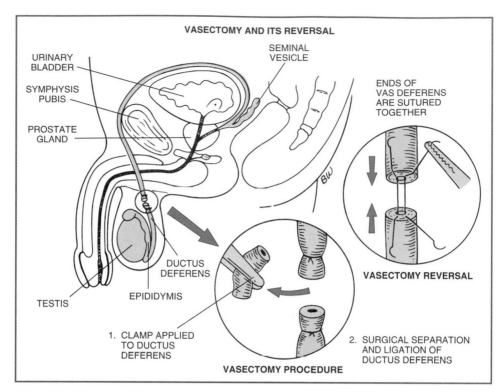

VASECTOMY AND ITS REVERSAL

Figure 5–6. Vasectomy: The surgeon cuts and removes a section of the vas deferens. This method of sterilization prevents sperm from entering the ejaculatory duct without otherwise interfering with normal sexual function. Vasectomy reversal: The ends of the vas deferens are sutured together. (From Taber's Cyclopedic Medical Dictionary, ed 18. FA Davis, Philadelphia, 1997, p 2066, with permission.)

5–139 Benign prostat/ic hyper/plasia (BPH) is an excessive increase of cells within the inner portion of the prostate. The condition is normal in men older than 60 years of age and is significant if the growing hyper/plasia obstructs urinary flow.

Determine the words in this frame that mean

excessive formation or growth: _____ / _____

pertaining to the prostate gland: _____ / _____

hyper/plasia
(hī-pĕr-PLĀ-zē-ă)
prostat/ic
(prŏs-TĂT-ik)

Review

Select the element(s) that match(es) the meaning.

carcin / o	-cele	a-
cyst / o	-cyte	dys-
hepat / o	-genesis	hyper-
hydr / o	-itis	neo-
muc / o	-megaly	
olig / o	-oid	
orchid / o	-pathy	
orchi / o	-pexy	
prostat / o	-rrhaphy	
spermat / o	-tome	
test / o		
vas / o		

a. _____ above, excessive

b. _____ bad, painful, difficult

c. _____ bladder

d. _____ cancer

e. _____ cell

f. _____ disease

g. _____ enlargement

h. _____ hernia, swelling

i. _____ inflammation

j. _____ instrument to cut

k. _____ liver

l. _____ mucus

m. _____ new

n. _____ producing, forming

o. _____ prostate gland

p. _____ resembling

q. _____ scanty, little

r. _____ sperm

s. _____ fixation

t. _____ suture

u. _____ testes

v. _____ vessel, vas deferens

w. _____ water

x. _____ without, not

Check your answers with the Review Answer Key on the following page.

Review Answer Key

a. hyper-

b. dys-

c. cyst/o

d. carcin/o

e. -cyte

f. -pathy

g. -megaly

h. -cele

i. -itis

j. -tome

k. hepat/o

l. muc/o

m. neo-

n. -genesis

o. prostat/o

p. -oid

q. olig/o

r. spermat/o

s. -pexy

t. -rrhaphy

u. test/o, orchi/o, orchid/o

v. vas/o

w. hydr/o

x. a-

REINFORCEMENT FRAME: If you are not satisfied with your level of comprehension, go back to Frame 5–94 to rework the frames.

Additional Pathological Conditions

Female Reproductive System

candidiasis (kăn-dĭ-DĪ-ă-sĭs): vaginal fungal infection caused by *Candida albicans*, characterized by a curdy or cheeselike discharge and extreme itching.

chlamydia (klă-MĬD-ē-ă): caused by infection with the bacterium *Chlamydia trachomatis*, the most prevalent and among the most damaging of all sexually transmitted diseases (STDs). In women, chlamydial infections cause cervicitis with a mucopurulent discharge and an alarming increase in pelvic infections. In men, chlamydial infections cause urethritis with a whitish discharge from the penis.

endometriosis (ĕn-dō-mē-trē-Ō-sĭs): Endometrial tissue is found in various abnormal sites throughout the pelvis or in the abdominal wall.

fibroids (FĪ-broyds): benign uterine tumors.

gonorrhea (gŏn-ō-RĒ-ă): sexually transmitted inflammation of the mucous membrane of either sex. Can be transmitted to the fetus during delivery.

leukorrhea (loo-kō-RĒ-ă): usually white or yellow mucous discharge from the cervical canal or the vagina.

oligomenorrhea (ŏl-ĭ-gō-mĕn-ō-RĒ-ă): scanty or infrequent menstrual flow.

pyosalpinx (pī-ō-SĂL-pĭnks): pus in the fallopian tube.

retroversion (rĕt-rō-VĔR-shŭn): a turning, or state of being turned back, especially an entire organ being tipped from its normal position (e.g., the uterus).

sterility (stĕr-ĬL-ĭ-tē): inability of the woman to become pregnant or for the man to impregnate a woman.

syphilis (SĬF-ĭ-lĭs): infectious, chronic, venereal disease occurring in both sexes, characterized by lesions that change to a chancre and may involve any organ or tissue. It usually exhibits cutaneous manifestations (Fig. 5–7). Relapses are frequent, it may exist without symptoms for years, and it can be transmitted from mother to fetus.

toxic shock syndrome: a rare and sometimes fatal disease caused by a toxin or toxins produced by certain strains of the bacterium *Staphylococcus aureus*. The disease usually occurs in young menstruating women, most of whom were using vaginal tampons for menstrual protection.

trichomoniasis (trĭk-ō-mō-NĪ-ă-sĭs): infestation with a parasite of genus *Trichomonas*; often causes vaginitis, urethritis, and cystitis.

Male Reproductive System

anorchism (ăn-ŌR-kĭzm): congenital absence of one or both testes.

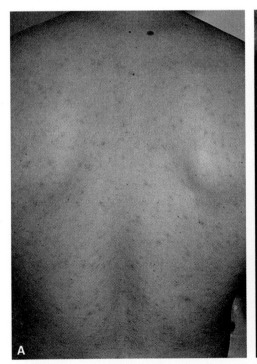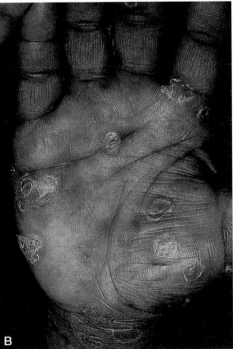

Figure 5–7. Syphilis: secondary syphilitic rash on (A) back and (B) palm. (From Taber's Cyclopedic Medical Dictionary, ed 18. FA Davis, Philadelphia, 1997, p 1891, with permission.)

balanitis (băl-ă-NĪ-tĭs): inflammation of the skin covering the glans penis.

benign prostatic hypertrophy (bē-NĪN prŏs-TĂT-ĭk hī-PĔR-trŏ-fē): enlargement of the prostate gland, a condition commonly seen in men over 50.

cryptorchidism (krĭpt-ŎR-kĭd-ĭzm): failure of testicles to descend into scrotum.

gonorrhea (gŏn-ō-RĒ-ă): contagious bacterial infection of the genital mucous membranes caused by the gonococcus, *Neisseria gonorrhoeae*.

herpes genitalis (HĔR-pēz jĕn-ĭ-TĂL-ĭs): infection of the genital and anorectal skin and mucosa with herpes simplex virus type 2 in both sexes. It is usually spread by sexual contact and is classed as a sexually transmitted disease (STD). This viral infection may be transmitted to the fetus during delivery and may be fatal.

impotence (ĬM-pŏ-tĕns): weakness, especially inability of the man to achieve or maintain erection.

phimosis (fī-MŌ-sĭs): stenosis or narrowness of preputial orifice so that the foreskin cannot be pushed back over the glans penis.

urethritis (ū-rē-THRĪ-tĭs): inflammation of the urethra caused by various conditions, including sexually transmitted infection such as chlamydia or gonorrhea.

Medical Record

The reports that follow are related to the medical specialties called gynecology and urology. A gynecologist treats diseases of the female reproductive organs, including the breasts. A urologist provides treatment of the urinary tract in both sexes and the genital tract in the man.

MEDICAL RECORD 5–1. Postmenopausal Bleeding

Dictionary Exercise

This exercise will help you master the terminology in the medical record. Underline the following terms in the reading exercise and use a medical dictionary to define the words. The pronunciations of medical terms in this report are included in the Audiocassette Exercise on pages 221–223.

axilla _____

D&C _____

diagnostic _____

gravida 4 _____

lesion _____

mastectomy _____

menstrual _____

metastases _____

neoplastic _____

para 4 _____

postmenopausal _____

Premarin _____

preulcerating _____

vaginal _____

Word Element Exercise

Break down the following words into their basic elements. The first one is completed for you.

dia/gnos/tic   neoplastic
postmenopausal   mastectomy
vaginal

VALIDATION FRAME: Check your answers In Appendix B, Answer Key.

Reading Exercise

Read the medical report out loud.

A 52-year-old gravida 4, para 4 woman had her last menstrual period at age 48. She was in our office last month for an evaluation because of postmenopausal bleeding. She has been taking Premarin and has had vaginal bleeding. The patient is currently admitted for gynecological laparoscopy (Fig. 5–8), and diagnostic D&C to rule out the possibility of neoplastic process.

Last year this patient was admitted to General Hospital for a simple mastectomy. The patient had a large preulcerating lesion of the left breast with metastases to the axilla, liver, and bone. Further medical evaluation will be performed next week.

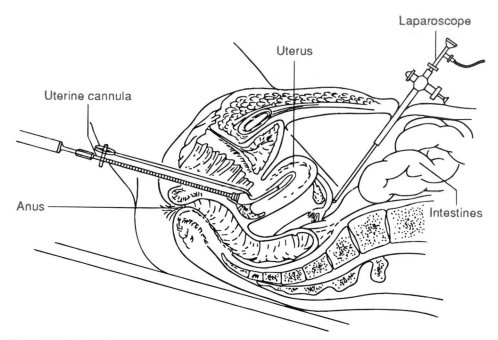

Figure 5–8. Gynecological laparascopy. (From Watson, J, and Jaffe, MS: Nurse's Manual of Laboratory and Diagnostic Tests, ed 2. FA Davis, Philadelphia, 1995, p 529, with permission.)

MEDICAL RECORD EVALUATION 5–1. Postmenopausal Bleeding

1. How many times has the patient been pregnant? How many children has the patient given birth to?

2. Why is the patient being admitted to the hospital?

3. What is a D&C?

4. What is the patient's past surgical history?

5. At what sites did the patient have malignant growth?

MEDICAL RECORD 5–2. Bilateral Vasectomy

Dictionary Exercise

This exercise will help you master the terminology in the medical record. Underline the following terms in the reading exercise and use a medical dictionary to define the words. The pronunciations of medical terms in this report are included in the Audiocassette Exercise on pages 221–223.

bilateral _____

cauterized _____

Darvocet-100 _____

hemostat _____

prn _____

semen _____

Q _____

vasectomy _____

supine _____

scrotum _____

testicle _____

vas _____

xylocaine _____

Reading Exercise

Read the bilateral vasectomy report (see Fig. 5–6) out loud.

The patient was placed on the table in the supine position and prepped, scrotum shaved, and draped in the usual fashion. The right testicle was grasped and brought to skin level. This area was then injected with 1% Xylocaine anesthesia. After a few minutes, a small incision was made and the right vas was located. A hemostat was then used and clamped on the right and left vas. A segment of the right vas was removed and both ends were cauterized and tied independently with 3–0 silk suture. The skin was closed with 2–0 chromic suture. The same procedure was performed on the left side. There were no complications or bleeding. The patient was discharged to home in care of his wife. Postoperative care instruction sheet was given along with prescription of Darvocet-N100 mg, 1 q4h PRN for pain. Patient will be seen for follow-up semen analysis in 6 weeks.

MEDICAL RECORD EVALUATION 5–2. Bilateral Vasectomy

1. What is the end result of a bilateral vasectomy?

2. What structure does vas refer to?

3. Was the patient awake during the surgery? What type of anesthesia was used?

4. What was used to prevent bleeding?

5. Did the patient have any complications during surgery?

6. What type of suture material was used to close the incision?

7. What was the patient given for pain relief at home?

8. Why is it important for the patient to go for a follow-up visit?

Abbreviations

Abbreviation	Meaning	Abbreviation	Meaning

FEMALE REPRODUCTIVE SYSTEM

CS	cesarean section	OB-GYN	obstetrics and gynecology
C-Section	cesarean section	OCPs	oral contraceptive pills
D&C	dilation and curettage	Pap smear	Papanicolau's smear
GC	gonorrhea	PID	pelvic inflammatory disease
Gyn	gynecology	PMP	previous menstrual period
HSV	herpes simplex virus	TAH	total abdominal hysterectomy
IUD	intrauterine device	TSS	toxic shock syndrome
IVF	in vitro fertilization	XX	female sex chromosomes
LMP	last menstrual period		

MALE REPRODUCTIVE SYSTEM

BPH	benign prostatic hyperplasia, benign prostatic hypertrophy	VD	venereal disease
GU	genitourinary	TUR, TURP	transurethral resection of the prostate
HSV	herpes simplex virus	XY	male sex chromosomes
STD	sexually transmitted diseases		

Audiocassette Exercise

The audiocassette tape helps you master the pronunciation of medical words. Listen to the tape for instructions to complete this exercise. You may also use this list without the audiotape to practice correct pronunciations and spelling of medical terms.

Frame	Word	Pronunciation	Spelling Exercise
Additional Pathological Conditions	[] anorchism	(ăn-ŌR-kizm)	_____
5–135	[] aplasia	(ă-PLĀ-zē-ă)	_____
5–105	[] aspermatism	(ă-SPĔR-mă-tĭzm)	_____
Reading Exercise	[] axilla	(ăk-SĬL-ă)	_____
Additional Pathological Conditions	[] balanitis	(băl-ă-NĪ-tĭs)	_____
5–123	[] benign	(bē-NĪN)	_____
5–139	[] benign prostatic hypertrophy	(bē-NĪN prŏs-TĂT-ĭk hī-PĔR-trŏ-fē)	_____
Reading Exercise	[] bilateral	(bī-LĂT-ĕr-ăl)	_____
5–107	[] bulbourethral gland	(bŭl-bō-ū-RĒ-thrăl GLĂND)	_____
5–123	[] cancerous	(KĂN-sĕr-ŭs)	_____
Additional Pathological Conditions	[] candidiasis	(kăn-dĭ-DĪ-ă-sĭs)	_____
Reading Exercise	[] cauterize	(KAW-tĕr-īz)	_____
Additional Pathological Conditions	[] chlamydia	(klă-MĬD-ē-ă)	_____
5–107	[] Cowper's gland	(KOU-pers GLĂND)	_____
Additional Pathological Conditions	[] cryptorchidism	(kript-ŌR-kĭd-ĕzm)	_____
Reading Exercise	[] diagnostic	(dī-ăg-NŎS-tĭc)	_____
5–133	[] dysplasia	(dĭs-PLĀ-zē-ă)	_____
Additional Pathological Conditions	[] endometriosis	(ĕn-dō-mē-trē-Ō-sĭs)	_____
5–107	[] epididymis	(ĕp-ĭ-DĬD-ĭ-mĭs)	_____
Additional Pathological Conditions	[] fibroids	(FĪ-broyds)	_____
Additional Pathological Conditions	[] gonorrhea	(gŏn-ō-RĒ-ă)	_____
Reading Exercise	[] gravida	(GRĂV-ĭ-dă)	_____
Reading Exercise	[] hemostat	(HĒ-mō-stăt)	_____
5–126	[] hepatocarcinoma	(hĕp-ă-tō-kăr-sĭ-NŌ-ma)	_____
5–120	[] hydrocele	(HĪ-drō-sēl)	_____
5–136	[] hyperplasia	(hī-pĕr-PLĀ-zē-ă)	_____
Additional Pathological Conditions	[] impotence	(ĬM-pŏ-tĕns)	_____
Additional Pathological Conditions	[] leukorrhea	(loo-kō-RĒ-ă)	_____
5–123	[] malignant	(mă-LĬG-nănt)	_____
Reading Exercise	[] mastectomy	(măs-TĔK-tō-mē)	_____

Frame	Word	Pronunciation	Spelling Exercise
Reading Exercise	[] metastases	(mĕ-TĂS-tă-sēz)	
5–110	[] mucoid	(MŪ-koyd)	
5–109	[] mucous	(MŪ-kŭs)	
5–108	[] mucus	(MŪ-kŭs)	
5–125	[] neoplasms	(NĒ-ō-plăzm)	
Reading Exercise	[] neoplastic	(nē-ō-PLĂS-tĭk)	
5–128	[] noncancerous	(nŏn-KĂN-sĕr-ŭs)	
5–106	[] oligospermia	(ŏl-ĭ-gō-SPĔR-mē-ă)	
5–112	[] orchidorrhaphy	(ōr-kĭ-DŌR-ă-fē)	
5–111	[] orchiopexy	(ōr-kē-ō-PĔK-sē)	
5–111	[] orchioplasty	(ŌR-kē-ō-plās-tē)	
5–111	[] orchiorrhaphy	(ōr-kē-ŌR-ră-fē)	
Reading Exercise	[] para	(PĂR-ă)	
Additional Pathological Conditions	[] phimosis	(fĭ-MŌ-sĭs)	
Reading Exercise	[] postmenopausal	(pōst-mĕn-ō-PAW-zăl)	
Reading Exercise	[] Premarin	(PRĔM-ă-rĭn)	
Reading Exercise	[] preulcerating lesion	(prē-ŬL-sĕr-ā-tĭng LĒ-zhŭn)	
5–121	[] prostatic cancer	(prŏs-TĂT-ik KĂN-sĕr)	
5–118	[] prostatitis	(prŏs-tă-TĪ-tĭs)	
5–117	[] prostatocystitis	(prŏs-tă-tō-sĭs-TĪ-tĭs)	
5–116	[] prostatocystotomy	(prŏs-tă-tō-sĭs-TŎT-ō-mē)	
5–114	[] prostatomegaly	(prŏs-tă-tō-MĔG-ă-lē)	
Additional Pathological Conditions	[] pyosalpinx	(pī-ō-SĂL-pĭnks)	
Additional Pathological Conditions	[] retroversion	(rĕt-rō-VĔR-zhun)	
5–95	[] scrotum	(SKRŌ-tŭm)	
5–99	[] spermatocyte	(spĕr-MĂT-ō-sīt)	
5–101	[] spermatogenesis	(spĕr-măt-ō-JĔN-ĕ-sĭs)	
5–103	[] spermatoid	(SPĔR-mă-toyd)	
5–100	[] spermatolith	(spĕr-MĂT-ō-lĭth)	
5–104	[] spermaturia	(spĕr-mă-TŪ-rē-ă)	
Additional Pathological Conditions	[] sterility	(stĕr-ĬL-ĭ-tē)	
Reading Exercise	[] supine	(SOO-pīn)	
Additional Pathological Conditions	[] syphilis	(SĬF-ĭ-lĭs)	
5–98	[] testectomy	(tĕs-TĔK-tō-mē)	
5–95	[] testes	(TĔS-tēz)	
5–96	[] testicle	(TĔS-tĭ-kl)	
5–95	[] testis	(TĔS-tĭs)	
5–98	[] testitis	(tĕs-TĪ-tĭs)	
5–96	[] testopathy	(tĕs-TŎP-ă-thē)	
5–95	[] testosterone	(tĕs-TŎS-tĕr-ōn)	

Frame	Word	Pronunciation	Spelling Exercise
Additional Pathological Conditions	[] toxic shock syndrome		_____
Additional Pathological Conditions	[] trichomoniasis	(trĭk-ō-mō-NĪ-ă-sĭs)	_____
Additional Pathological Conditions	[] urethritis	(ū-rē-THRĪ-tĭs)	_____
Reading Exercise	[] vaginal	(VĂJ-ĭn-ăl)	_____
5–107	[] vas deferens	(VĂS DĔF-ĕr-ĕnz)	_____
5–138	[] vasalgia	(vă-SĂL-jē-ă)	_____
5–137	[] vasectomy	(vă-SĔK-tō-mē)	_____

Unit Exercises

DEFINITIONS

Review Unit Summary (pages 231–233) before completing this exercise. Write the definition for each element.

SUFFIXES, PREFIXES, AND ABBREVIATIONS

Element	Meaning

SURGICAL SUFFIXES

1. -pexy _____
2. -plasty _____
3. -rrhaphy _____
4. -tome _____
5. -tomy _____

OTHER SUFFIXES

6. -cele _____
7. -logist _____
8. -logy _____
9. -megaly _____
10. -oid _____
11. -pathy _____
12. -plasia _____
13. -plasm _____
14. -rrhage _____
15. -rrhagia _____
16. -rrhea _____
17. -spasm _____

PREFIXES AND ABBREVIATIONS

18. a- _____
19. hyper- _____
20. CA _____
21. CS _____
22. C-Section _____
23. D&C _____
24. OB-GYN _____
25. PID _____

COMBINING FORMS RELATED TO THE FEMALE REPRODUCTIVE SYSTEM

26. cervic/o _____
27. colp/o _____
28. gynec/o _____

Element	Meaning
29. hyster/o	_____
30. mast/o	_____
31. men/o	_____
32. metr/o	_____
33. oophor/o	_____
34. salping/o	_____

COMBINING FORMS RELATED TO THE MALE REPRODUCTIVE SYSTEM

Element	Meaning
35. orchi/o, orchid/o, test/o	_____
36. prostat/o	_____
37. spermat/o	_____
38. vas/o	_____

OTHER COMBINING FORMS

Element	Meaning
39. adip/o, lip/o	_____
40. carcin/o	_____
41. cyst/o	_____
42. hemat/o, hem/o	_____
43. hydr/o	_____
44. muc/o	_____
45. olig/o	_____

VALIDATION FRAME: Check your answers in the Index of Medical Word Elements, Appendix A. If you scored less than _____ %,* review Unit Summary (pages 231–233) and retake this exercise.

To obtain a percentage score, multiply the number of correct answers times 2.22.

Number of Correct Answers: _____   **Percentage Score:** _____

*Enter the percentage required by your instructor to complete this course.

Vocabulary

Match the medical term(s) below with the definitions in the numbered list.

amenorrhea
aplasia
aspermatism
cervix uteri
dysmenorrhea
epididymis
estrogen
gravida 4

hydrocele
oophoritis
para 4
pelvic inflammatory disease (PID)
postmenopausal
progesterone
prostatic cancer

prostatomegaly
testopathy
testosterone
uterus
vas deferens
vasectomy
uterus

1. _____ Enlargement of the prostate gland.

2. _____ Any disease of the testes.

3. _____ Male hormone produced by testes.

4. _____ Absence or abnormal stoppage of the menses.

5. _____ Female hormone(s) produced by the ovaries.

6. _____ Inflamed condition of the ovaries.

7. _____ Condition in which there is a lack of male sperm.

8. _____ Woman in her fourth pregnancy.

9. _____ Organ that nourishes the embryo.

10. _____ Malignant neoplasm of the prostate.

11. _____ Tube that temporarily stores sperm.

12. _____ Collection of fluid in a saclike cavity.

13. _____ Duct that transports sperm from the testes to the urethra.

14. _____ Woman who has delivered four infants.

15. _____ Neck of the uterus.

16. _____ Painful menstruation.

17. _____ Occurring after menopause.

18. _____ Failure or lack of formation or growth.

19. _____ A procedure to sterilize the male by cutting the vas deferens, which prevents the release of sperm.

20. _____ Collective term for any extensive bacterial infection of the pelvic organs especially the uterus, uterine tubes, or ovaries.

VALIDATION FRAME: Check your answers in Appendix B, Answer Key. If you scored less than _____ %, review the vocabulary and retake the exercise.

To obtain a percentage score, multiply the number of correct answers times 5.

Number of Correct Answers: _____   **Percentage Score:** _____

Additional Pathological Conditions

Match these medical term(s) with the definitions in the numbered list.

anorchism
balanitis
benign prostatic hypertrophy
candidiasis
chlamydia
cryptorchidism
endometriosis

fibroids
gonorrhea
impotence
leukorrhea
oligospermia
phimosis
pyosalpinx

retroversion
sterility
syphilis
toxic shock syndrome
trichomoniasis
urethritis

1. _____ Failure of testicles to descend into scrotum.

2. _____ Pus in the fallopian tube.

3. _____ Inability of the woman to become pregnant or for the man to impregnate a woman.

4. _____ Congenital absence of one or both testes.

5. _____ Vaginal fungal infection caused by *Candida albicans* and marked by a curdy discharge and extreme itching.

6. _____ Caused by infection with the bacterium *Chlamydia trachomatis* and occurring in both sexes.

7. _____ Inflammation of the skin covering the glans penis.

8. _____ Enlargement of the prostate gland; commonly seen in men older than 50 years of age.

9. _____ Usually white or yellow mucous discharge from the cervical canal or vagina.

10. _____ Condition in which endometrial tissue is found in various abnormal sites throughout the pelvis or in the abdominal wall.

11. _____ Benign uterine tumors.

12. _____ Sexually transmitted inflammation of the mucous membranes of either sex; can be transmitted to the fetus during the birth process.

13. _____ Infectious, chronic, venereal disease in both sexes, characterized by lesions that may involve any organ or tissue. It usually exhibits cutaneous manifestations, relapses are frequent, and it may exist without symptoms for years; can be transmitted from mother to fetus.

14. _____ Rare and sometimes fatal disease caused by a toxin or toxins produced by certain strains of the bacterium *Staphylococcus aureus*; occurs in menstruating women who use vaginal tampons.

15. _____ Infestation with a parasite of genus *Trichomonas*, often causing vaginitis, urethritis, and cystitis.

16. _____ Inflammation of the urethra.

17. _____ Stenosis of preputial orifice so that the foreskin does not retract over the glans penis.

18. _____ Inability of the man to achieve a penile erection.

19. _____ Reduced number of spermatozoa in the semen.

20. _____ Tipping back of an organ (e.g., the uterus) from its normal position.

VALIDATION FRAME: Check your answers in Appendix B, Answer Key. If you scored less than _____ %, review the vocabulary and retake the exercise.
To obtain a percentage score, multiply the number of correct answers times 5.

Number of Correct Answers: _____   **Percentage Score:** _____

Unit Summary

COMBINING FORMS RELATED TO THE FEMALE REPRODUCTIVE SYSTEM

Combining Form	Pronunciation	Meaning
cervic/o	sĕr-vĭ-kō	neck, cervix (neck of the uterus) uteri
colp/o vagin/o	kŏl-pō vă-jĭn-ō	vagina
episi/o vulv/o	ĕ-pĭs-ē-ō vŭl-vō	vulva
gynec/o	gī-nĕ-kō	woman, female
hyster/o metr/o uter/o	hĭs-tĕr-ō mĕt-rō ū-tĕr-ō	uterus
lapar/o	lăp-ăr-ō	abdomen
mamm/o mast/o	măm-ō măs-tō	breast
men/o	mĕn-ō	menses, menstruation
nat/o	năt-ō	birth
oophor/o	ō-ŏf-ōr-ō	ovary
salping/o	săl-pĭng-gō	fallopian (uterine) tube
eustachian	ū-stāk-ē-ăn	(auditory) tube

COMBINING FORMS RELATED TO THE MALE REPRODUCTIVE SYSTEM

Combining Form	Pronunciation	Meaning
balan/o	băl-ă-nō	glans penis
orchid/o orchi/o orch/o test/o }	ŏr-kĭ-dō ŏr-kē-ō ŏr-kō tĕst-tō	testis, testicle
prostat/o	prŏs-tă-tō	prostate gland
spermat/o	spĕr-mă-tō	sperm
vas/o	vă-sō	vas deferens, vessel

OTHER COMBINING FORMS IN UNIT 5

Combining Form	Pronunciation	Meaning
adip/o, lip/o	ăd-ĭ-pō, lĭ-pō	fat
carcin/o	kăr-sĭn-ō	cancer
cyst/o	sĭs-tō	bladder

Combining Form	Pronunciation	Meaning
hemat/o, hem/o	hēm-ă-to, hēm-ō	blood
hydr/o	hī-drō	water
muc/o	mū-kō	mucus
olig/o	ŏl-ĭ-gō	scanty, little

SUFFIXES AND PREFIXES

Suffix (Prefix)	Pronunciation	Meaning
ADJECTIVE ENDING SUFFIXES		
-al	ăl	
-ic	ĭk	pertaining to
-ous	ŭs	
SURGICAL SUFFIXES		
-ectomy	ĕk-to-mē	excision, removal
-pexy	pĕks-ē	fixation
-plasty	plăs-tē	plastic surgery
-rrhaphy	ră-fē	suture
-tome	tōm	instrument to cut
-tomy	tō-mē	incision, cut into
OTHER SUFFIXES		
-algia	ăl-jē-ă	
-dynia	dĭn-ē-ă	pain
-cele	sēl	hernia, swelling
-genesis	jĕn-ĕ-sĭs	producing, forming
-itis	ī-tĭs	inflammation
-lith	lĭth	stone, calculus
-logy	lō-jē	study of
-logist	lō-jĭst	specialist in the study of
-megaly	mĕg-ă-lē	enlargement
-oid	oyd	resembling
-oma	ō-mă	tumor
-pathy	pă-thē	disease
-plasia	plā-zē-ă	
plasm	plăzm	formation, growth
-ptosis	tō-sĭs	prolapse, falling, dropping
-rrhage	rĭj	
-rrhagia	ră-jē-ă	bursting forth (of)

Suffix (Prefix)	Pronunciation	Meaning
-rrhea	rē-ă	flow, discharge
-scope	skōp	instrument to view
-spasm	spăzm	involuntary contraction, twitching
-uria	ū-rē-ă	urine, urination
PREFIXES		
a-, an-	ă, ăn	without, not
dys-	dĭs	bad, painful, difficult
hyper-	hī-pĕr	excessive
neo-	nē-ō	new
post-	pōst	after, behind
pre-	prē	before

UNIT 6

Respiratory System

The respiratory system consists of the upper and lower respiratory tracts. The upper respiratory tract includes the nose, pharynx, larynx, and trachea. The lower respiratory tract consists of the left and right bronchi and the lungs, where the exchange of oxygen (O_2) and carbon dioxide (CO_2) takes place during the respiratory cycle (Fig. 6–1).

The combining forms related to the respiratory system are summarized here. Review this information before you begin to work the frames.

COMBINING FORMS

Combining Form	Meaning	Example	Pronunciation
bronch/o	bronchus (airway)	bronch/o/scope instrument to view or examine	BRŎNG-kō-skōp
bronchi/o		bronchi/ectasis expansion, dilation	brŏng-kē-ĔK-tă-sĭs
epiglott/o	epiglottis	epiglott/itis inflammation	ĕp-ĭ-glŏt-Ī-tĭs
nas/o	nose	nas/al pertaining to	NĀ-zăl
rhin/o		rhin/o/plasty surgical repair	RĪ-nō-plăs-tē
or/o	mouth	or/o/pharynx throat	ōr-ō-FĂR-ĭnks
ox/o	oxygen	hyp*/ox/emia deficient blood	hī-PŎKS-ē-mē-ă
pharyng/o	pharynx (throat)	pharyng/itis inflammation	făr-ĭn-JĪ-tĭs
pleur/o	pleura	pleur/algia pain	ploo-RĂL-jē-ă
pneum/o	air, lung	pneum/o/thorax chest	nū-mō-THŌ-răks
pneumon/o		pneumon/ectomy excision	nū-mŏn-ĔK-tō-mē
~~pulmun/o~~ *pulmon/o*	lung	pulmon/ary pertaining to	PŬL-mō-nĕ-rē
sinus/o	sinus, cavity	sinus/itis inflammation	sī-nŭs-Ī-tĭs

*hyp- variation of the prefix hypo-, often used before a vowel.

234

Combining Form	Meaning	Example	Pronunciation
thorac/o	chest	thorac/o/tomy incision, cut into	thō-răk-ŎT-ō-mē
tonsill/o	tonsils	tonsill/ectomy excision	tŏn-sĭl-ĔK-tō-mē
trache/o	trachea (windpipe)	trache/o/stomy forming a new opening or mouth	trā-kē-ŎS-tō-mē

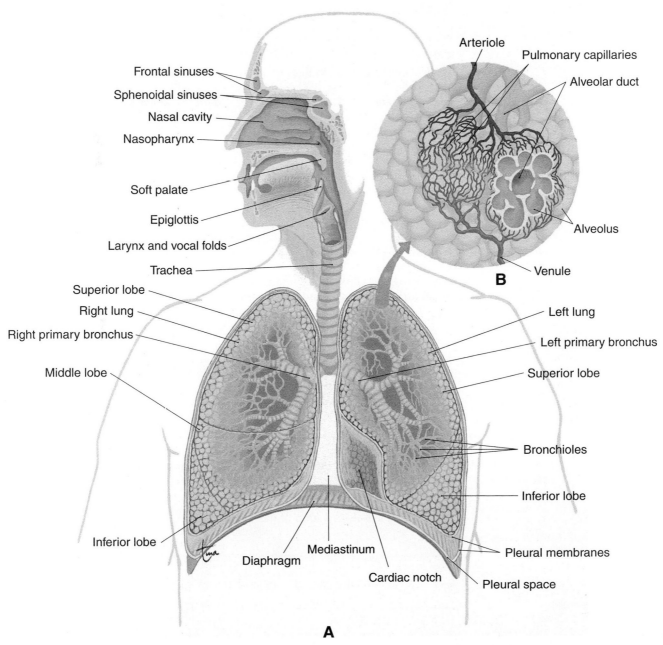

Figure 6–1. (A) Frontal view of the respiratory system. (B) Microscopic view of alveoli and pulmonary capillaries. (From Scanlon, VC, and Sanders, T: Understanding Human Structure and Function. FA Davis, Philadelphia, 1997, p 268, with permission.)

UPPER RESPIRATORY TRACT

6-1   Use the Index of Medical Word Elements, Part A of Appendix A, to define the word elements used in this unit.

Medical Word Element	Meaning
-cele	_____
hydr/o	_____
laryng/o	_____
-phagia	_____
-scope	_____
-stenosis	_____

6-2   Use the Index of Medical Word Elements, Part B of Appendix A, to identify medical elements used in this unit.

English Term	Medical Word Element
air	_____ / _____
nose	_____ / _____ or
	_____ / _____
paralysis	_____
trachea	_____ / _____
treatment	_____

---

rhin/itis, nas/itis
(rī-NĪ-tĭs), (nā-ZĪ-tis)
nas/o/scope
NĀ-zō-skōp)
rhin/o/scope
(RĪ-nō-skōp)

6-3   The external openings of the nose are referred to as the nostrils or nares (singular: naris). **Nas/o** and **rhin/o** are combining forms that refer to the nose.

Form medical terms meaning

inflammation of the nose: _____ / _____ or _____ / _____

instrument to view the nose: _____ / _____ / _____ or

_____ / _____ / _____

---

nose

6-4   Peri/nas/al is a directional word meaning around the _____ .

---

rhin/itis
(rī-NĪ-tĭs)

6-5   A simple cold is a form of nas/itis or _____ / _____ .

---

rhin/o/scope
(RĪ-nō-skōp)

6-6   To examine the nares, the physician uses a nas/o/scope or _____ / _____ / _____ .

---

nose

6-7   A rhin/o/logist is a physician who specializes in diseases of the _____ .

6–8 As a general rule **nas/o** *is not* used to build surgical terms, but if you are in doubt about which element to use, consult a medical dictionary.

Form surgical words meaning

surgical repair of the nose: _____ / _____ / _____

incision of the nose: _____ / _____ / _____

rhin/o/plasty
(RĪ-nō-plăs-tē)
rhin/o/tomy
(rī-NŎT-ō-mē)

6–9 Air enters the nose and passes through the **(1) nasal cavity**, where fine hairs catch many of the dust particles that we inhale.

Label the nasal cavity in Figure 6–2.

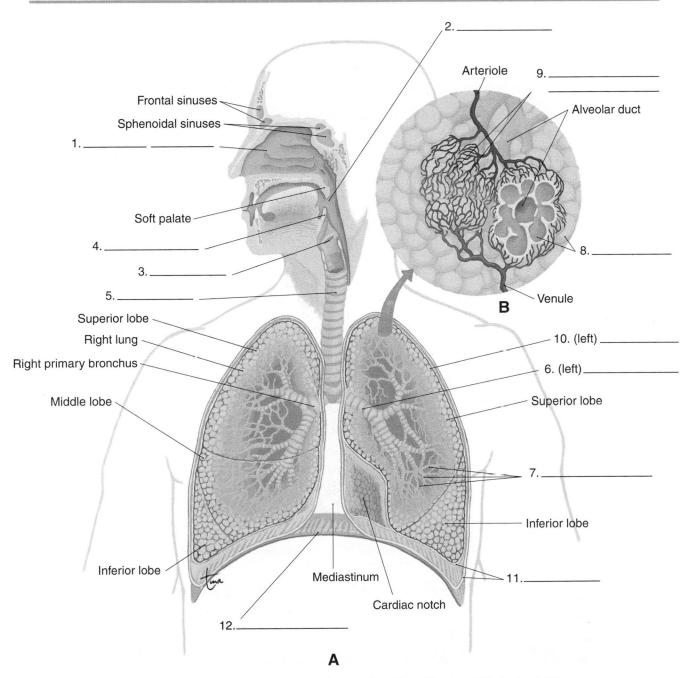

Figure 6–2. The respiratory system. (Adapted from Scanlon, VC, and Sanders, T: Understanding Human Structure and Function. FA Davis, Philadelphia, 1997, p 268, with permission.)

nas/o rhin/o aer/o	**6–10** The combining forms for the nose are _____ / _____ or _____ / _____ . **Pneum/o, pneumon/o**, and _____ / _____ are combining forms for air.
aer/o/phagia (ĕr-ō-FĂ-jē-ă)	**6–11** While sucking on a nipple to drink milk, water, or any liquid substance, babies have a tendency to swallow air. Usually this causes gaseous discomfort until the baby is burped. Use -phagia to form a medical term meaning swallow air. _____ / _____ / _____
air	**6–12** The suffix -therapy is used in words to mean treatment. Aer/o/therapy is the treatment of diseases by the use of _____ .
water	**6–13** Hydr/o/therapy is the treatment of diseases by means of _____ .
air water	**6–14** Using both air and water to treat a disease or injury is also a form of therapy. Aer/o/hydr/o/therapy is treatment by application of _____ and __
aer / o / therapy (ĕr-ō-THĔR-ă-pē) hydr / o / therapy hī-drō-THĔR-ă-pē) aer / o / hydr / o / therapy (ĕr-ō-hī-drō-THĔR-ă-pē)	**6–15** Develop medical words meaning treatment by air: _____ / _____ / _____ treatment by water: _____ / _____ / _____ treatment by air and water: _____ / _____ / _____ / _____ / _____
	6–16 After passing through the nasal cavity, air reaches the **(2) pharynx** or **throat**. Label the pharynx in Figure 6–2.
pharyng/o myc -osis	**6–17** From pharyng/o/myc/osis, determine the elements meaning pharynx: _____ / _____ fungus: _____ abnormal condition: _____

6-18 Pharyng/o/myc/osis is a fungal disease of the

pharynx
(FĂR-ĭnks)

_____ .

6-19 The suffix -plegia is used in words to mean paralysis. Pharyng/o/plegia and pharyng/o/paralysis are words used to express a muscle paralysis of the

pharynx
(FĂR-ĭnks)

_____ .

6-20 Smoking, drinking alcohol, and chewing tobacco can cause **CA** of the pharynx. Patients with **CA** of the pharynx may require some type of plastic surgery.

When you see **CA** in a medical chart you will know it is an abbreviation for

cancer
(KĂN-sĕr)

_____ .

6-21 Use **pharyng/o** to form medical words meaning

pharyng/itis
(făr-ĭn-JĪ-tĭs)
pharyng/o/plasty
(făr-ĬN-gō-plăs-tē)
pharyng/o/tomy
(făr-ĭn-GŎT-ō-mē)
pharyng/o/tome
(făr-ĬN-gō-tōm)
pharyng/o/spasm
(far-ĬN-gō-spăzm)

inflammation of the pharynx: _____ / _____

surgical repair of the pharynx: _____ / _____ / _____

incision of the pharynx: _____ / _____ / _____

instrument to incise the pharynx: _____ / _____ / _____

twitching of the pharynx: _____ / _____ / _____

6-22 Build a word meaning a hernia or swelling of the pharynx:

pharyng/o/cele
(făr-ĬN-gō-sēl)

_____ / _____ / _____

6-23 Pharyng/o/stenosis is a narrowing, or _____ , of

stricture
(STRĬK-chŭr)

pharynx
(FĂR-ĭnks)

the _____ .

6-24 The **(3) larynx** or **voice box** is responsible for sound production and makes speech possible.

Label the larynx in Figure 6–2.

6-25 From laryng/itis (inflammation of the larynx), construct the combining

laryng/o

form of the larynx: _____ / _____ .

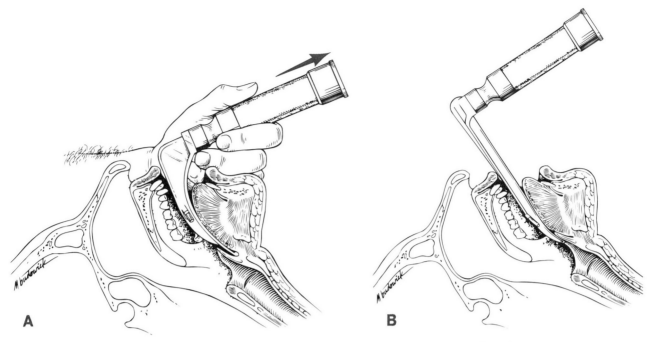

A   **B**

Figure 6–3. Direct laryngoscopy with curved (MacIntosh) blade in vallecula (*left*). Direct laryngoscopy with straight (Miller) blade directly lifting epiglottis (*right*). (From Finucane, BT, and Santora, AH: Principles of Airway Management. FA Davis, Philadelphia, 1988, pp 131 and 137, with permission.)

---

laryng/o/scope (lăr-ĬN-gō-skōp)	**6–26** Combine **laryng/o** + -scope (Fig. 6–3) to form a word meaning instrument to view the larynx: _____ / _____ / _____

---

laryng/ectomy (lăr-ĭn-JĔK-tō-mē)	**6–27** When cancer of the larynx is detected in its early stages, a partial laryng/ectomy may be recommended. For extensive cancer of the larynx, the entire larynx is removed. In either case, when an excision of the larynx is performed, the surgery is called _____ / _____ .

---

laryng/o/spasm (lăr-ĬN-gō-spazm)	**6–28** Spasms of the larynx impede breathing. The medical word meaning spasm of the larynx is _____ / _____ / _____ .

-stenosis
(stĕ-NŌ-sĭs)
laryng/o
(lăr-ĬN-gō)
	6–29 Laryng/o/stenosis is a stricture of the larynx.
	
	Determine the elements that mean
	
	    narrowing or stricture: _____
	
	    larynx: _____ / _____

laryng/itis
(lăr-ĭn-JĪ-tĭs)

6–30 Formulate medical words meaning

inflammation of the larynx: _____ / _____

instrument to view or examine the larynx:

_____ / _____ / _____

laryng/o/scope
(lăr-ĬN-gō-skōp)
laryng/o/scopy
(lăr-ĭn-GŎS-kō-pē)

visual examination of the larynx: _____ / _____ / _____

a stricture or narrowing of the larynx:

laryng/o/stenosis
(lăr-ĭn-gō-stĕ-NŌ-sĭs)

_____ / _____ / _____

6–31 At the top of the larynx is a small leaf-shaped cartilage called the **(4) epiglottis**.

During swallowing, the epiglottis closes off the larynx so that food and liquid are directed into the esophagus. If anything but air passes into the larynx, a cough reflex attempts to expel the material to avoid a serious blockage of breathing.

Label the epiglottis in Figure 6–2.

6–32 Air passes from the larynx to the (5) **trachea** or **windpipe**, whose purpose is to convey air to and from the lungs.

Label the trachea in Figure 6–2.

trache/o

-pathy

6–33 From trache/o/pathy, determine the elements meaning

trachea: _____ / _____

disease: _____

trache/o/stomy
(trā-kē-ŎS-tō-mē)

6–34 In a life-threatening situation, when breathing ceases because of trache/al (pertaining to the trachea) obstruction, a trache/o/stomy is performed to permit an airway.

The word meaning formation of a new opening or mouth into the trachea is

_____ / _____ / _____ .

trache/o/plasty
(TRĀ-kē-ō-plăs-tē)
trache/o/stenosis
(trā-kē-ō-stĕn-Ō-sĭs)
trache/o/tomy
(trā-kē-ŎT-ō-mē)
trache/o/malacia
(trā-kē-ō-mă-LĀ-shē-ă)

6–35 Develop medical words meaning

surgical repair of the trachea: _____ / _____ / _____

stricture or narrowing of the trachea: _____ / ____ / _____

incision of the trachea: _____ / _____ / _____

softening of the trachea: _____ / _____ / _____

trachea
(TRĀ-kē-ă)

larynx
(LĂR-inks)

6–36 Trache/o/laryng/o/tomy is an incision of the _____

and _____ .

---

cartilage
(KĂR-tĭ-lĭj)

6–37 The trachea is composed of smooth muscle embedded with C-shaped cartilage rings (see Fig. 6–2). These rings provide the necessary rigidity to keep the air passage open at all times. The combining form **chondr/o** refers to

cartilage. Chondr/itis is an inflammation of _____ .

---

chondr/o/plasty
(KŎN-drō-plăs-tē)
chondr/o/pathy
(kŏn-DRŎP-ă-thē)
chondr/oma
(kŏn-DRŌ-mă)

6–38 Form medical words meaning

surgical repair of cartilage: _____ / _____ / _____

disease of cartilage: _____ / _____ / _____

tumor composed of cartilage: _____ / _____

6–39 Use the Index of Medical Word Elements, Part B of Appendix A, to identify the word elements denoting the following English terms.

English Term	Medical Word Element
liver	_____ / _____
muscle	_____ / _____
new	_____
stomach	_____ / _____
suture	_____

---

suture, muscle
(SŪ-chŭr)

6–40 The combining form **my/o** refers to muscle. My/o/rrhaphy is a

_____ of _____ .

---

my/o/rrhaphy
(mī-ŌR-ă-fē)

6–41 When the surgeon sutures a muscle, the procedure is called

_____ / _____ / _____ .

---

my/o/plasty
(MĪ-ō-plăs-tē)
my/oma
(mī-Ō-mă)
my/o/pathy
(mī-ŎP-ă-thē)
my/o/rrhaphy
(mī-ŌR-ă-fē)

6–42 Develop medical words meaning

surgical repair of muscle: _____ / _____ / _____

tumor of muscle: _____ / _____

disease of the muscle: _____ / _____ / _____

suture of muscle: _____ / _____ / _____

liver	**6-43** Recall that a carcin/oma is a cancerous tumor. This type of cancer develops from epithelial tissue. For example, hepat/o/carcin/oma is a malignant tumor of the _____ .

6-44   Define *epithelial tissue* using your medical dictionary.

_____

_____

_____

new
 	
formation, growth
	6-45 Tumors are also called neo/plasms. They are growths or masses of tissue that may be either malignant or benign.
	
	Analyze neo/plasm by defining the elements.
	
	    neo- means _____ .
	
	    -plasm means _____ or _____ .

chondr/oma (kŏn-DRŌ-mă)	**6-46** Benign tumors are named by adding -oma to the type of tissue in which the tumor occurs. For example, a benign tumor of cartilage is called _____ / _____ .

gastr/oma
(găs-TRŌ-mă)
hepat/oma
(hĕp-ă-TŌ-mă)
my/oma
(mī-Ō-mă)
	6-47 Practice forming medical words meaning
	
	    tumor of the stomach: _____ / _____
	
	    tumor of the liver: _____ / _____
	
	    tumor of muscle: _____ / _____

Review

Select the medical word element(s) that match(es) the meaning of each term listed below.

aer/o	-malacia	neo-
carcin/o	-oma	peri-
chondr/o	-phagia	
hydr/o	-plasia	
laryng/o	-plasm	
my/o	-plasty	
nas/o	-plegia	
pharyng/o	-scope	
rhin/o	-scopy	
trache/o	-spasm	
	-stenosis	
	-stomy	
	-therapy	
	-tome	
	-tomy	

a. _____ air

b. _____ around

c. _____ cancer

d. _____ cartilage

e. _____ formation, growth

f. _____ forming a new opening, mouth

g. _____ incision, cut into

h. _____ instrument to cut

i. _____ instrument to view

j. _____ involuntary contraction, twitching

k. _____ larynx (voice box)

l. _____ muscle

m. _____ new

n. _____ nose

o. _____ paralysis

p. _____ pharynx (throat)

q. _____ softening

r. _____ stricture, narrowing

s. _____ surgical repair

t. _____ swallow, eat

u. _____ trachea (windpipe)

v. _____ treatment

w. _____ tumor

x. _____ visual examination

y. _____ water

Check your answers with the Review Answer Key on the following page.

Review Answer Key

a. aer/o

b. peri-

c. carcin/o

d. chondr/o

e. -plasm, -plasia

f. -stomy

g. -tomy

h. -tome

i. -scope

j. -spasm

k. laryng/o

l. my/o

m. neo-

n. nas/o, rhin/o

o. -plegia

p. pharyng/o

q. -malacia

r. -stenosis

s. -plasty

t. -phagia

u. trache/o

v. -therapy

w. -oma

x. -scopy

y. hydr/o

REINFORCEMENT FRAME: If you are not satisfied with your level of comprehension, go back to Frame 6–1 and rework the frames.

LOWER RESPIRATORY TRACT

6-48 The trachea divides into two branches called **bronchi** (singular, **(6) bronchus**). Each bronchus branches to a separate lung and subdivides into increasingly smaller bronchi. The smallest branches of the bronchi are referred to as the **(7) bronchioles**.

Label the structures in Figure 6-2 as you learn about the respiratory system.

---

bronchi
(BRŎNG-kē)

6-49 **Bronch/o** and **bronchi/o** are combining forms that refer to the bronchi (singular, bronchus). Bronch/itis is an inflammation of the bronchus or _____ (plural).

---

bronchi
(BRŎNG-kē)

6-50 Change bronchus to a plural form:

_____

---

bronch/itis
(brŏng-KĪ-tĭs)
bronch/o/spasm
(BRŎNG-kō-spăzm)
bronch/o/stenosis
(brŏng-kō-stĕn-Ō-sĭs)

6-51 Use **bronch/o** to build medical words meaning

inflammation of the bronchi: _____ / _____

spasm of the bronchus: _____ / ___ / _____

stricture of the bronchi: _____ / ___ / _____

---

bronch/o/spasm
(BRŎNG-kō-spăzm)

6-52 Patients with asthma suffer from wheezing caused by spasms of the bronchi. This condition is called bronchi/o/spasm or

_____ / ___ / _____ .

---

bronchi/ectasis
(brŏng-kē-ĔK-tă-sĭs)

6-53 A dilation of the bronchi is called bronchi/ectasis.

Chronic pneumon/ia or flu may result in a dilation of the bronchi. The medical term for this condition is called _____ / _____ .

---

blood

6-54 You have already learned that a hem/o/rrhage is a bursting forth (of) _____ .

---

hem/o/rrhage
(HĔM-ĕ-rĭj)
bronch/o/rrhagia
(brŏng-kōr-Ā-jē-ă)

6-55 Bronch/o/rrhagia literally means a bursting forth (of the) bronchus, but it actually is a bronchi/al hem/o/rrhage, and is one of the symptoms of lung cancer.

Identify the words in this frame meaning

bursting forth (of) blood: _____ / ___ / _____

bronchial hemorrhage: _____ / ___ / _____

6–56 Use the Index of Medical Word Elements, Part A of Appendix A, to define the word elements used in this unit.

Medical Word Element	Meaning
-cele	_____
-centesis	_____
-malacia	_____
macro-	_____
micro-	_____
myc/o	_____
pneum/o	_____
pneumon/o	_____

micr/o/scope
(MĪ-krō-skōp)

6–57 Macro/scopic structures are visible to the naked eye. Micro/scopic structures are visible only by the use of a micro/scope. Micro/scopic capillaries are visible only by the use of an instrument called a

_____ / _____ / _____ .

6–58 At the end of the bronchial tree there is a cluster of very small, grapelike air sacs known as **(8) alveoli** (singular form, **alveolus**). An alveolus is surrounded by a network of microscopic **(9) pulmonary capillaries**. It is through these walls that an exchange of carbon dioxide (CO_2) and oxygen (O_2) takes place.

Label the alveoli and pulmonary capillaries in Figure 6–2.

alveoli
(ăl-VĒ-ō-lī)

6–59 Clusters of air sacs at the end of the bronchial tree are called

_____ (plural).

O_2

CO_2

6–60 During respiration, the exchange of CO_2 and O_2 takes place in the alveoli.

The chemical symbol for oxygen is _____ .

The chemical symbol for carbon dioxide is _____ .

6–61 Each bronchus (plural, **bronchi**) leads to a separate **(10) lung**. The structures of the bronchi and the alveoli are part of the lungs, which are the organs of respiration.

Label the lungs in Figure 6–2.

6–62 Define *respiration*, using your medical dictionary.

_____

_____

_____

6-63 **Pneum/o** and **pneumon/o** are the combining forms that refer to the lung(s) or air.

Pneumon/itis is an _____ of the _____ .

inflammation, lung(s)
(ĭn-flă-MĀ-shŭn)

6-64 Pneumon/ia, an acute inflammation and infection of the lungs in which the alveoli fill with secretions, is the fifth leading cause of death in the United States.

Analyze pneumon/ia by defining the elements.

pneumon/o means _____ or _____ .

-ia means _____ (noun ending).

lung(s), air
condition

6-65 In patients with lung cancer, it may be necessary to remove part or all of the lung.

Use **pneumon/o** to form the surgical procedure meaning excision of the lung:

_____ / _____ .

pneumon/ectomy
(nū-mŏn-ĔK-tō-mē)

6-66 Sometimes a disease causes the lung tissue to soften.

Use **pneumon/o** to develop a word meaning softening of the lungs:

_____ / ____ / _____ .

pneumon/o/malacia
(nū-mō-nō-mă-LĀ-sē-ă)

6-67 Use **pneumon/o** to build medical words meaning

abnormal condition of the lungs: _____ / _____

disease of the lung: _____ / ____ / _____

excision of a lung: _____ / _____

pneumon/osis
(nū-mŏn-Ō-sĭs)
pneumon/o/pathy
(nū-mō-NŎP-ăth-ē)
pneumon/ectomy
(nū-mŏn-ĔK-tō-mē)

6-68 The suffix -centesis is used in words to denote a surgical puncture.

Pneum/o/centesis is a surgical puncture to aspirate the _____ .

lung(s)

6-69 Define *aspirate*, using your medical dictionary.

_____

_____

6-70 An abscess, which is an abnormal localized collection of fluid that is sometimes caused in the lung by pneumonia, may require pneum/o/centesis. Form another word that means surgical puncture of a lung:

_____ / ____ / _____ .

pneumon/o/centesis
(nū-mō-nō-sĕn-TĒ-sis)

lung(s), air

black

abnormal condition

6–71   Pneumon/o/melan/osis is an abnormal condition of black lung caused by inhalation of black dust; it is common among coal miners.

Analyze pneumon/o/melan/osis by defining the elements.

pneumon/o means _____ or _____ .

melan/o means _____ .

-osis means _____ _____ .

---

oxygen

carbon dioxide

6–72   The lungs are divided into five lobes: three lobes in the right lung and two lobes in the left lung. Both lungs supply the blood with O_2 inhaled from outside the body and dispose of waste CO_2 in the exhaled air.

The symbol O_2 means _____ ; the symbol CO_2 means

_____ _____ .

---

excision or removal
(ĕk-SĬ-zhŭn)

6–73   A person with lung cancer may undergo a lob/ectomy, which is a(n) _____ of a lobe.

---

lob/o

6–74   From lob/ar (pertaining to the lobe), construct the combining form for lobe. _____ / _____

---

lob/itis
(lō-BĪ-tĭs)
lob/o/tomy
(lō-BŎT-ō-mē)
lob/ectomy
(lō-BĔK-tō-mē)

6–75   Develop medical words meaning

inflammation of a lobe: _____ / _____

incision of the lobe: _____ / _____ / _____

excision of a lobe: _____ / _____

6–76   Each lung is enclosed in a double-folded membrane called the **(11) pleura**.

Label the pleura in Figure 6–2.

---

inflammation

6–77   Pleur/itis is an _____ of the pleura.

---

pleur/o

6–78   From pleur/o/dynia, identify the combining form for pleura:

_____ / _____ .

---

pleur/o/dynia
(ploo-rō-DĬN-ē-ă)
pleur/algia
(ploo-RĂL-jē-ă)

6–79   A pain in the pleura is known as _____ / _____ / _____

or _____ / _____ .

pneumon/o or pneum/o	**6-80** Pleur/o/pneumon/ia is pleurisy complicated with pneumonia. The combining form for lung or air is _____ / _____ .

pleur/itis ploo-RĪ-tĭs) pleur/o/cele (PLOO-rō-sēl)	**6-81** Form medical words meaning inflammation of the pleura: _____ / _____ hernia or swelling of the pleura: _____ / _____ / _____

inflammation, pleura (PLOO-ră)	**6-82** Pleurisy is an inflammation of the pleura. Pleur/itis is also an _____ of the _____ .

inflammation, pleura (PLOO-ră)	**6-83** Whenever you see pleurisy or pleur/itis, you will know it means _____ of the _____ .

pleur/o/dynia (ploo-rō-DĬN-ē-ă)	**6-84** The pleura often gets inflamed in pneumonia, causing pleur/algia or _____ / _____ / _____ .

6-85 Use the Index of Medical Word Elements, Part B of Appendix A, to identify medical elements in this unit.

English Term	*Medical Word Element*
bad, painful, difficult	_____
fungus	_____ / _____
good, normal	_____
straight	_____ / _____
without, not	_____

thorac/o/tomy (thō-răk-ŎT-ō-mē)	**6-86** The combining form **thorac/o** refers to the chest. Form a word meaning an incision of the chest: _____ / _____ / _____ .

thorac/o/centesis (thō-răk-ō-sĕn-TĒ-sĭs)	**6-87** To remove fluid from the thorac/ic (pertaining to the chest) cavity, a surgical puncture of the chest is performed. This procedure is called _____ / _____ / _____ .

thorac/o/centesis (thō-răk-ō-sĕn-TĒ-sĭs)	**6–88** Fluid often builds up around the lung(s) in patients with cancer or pneumonia. To remove fluid from the thorac/ic cavity, the physician performs the surgical procedure called _____ / _____ / _____ .
breathing	**6–89** The suffix -pnea refers to _____ .
breathing	**6–90** A/pnea literally means without _____ ; except in death, it is a temporary condition.
a/pnea (ăp-NĒ-ă)	**6–91** A baby whose mother used cocaine during pregnancy is more likely to develop life-threatening a/pnea. Form a word meaning temporary stopping of breathing: _____ / _____ .
dys/pnea (dĭsp-NĒ-ă)	**6–92** Use dys- to form a word meaning painful or difficult breathing: _____ / _____ .
dys/pnea (dĭsp-NĒ-ă)	**6–93** Dys/pnea is normal when it is due to vigorous work or athletic activity. Dys/pnea can also occur as a result of various disorders of the respiratory system, such as pleurisy. Thus, a person with pleurisy may suffer from _____ / _____ .
dys/pnea (dĭsp-NĒ-ă)	**6–94** Asthma (Fig. 6–4) is a respiratory condition marked by recurrent attacks of labored breathing accompanied by wheezing. Asthma patients who have difficult breathing are experiencing _____ / _____ .
eu- -pnea	**6–95** Eu/pnea is normal breathing, as distinguished from dys/pnea and a/pnea. From eu/pnea, determine the elements meaning good or normal: _____ breathing: _____

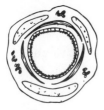
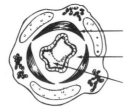

Spasm of smooth muscle

Mucosal edema

Retained secretions

A   B

Figure 6–4. (A) Cross-sectional view of a healthy airway and (B) from a patient with asthma. A combination of airway secretions, edema, and bronchospasm contributes to a reduction in the airway diameter. (From Wilkins, RL, and Dexter, JR: Respiratory Disease: Principles of Patient Care. FA Davis, Philadelphia, 1993, p 16, with permission.)

a/pnea
(ăp-NĒ-ă)
dys/pnea
(dĭsp-NĒ-ă)
eu/pnea
(ūp-NĒ-ă)

6–96   Here is a little more practice forming words with -pnea.

Construct medical words meaning

without breathing: _____ / _____

difficult or labored breathing: _____ / _____

normal breathing: _____ / _____

tachy/pnea
(tăk-ĭp-NĒ-ă)

6–97   Combine tachy and pnea to form a word meaning rapid or fast breathing: _____ / _____ .

-pnea

orth/o

6–98   Orth/o/pnea is a respiratory condition in which there is breathing discomfort in any posture except in the erect sitting or standing position.

Identify the element that means

breathing: _____

straight or straightening: _____ / _____

brady/pnea
(brăd-ĭp-NĒ-ă)

6–99   Use brady- and -pnea to form a word meaning slow breathing: _____ / _____ .

6–100   The **(12) diaphragm** is a muscular partition that separates the lungs from the abdominal cavity.

Label the diaphragm in Figure 6–2.

VALIDATION FRAME: Check your labeling of Figure 6–1 with Appendix B, Answer Key.

descends

ascends

6–101   Examine Figure 6–5 and use the words "ascends" or "descends" to complete this frame.
During inspiration (or inhalation), the diaphragm

_____ .

During expiration (or exhalation), the diaphragm

_____ .

inhalation
(ĭn-hă-LĀ-shŭn)
exhalation
(ĕks-hă-LĀ-shŭn)

6–102   Identify the words in Figure 6–3 that mean the process of breathing air

into the lungs: _____

out of the lungs: _____

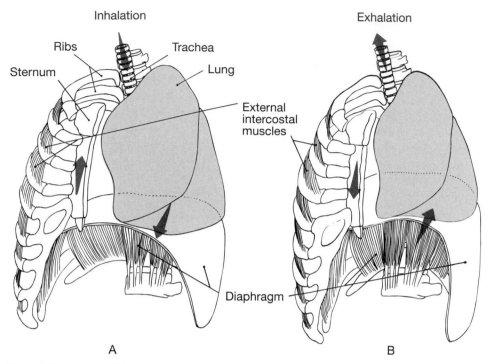

Figure 6–5. Actions of the respiratory muscles. (A) Inhalation: diaphragm contracts downward; external intercostal muscles pull rib cage upward and outward; lungs are expanded. (B) Normal exhalation: diaphragm relaxes upward; rib cage falls down and in as external intercostal muscles relax; lungs are compressed. (From Scanlon, VC, and Sanders, T: Understanding Human Structure and Function. FA Davis, Philadelphia, 1997, p 271, with permission.)

air	**6–103** **Aer/o** is the combining form for _____ .
aer/o/phobia (ĕr-ō-FŌ-bē-ă)	**6–104** Aer/o/phobia is a fear of air, drafts of air, airborne influences, or "bad air" (body odor). The medical word meaning fear of air is _____ / _____ / _____ .
hem/o/phobia (hē-mō-FŌ-bē-ă)	**6–105** Combine **hem/o** and -phobia to form a word meaning fear of blood: _____ / _____ / _____ .

muc/o
 	
myc/o
	6–106 Although the combining forms **muc/o** and **myc/o** look somewhat alike, they both have different meanings.
	
	Write the combining form that means
	
	   mucus: _____ / _____
	
	   fungus: _____ / _____

lung, air fungus abnormal condition	**6–107** Analyze pneumon/o/myc/osis by defining the elements. **pneumon/o** refers to _____ or _____ . **myc** refers to a _____ . -osis refers to an _____ _____ .

bronchi/al (BRŎNG-kē-ăl) bronch/itis (brŏng-KĪ-tĭs)	**6–108** Bronch/itis, an inflammation of mucous membrane of the bronchi/al tubes, is a viral condition that alters air flow to the lungs and is considered an upper respiratory infection (URI). Build a medical word that means pertaining to the bronchi: ⎯⎯⎯⎯⎯⎯ / ⎯⎯⎯⎯ inflammation of the bronchi: ⎯⎯⎯⎯⎯⎯ / ⎯⎯⎯⎯⎯⎯
upper respiratory infection stridor (STRĪ-dōr)	**6–109** Croup, a severe inflammation and obstruction of the upper respiratory tract, is most frequently associated with infants and children up to 3 years of age. It usually occurs after a URI and is characterized by a distinct barking cough or stridor. Define the abbreviation URI. ⎯⎯⎯⎯⎯⎯ ⎯⎯⎯⎯⎯⎯⎯⎯ ⎯⎯⎯⎯⎯⎯⎯⎯ . A common symptom of croup is a barking cough known as ⎯⎯⎯⎯⎯⎯⎯⎯ .
laryng/itis (lăr-ĭn-JĪ-tĭs)	**6–110** The larynx contains the organ of sound called the vocal cords. When the vocal cords become inflamed from overuse or infection, laryng/itis occurs, causing hoarseness and difficulty speaking. The medical term for an inflamed larynx is ⎯⎯⎯⎯⎯⎯ / ⎯⎯⎯⎯⎯⎯ .
bronch/o pneumon -ia	**6–111** Pneumon/ia is a lung inflammation caused by bacteria, a virus, or chemical irritants. Some pneumon/ias affect only one lobe of the lung (lobar pneumon/ia). Others, such as bronch/o/pneumon/ia involve the bronchioles and the alveoli. Identify the elements in bronch/o/pneumon/ia that mean bronchus: ⎯⎯⎯⎯⎯⎯ / ⎯⎯ lung, air: ⎯⎯⎯⎯⎯⎯⎯⎯ condition: ⎯⎯⎯⎯
bronch / o / pneumon / ia (brong-kō-nū-MŌ-nē-ă)	**6–112** A pneumon/ia that involves the bronchi/oles and alveoli is called ⎯⎯⎯⎯⎯⎯ / ⎯⎯ / ⎯⎯⎯⎯⎯⎯ / ⎯⎯⎯ .
-oles	**6–113** In Frame 6–112, the element that means small is ⎯⎯⎯⎯⎯ .
PCP *Pneumocystis carinii* (nū-mō-SĬS-tĭs kă-RĪ-nē-ī)	**6–114** Another type of pneumon/ia, *Pneumocystis carinii* pneumon/ia (PCP), presents itself with a nonproductive cough, slight or no fever, and dys/pnea. This type of pneumon/ia is seen in debilitated children and patients with AIDS. The abbreviation for *Pneumocystis carinii* pneumon/ia is ⎯⎯⎯⎯⎯ . A type of pneumonia seen in patients with AIDS is ⎯⎯⎯⎯⎯⎯ ⎯⎯⎯⎯⎯⎯ .

dys/pnea (dĭsp-NĒ-ă)	**6–115** The medical term in Frame 6–114 that means labored or difficult breathing is _____ / _____ .
emphysema (ĕm-fĭ-SĒ-mă)	**6–116** Emphysema, a chronic disease characterized by overexpansion and destruction of the alveoli, is often associated with cigarette smoking. Destruction of alveoli occurs in the respiratory disease called _____ .
COLD **emphysema** (ĕm-fĭ-SĒ-mă)	**6–117** Chronic obstructive lung disease (COLD) is a group of respiratory disorders characterized by a chronic, partial obstruction of the bronchi and lungs. The three major disorders included in COLD are bronch/itis, asthma, and emphysema. The abbreviation for chronic lung disease is _____ . Three major pathological conditions associated with COLD are bronch/itis, asthma, and _____ .
bronch/itis (brong-KĪ-tĭs)	**6–118** Chronic bronch/itis, an inflammation of the mucous membranes lining the bronchial airways, is characterized by increased mucus production resulting in a chronic productive cough. Cigarette smoking, environmental irritants, allergic response, and infectious agents are causative factors. The medical term for inflammation of the bronchi is _____ / _____ .
metastasize or metastasis (mĕ-TĂS-tă-sīz), (mĕ-TĂS-tă-sĭs)	**6–119** Lung cancer, associated with smoking, is the leading cause of cancer-related deaths in men and women in the United States. It usually spreads rapidly and metastasizes to other parts of the body, making it difficult to diagnose and treat in its early stages. When cancer spreads to other parts of the body, the medical term used to describe that condition is _____ .
tuberculosis (tū-bĕr-kū-LŌ-sĭs) **tubercles** (TŪ-bĕr-klz)	**6–120** Tuberculosis (TB), an infectious disease, produces small lesions or tubercles in the lungs. If left untreated, it infects the bones and organs of the entire body. A recent increase in the disease is attributed to the rise in AIDS. The abbreviation TB refers to _____ . The name tuberculosis is derived from small lesions that appear in the lungs called _____ .

Review

Select the medical word element(s) that match(es) the meaning of each of the following terms.

aer/o	-cele	a-
bronch/o	-centesis	dys-
bronchi/o	-ectasis	eu-
lob/o	-osis	macro-
melan/o	-phobia	micro-
myc/o	-pnea	
orth/o	-rrhage	
pleur/o	-rrhagia	
pneum/o	-scope	
pneumon/o	-spasm	
thorac/o	-stenosis	

a. _____ abnormal condition

b. _____ air

c. _____ bad, painful, difficult

d. _____ black

e. _____ breathing

f. _____ bronchus

g. _____ bursting forth (of)

h. _____ chest

i. _____ expansion, dilation

j. _____ fear

k. _____ fungus

l. _____ good, normal

m. _____ hernia, swelling

n. _____ instrument to view

o. _____ involuntary contraction, twitching

p. _____ large

q. _____ lobe

r. _____ lung, air

s. _____ pleura

t. _____ small

u. _____ straight

v. _____ stricture, narrowing

w. _____ surgical puncture

x. _____ without, not

Check your answers with the Review Answer Key on the following page.

Review Answer Key

a. -osis

b. aer/o

c. dys-

d. melan/o

e. -pnea

f. bronch/o, bronchi/o

g. -rrhage, -rrhagia

h. thorac/o

i. -ectasis

j. -phobia

k. myc/o

l. eu-

m. -cele

n. -scope

o. -spasm

p. macro-

q. lob/o

r. pneum/o, pneumon/o

s. pleur/o

t. micro-

u. orth/o

v. -stenosis

w. -centesis

x. a-

REINFORCEMENT FRAME: If you are not satisfied with your level of comprehension, go back to Frame 6–48 and rework the frames.

Additional Pathological Conditions

acidosis (ăs-i-DŌ-sĭs): excessive acidity of body fluids. Respiratory acidosis is caused by abnormally high levels of carbon dioxide (CO_2) in the body.

adult respiratory distress syndrome (ARDS) (ă-DŬLT rĕs-PĪR-ă-tō-rē dĭs-TRĔS SĬN-drōm): form of restrictive lung disease that follows severe infection or trauma in young and previously healthy individuals. There is respiratory failure with hypoxemia.

atelectasis (ăt-ĕ-LĔK-tă-sĭs): collapse of lung tissue, preventing the respiratory exchange of oxygen and carbon dioxide. Can be caused by a variety of conditions including obstruction of foreign bodies, excessive secretions, or pressure upon the lung from a tumor.

coryza (kō-RĪ-ză): acute inflammation of the nasal passages accompanied by profuse nasal discharge; a cold.

croup (KROOP): acute respiratory condition found in infants and children characterized by a resonant barking cough or stridor and severe dyspnea.

cystic fibrosis (CF) (SĬS-tĭk fĭ-BRŌ-sĭs): inherited disease of the exocrine glands with production of thick mucus that causes severe congestion within the lungs and digestive systems. Average life expectancy is approximately 20 years.

empyema (ĕm-pĭ-Ē-mă): Pus in a body cavity, especially in the pleural cavity (pyothorax). Usually the result of a primary infection in the lungs.

epiglottitis (ĕp-ĭ-glŏt-Ī-tĭs): acute epiglottitis is a severe, life-threatening infection of the epiglottis and surrounding area that occurs most often in children between 2 and 12 years of age. In the classic form, a sudden onset of fever, dysphagia, inspiratory stridor, and severe respiratory distress occur that often requires intubation or tracheotomy to open the obstructed airway.

epistaxis (ĕp-ĭ-STĂK-sĭs): hemorrhage from the nose; nosebleed.

hypoxia (hī-PŎKS-ē-ă): deficiency of oxygen.

influenza (ĭn-floo-ĔN-ză): acute, contagious respiratory infection characterized by sudden onset of fever, chills, headache, and muscle pain.

lung cancer (LŬNG KĂN-sĕr): pulmonary malignancy attributable to cigarette smoking. Survival rates are low owing to its rapid metastasis and late detection.

pertussis (pĕr-TŬS-ĭs): acute infectious disease characterized by a "whoop"-sounding cough. Immunization of infants as part of the DPT vaccine prevents contraction; whopping cough.

pleural effusion (PLOO-răl ĕ-FŪ-zhŭn): abnormal presence of fluid in the pleural cavity. The fluid may contain blood (hemothorax) or pus (pyothorax).

pneumothorax (nū-mō-THŌ-răks): collection of air or gas in the pleural cavity that enters through a perforated lung or chest wall.

rales (RĀHLZ): abnormal crackling sound heard on inspiration that is noted by use of a stethoscope. It is produced by passage of air that contains moisture and often indicates a pneumonia condition.

rhonchi (RONG-kē): abnormal chest sounds resembling snoring, produced in airways with accumulated fluids.

sudden infant death syndrome (SIDS): the completely unexpected and unexplained death of an apparently well, or virtually well, infant. The most common cause of death between the second week and first year of life; crib death.

stridor (STRĪ-dōr): harsh, high-pitched breathing sound resembling the blowing of wind, caused by obstruction of air passages.

wheezes (HWĒZ-ĕz): whistling or sighing sound resulting from narrowing of the lumen of a respiratory passageway that is noted by use of a stethoscope. Occurs in asthma, croup, hay fever, obstructive emphysema, and other obstructive respiratory conditions.

Medical Record

The following reports are from a specialty within internal medicine called pulmonary medicine. The pulmonologist specializes in respiratory system diseases with a particular emphasis on those that affect the lungs.

MEDICAL RECORD 6–1. Papillary Carcinoma

Dictionary Exercise

Underline the following terms in the reading exercise. Use a medical dictionary and Appendix E, Abbreviations, to write a definition of each word in the list. This exercise helps you master the terminology in the medical record.

anesthesia _____

biopsy _____
_____

carcinoma _____

cm _____

diagnosis _____
_____

expire _____

hemorrhage _____

lymph node _____

meatus _____

metastatic _____

nasal cavity _____

necropsy _____

needle biopsy _____

nodular _____

papillary _____

pathologic _____

pneumonia _____
_____

polyp _____

polypectomy _____

polypoid _____

pulmonary _____

snare _____

submaxillary region _____

superficial _____

Word Element Exercise

Break down the following words into their basic elements.

carcinoma   hemorrhage
polypoid   nasal
polypectomy   pneumonia

VALIDATION FRAME: Check your answers in Appendix B, Answer Key.

Reading Exercise

Read the case study out loud.

A 55-year-old white man was seen 2 years ago because of upper airway obstruction due to large polyps in the right nasal cavity. On examination, a large polypoid mass was observed to fill most of the right nasal cavity. The mass originated in the middle meatus. With the use of a nasal snare, polypectomy was performed to remove several sections. There was a slight hemorrhage. On the next day, a 4×3 cm oval soft mass was excised from beneath the left submaxillary region, with the patient under local anesthesia. The mass was just beneath the superficial fascia and appeared to be an enlarged lymph node unconnected with the nasal disease.

The pathological diagnosis of the nasal growth was low-grade papillary carcinoma. The diagnosis of the lymph node was metastatic carcinoma. A chest film was taken that indicated the presence of pulmonary densities attributed to unresolved pneumonia. Also, a needle biopsy of the enlarged liver nodes yielded no results.

After discharge from the hospital, the patient expired at home and no necropsy was obtained.

MEDICAL RECORD EVALUATION 6–1. Papillary Carcinoma

1. What type of patients are at risk for nasal polyps?

2. When is a polypectomy indicated?

3. Were the patient's nasal polyps cancerous?

4. What contributed to the patient's expiration?

5. Why was a biopsy of the liver performed?

MEDICAL RECORD 6–2. Lobar Pneumonia

Dictionary Exercise

Underline the following terms in the reading exercise. Use a medical dictionary to write a definition of each word in the list. This exercise helps you master the terminology in the medical record.

asthma _____

excursion _____

lobe _____

nasal polyps _____

polypectomy _____

percussion _____

phlegm _____

pneumonia _____

resonance _____

tactile fremitus _____

Reading Exercise

Read the medical report out loud.

Emergency Room Number: 543985720

Chief Complaint: Cough and fever.

History of Present Illness: Patient reports with 7 days' history of sinus drainage, cough, and yellow phlegm.

Review of Systems: She denies ear pain, sore throat, abdominal pain, dysuria, frequency or infrequency of urination.

Past Medical History: History of asthma. History of nasal polyps with nasal polypectomy performed at the beginning of this year.

Social/Family History: Noncontributory.

Physical Examination: Temperature 39°C, pulse 128/minute; respiratory rate 28/minute; blood pressure 112/68 mmHg. Ears are clear, all pharynx unremarkable, some sinus tenderness to percussion. Neck is supple. Chest shows diminished excursion noted on the right side with each inspiratory effort; diminished resonance to percussion and increased tactile fremitus noted over right middle lobe anteriorly. Lungs have clear breath sounds over all left lung fields and right upper lobe; bronchial breath sounds noted over right middle lobe.

Diagnosis: Right middle lobe pneumonia.

MEDICAL RECORD EVALUATION 6–2. Lobar Pneumonia

1. What physical examination techniques are useful in this case?

2. What explains the unilateral chest expansion?

3. What explains the decrease in resonance and increase in tactile fremitus?

4. What is the significance of bronchial breath sounds in this case?

5. What laboratory data are useful to confirm the diagnosis?

Abbreviations

Abbreviation	Meaning	Abbreviation	Meaning
ARDS	adult respiratory distress syndrome	PND	paroxysmal nocturnal dyspnea
COLD	chronic obstructive lung disease	RD	respiratory disease
CPR	cardiopulmonary resuscitation	SOB	shortness of breath
HMD	hyaline membrane disease	TB	tuberculosis
IPPB	intermittent positive-pressure breathing	URI	upper respiratory infection
IRDS	infant respiratory distress syndrome	VC	vital capacity

Audiocassette Exercise

The audiocassette tape helps you master the pronunciation of medical words. Listen to the tape for instructions for this exercise. You may also use this list without the audiotape to practice correct pronunciation and spelling of the terms.

Frame Exercise	Word	Pronunciation	Spelling
Additional Pathological Conditions	[] acidosis	(ăs-ĭ-DŌ-sĭs)	_____
Additional Pathological Conditions	[] adult respiratory distress syndrome	(ă-DŬLT rĕs-PĪR-ă-tō-rē dĭs-TRĔS SĬN-drōm)	_____
6–14	[] aerohydrotherapy	(ĕr-ō-hī-drō-THĔR-ă-pē)	_____
6–11	[] aerophagia	(ĕr-ō-FĀ-jē-ă)	_____
6–104	[] aerophobia	(ĕr-ō-FŌ-bē-ă)	_____
6–12	[] aerotherapy	(ĕr-ō-THĔR-ă-pē)	_____
6–58	[] alveoli	(ăl-vē-Ō-lī)	_____
Reading Exercise	[] anesthesia	(ăn-ĕs-THĒ-zē-ă)	_____
6–90	[] apnea	(ăp-NĒ-ă)	_____
6–69	[] aspirate	(ĂS-pĭ-rāt)	_____
6–94	[] asthma	(ĂZ-mă)	_____
Additional Pathological Conditions	[] atelectasis	(ăt-ĕ-LĔK-tă-sĭs)	_____
Reading Exercise	[] biopsy	(BĪ-ŏp-sē)	_____
6–48	[] bronchi	(BRŎNG-kī)	_____
6–55	[] bronchial	(BRŎNG-kē-ăl)	_____
6–53	[] bronchiectasis	(brŏng-kē-ĔK-tă-sĭs)	_____
6–48	[] bronchiole	(BRŎNG-kē-ōl)	_____
6–52	[] bronchiospasm	(BRŎNG-kē-ō-spăzm)	_____
6–49	[] bronchitis	(brŏng-KĪ-tĭs)	_____
6–55	[] bronchorrhagia	(brŏng-kōr-Ă-jē-ă)	_____
6–51	[] bronchospasm	(BRŎNG-kō-spăzm)	_____
6–51	[] bronchostenosis	(brŏng-kō-stĕn-Ō-sĭs)	_____
6–48	[] bronchus	(BRŎNG-kŭs)	_____
6–43	[] carcinoma	(kăr-sĭ-NŌ-mă)	_____
6–37	[] chondritis	(kŏn-DRĪ-tĭs)	_____
6–38	[] chondroma	(kŏn-DRŌ-mă)	_____
6–38	[] chondropathy	(kŏn-DRŎP-ă-thē)	_____
6–38	[] chondroplasty	(KŎN-drō-plăs-tē)	_____
6–117	[] chronic obstructive lung disease		_____
Additional Pathological Conditions	[] coryza	(kŏ-RĪ-ză)	_____
6–109	[] croup	(KROOP)	_____
6–100	[] diaphragm	(DĪ-ă-frăm)	_____
6–92	[] dyspnea	(dĭsp-NĒ-ă)	_____
6–116	[] emphysema	(ĕm-fĭ-SĒ-mă)	_____

Frame Exercise	Word	Pronunciation	Spelling
Additional Pathological Conditions	[] empyema	(ĕm-pī-Ē-mă)	_____
6–31	[] epiglottis	(ĕp-ĭ-GLŎT-ĭs)	_____
Reading Exercise	[] epiglottitis	(ĕp-ĭ-glŏt-Ī-tĭs)	_____
Additional Pathological Conditions	[] epistaxis	(ĕp-ĭ-STĂK-sĭs)	_____
6–95	[] eupnea	(ūp-NĒ-ă)	_____
Reading Exercise	[] excursion	(ĕks-KŬR-zhŭn)	_____
6–101	[] expiration	(ĕks-pĭ-RĀ-shŭn)	_____
Reading Exercise	[] expired	(ĕk-SPĪRD)	_____
Reading Exercise	[] fascia	(FĂSH-ē-ă)	_____
6–47	[] gastroma	(găs-TRŌ-mă)	_____
6–105	[] hemophobia	(hē-mō-FŌ-bē-ă)	_____
6–55	[] hemorrhage	(HĔM-ĕ-rĭj)	_____
6–43	[] hepatocarcinoma	(hĕp-ă-tō-kăr-sĭn-Ō-mă)	_____
6–47	[] hepatoma	(hĕp-ă-TŌ-mă)	_____
6–13	[] hydrotherapy	(hī-drō-THĔR-ă-pē)	_____
Additional Pathological Conditions	[] hypoxia	(hī-PŎKS-ē-ă)	_____
Additional Pathological Conditions	[] influenza	(ĭn-floo-ĔN-ză)	_____
6–101	[] inspiration	(ĭn-spĭr-Ā-shŭn)	_____
6–27	[] laryngectomy	(lăr-ĭn-JĔK-tō-mē)	_____
6–25	[] laryngitis	(lăr-ĭn-JĪ-tĭs)	_____
6–26	[] laryngoscope	(lăr-ĬN-gō-skōp)	_____
6–30	[] laryngoscopy	(lăr-ĭn-GŎS-kō-pē)	_____
6–28	[] laryngospasm	(lăr-ĬN-gō-spăzm)	_____
6–29	[] laryngostenosis	(lăr-ĭng-gō-stĕn-Ō-sĭs)	_____
6–24	[] larynx	(LĂR-ĭnks)	_____
6–74	[] lobar	(LŌ-băr)	_____
Reading Exercise	[] lobar pneumonia	(LŌ-băr nū-MŌ-nē-ă)	_____
6–74	[] lobe	(LŌB)	_____
6–73	[] lobectomy	(lō-BĔK-tō-mē)	_____
6–75	[] lobitis	(lō-BĪ-tĭs)	_____
6–75	[] lobotomy	(lō-BŎT-ō-mē)	_____
6–57	[] macroscopic	(măk-rō-SKŎP-ĭk)	_____
Reading Exercise	[] meatus	(mē-Ā-tŭs)	_____
Reading Exercise	[] metastatic	(mĕt-ă-STĂT-ĭk)	_____
6–57	[] microscope	(MĪ-krō-skōp)	_____
6–57	[] microscopic	(mī-krō-SKŎP-ĭk)	_____
6–42	[] myoma	(mī-Ō-mă)	_____
6–42	[] myopathy	(mī-ŎP-ă-thē)	_____
6–42	[] myoplasty	(MĪ-ō-plăs-tē)	_____
6–40	[] myorrhaphy	(mī-ŌR-ă-fē)	_____

Frame Exercise	Word	Pronunciation	Spelling
6–3	[] nares	(NĀ-rēz)	_____
6–3	[] naris	(NĀ-rĭs)	_____
Reading Exercise	[] nasal polyps	(NĀ-zl PŎL-ĭps)	_____
6–3	[] nasitis	(nā ZĪ-tĭs)	_____
6–3	[] nasoscope	(NĀ-zō-skōp)	_____
Reading Exercise	[] necropsy	(NĔK-rŏp-sē)	_____
6–45	[] neoplasm	(NĒ-ō-plăzm)	_____
Reading Exercise	[] nodular	(NŎD-ū-lăr)	_____
6–98	[] orthopnea	(or-THŎP-nē-ă)	_____
Reading Exercise	[] papillary	(PĂP-ĭ-lăr-ē)	_____
Reading Exercise	[] percussion	(pĕr-KŬSH-ŭn)	_____
6–4	[] perinasal	(pĕr-ĭ-NĀ-zl)	_____
Additional Pathological Conditions	[] pertussis	(pĕr-TŬS-ĭs)	_____
6–21	[] pharyngitis	(făr-ĭn-JĪ-tĭs)	_____
6–21	[] pharyngocele	(făr-ĬN-gō-sēl)	_____
6–17	[] pharyngomycosis	(făr-ĭn-gō-mī-KŌ-sĭs)	_____
6–19	[] pharyngoparalysis	(făr-ĭn-gō-pă-RĂL-ĭ-sĭs)	_____
6–21	[] pharyngoplasty	(făr-ĭn-gō-PLĂS-tē)	_____
6–19	[] pharyngoplegia	(făr-ĭn-gō-PLĒ-jă)	_____
6–21	[] pharyngospasm	(făr-ĬN-gō-spăzm)	_____
6–23	[] pharyngostenosis	(fă-rĭng-gō-stē-NŌ-sĭs)	_____
6–21	[] pharyngotome	(făr-ĬN-gō-tōm)	_____
6–21	[] pharyngotomy	(făr-ĭn-GŎT-ō-mē)	_____
6–18	[] pharynx	(FĂR-ĭnks)	_____
Reading Exercise	[] phlegm	(FLĔM)	_____
6–76	[] pleura	(PLOO-ră)	_____
Additional Pathological Conditions	[] pleural effusion	(PLOO-răl ĕ-FŪ-zhŭn)	_____
6–79	[] pleuralgia	(ploo-RĂL-jē-ă)	_____
6–82	[] pleurisy	(PLOO-rĭs-ē)	_____
6–77	[] pleuritis	(ploo-RĪ-tĭs)	_____
6–81	[] pleurocele	(PLOO-rō-sēl)	_____
6–78	[] pleurodynia	(ploo-rō-DĪN-ē-ă)	_____
6–80	[] pleuropneumonia	(ploo-rō-nū-MŌ-nē-ă)	_____
6–68	[] pneumocentesis	(nū-mō-sĕn-TĒ-sĭs)	_____
6–114	[] *Pneumocystis carinii* pneumonia	(nū-mō-SĬS-tĭs kă-RĪ-nē-ī nū-MŌ-nē-ă)	_____
6–65	[] pneumonectomy	(nū-mŏn-ĔK-tō-mē)	_____
6–64	[] pneumonia	(nū-MŌ-nē-ă)	_____
6–63	[] pneumonitis	(nū-mō-NĪ-tĭs)	_____
6–70	[] pneumonocentesis	(nū-mō-nō-sĕn-TĒ-sĭs)	_____
6–66	[] pneumonomalacia	(nū-mō-nō-mā-LĀ-shē-ă)	_____

Frame Exercise	Word	Pronunciation	Spelling
6–71	[] pneumonomelanosis	(nū-mō-nō-měl-ăn-Ō-sĭs)	_____
6–107	[] pneumonomycosis	(nū-mōn-ō-mī-KŌ-sĭs)	_____
6–67	[] pneumonopathy	(nū-mō-NŎP-ăth-ē)	_____
6–67	[] pneumonosis	(nū-mō-NŌ-sĭs)	_____
Additional Pathological Conditions	[] pneumothorax	(nū-mō-THŌ-răks)	_____
Reading Exercise	[] polyp	(PŎL-ĭp)	_____
Reading Exercise	[] polypectomy	(pŏl-ĭ-PĔK-tō-mē)	_____
Reading Exercise	[] polypoid	(PŎL-ē-poyd)	_____
6–58	[] pulmonary	(PŬL-mō-ně-rē)	_____
Additional Pathological Conditions	[] rales	(RĀHLZ)	_____
Reading Exercise	[] resonance	(RĔZ-ō-năns)	_____
6–3	[] rhinitis	(rī-NĪ-tĭs)	_____
6–7	[] rhinologist	(rī-NŎL-ō-jĭst)	_____
6–8	[] rhinoplasty	(RĪ-nō-plăs-tē)	_____
6–3	[] rhinoscope	(RĪ-nō-skop)	_____
6–8	[] rhinotomy	(rī-NŎT-ō-mē)	_____
Additional Pathological Conditions	[] rhonchi	(RONG-kē)	_____
Reading Exercise	[] snare	(SNĀR)	_____
6–109	[] stridor	(STRĪ-dōr)	_____
Reading Exercise	[] submaxillary	(sŭb-MĂK-sĭ-lăr-ē)	_____
Reading Exercise	[] superficial	(soo-pĕr-FĬSH-ăl)	_____
Reading Exercise	[] tactile fremitus	(TĂK-tĭl FRĔM-ĭ-tŭs)	_____
6–87	[] thoracic	(thō-RĂS-ĭk)	_____
6–87	[] thoracocentesis	(thō-răk-ō-sĕn-TĒ-sĭs)	_____
6–86	[] thoracotomy	(thō-răk-ŎT-ō-mē)	_____
6–32	[] trachea	(TRĀ-kē-ă)	_____
6–34	[] tracheal	(TRĀ-kē-ăl)	_____
6–36	[] tracheolaryngotomy	(trā-kē-ō-lăr-ĭn-GŎT-ō-mē)	_____
6–35	[] tracheomalacia	(trā-kē-ō-mă-LĀ-shē-ă)	_____
6–33	[] tracheopathy	(trā-kē-ŎP-ăth-ē)	_____
6–35	[] tracheoplasty	(TRĀ-kē-ō-plăs-tē)	_____
6–35	[] tracheostenosis	(trā-kē-ō-stĕn-Ō-sĭs)	_____
6–34	[] tracheostomy	(trā-kē-ŎS-tō-mē)	_____
6–35	[] tracheotomy	(trā-kē-ŎT-ō-mē)	_____
6–120	[] tuberculosis	(tū-bĕr-kū-LŌ-sĭs)	_____
6–108	[] upper respiratory infection		_____
Additional Pathological Conditions	[] wheezes	(HWĒZ-ĕz)	_____

Unit Exercises

DEFINITIONS

Review Unit 6 Summary (pages 275–277) before completing this exercise. Write the definition for each element.

SUFFIXES AND PREFIXES

Element	Meaning
SURGICAL SUFFIXES	
1. -centesis	_____
2. -plasty	_____
3. -rrhaphy	_____
4. -tome	_____
5. -tomy	_____
6. -cele	_____
7. -ectasis	_____
8. -logist	_____
9. -malacia	_____
10. -phagia	_____
11. -phobia	_____
12. -plasm	_____
13. -plegia	_____
15. -rrhagia	_____
16. -stenosis	_____
PREFIXES	
17. epi-	_____
18. neo-	_____

COMBINING FORMS RELATED TO THE RESPIRATORY SYSTEM

Element	Meaning
19. bronch/o, bronchi/o	_____
20. chondr/o	_____
21. nas/o	_____
22. pharyng/o	_____
23. pleur/o	_____
24. pneum/o, pneumon/o	_____
25. rhin/o	_____
26. thorac/o	_____
27. trache/o	_____

OTHER COMBINING FORMS IN UNIT 6

Element	Meaning
28. aer/o	_____
29. cacin/o	_____
30. hem/o	_____
31. melan/o	_____
32. muc/o	_____
33. myc/o	_____
34. or/o	_____
35. orth/o	_____

VALIDATION FRAME: Check your answers in the Index of Medical Word Elements, Part A of Appendix A. If you scored less than _____ %,* review Unit 6 Respiratory System Summary (pages 275–277) and retake this exercise.

To obtain a percentage score, multiply the number of correct answers times 2.86.

Number of Correct Answers: _____   **Percentage Score:** _____

*Enter the percentage required by your instructor to complete this course.

Vocabulary

Match the medical word(s) below with the definitions in the numbered list.

aerophagia
anesthesia
apnea
aspiration
asthma
chondroma
chronic obstructive lung disease (COLD)

croup
diagnosis
hepatocarcinoma
meatus
necropsy
neopathy
pharyngoplegia

pleurisy
Pneumocystis carinii
polyp
rhinoplasty
snare
tuberculosis (TB)

1. _____ Autopsy, postmortem examination.

2. _____ Passage or opening.

3. _____ Respiratory condition marked by recurrent attacks of difficult or labored breathing accompanied by wheezing.

4. _____ Upper respiratory infection with stridor that occurs most frequently in children.

5. _____ Tumor with a pedicle.

6. _____ The use of scientific methods and medical skill to establish the cause and nature of a person's illness.

7. _____ Temporary cessation of breathing.

8. _____ Swallowing air.

9. _____ Using suction to remove fluids from a body cavity.

10. _____ Cartilaginous tumor.

11. _____ Cancerous tumor of the liver.

12. _____ New disease.

13. _____ Paralysis of muscles of the pharynx.

14. _____ Inflammation of the pleura.

15. _____ Type of pneumonia seen in patients with AIDS and in debilitated children.

16. _____ Device for excision of polyps and tumors by tightening wire loops around them.

17. _____ Surgical repair or plastic surgery of the nose.

18. _____ Presence of small lesions or tubercles in the lungs.

19. _____ Group of respiratory disorders characterized by chronic, partial obstruction of bronchi and lungs.

20. _____ Loss of feeling or sensation.

VALIDATION FRAME: Check your answers in Appendix B, Answer Key. If you scored less than _____ %, review the vocabulary and retake the exercise.

To obtain a percentage score, multiply the number of correct answers times 5.

Number of Correct Answers: _____   **Percentage Score:** _____

Additional Pathological Conditions

Match these medical word(s) with the definitions in the numbered list.

acidosis
adult respiratory distress syndrome (ARDS)
atelectasis
coryza
croup
cystic fibrosis (CF)
empyema

epiglottitis
epistaxis
hypoxia
influenza
lung cancer
pertussis
pleural effusion

pneumothorax
rales
rhonchi
sudden infant death syndrome (SIDS)
stridor
wheezes

1. _____ High-pitched breathing sound resembling the blowing of wind caused by obstruction of air passages.

2. _____ Nosebleed.

3. _____ Contagious respiratory infection characterized by onset of fever, chills, headache and muscle pain.

4. _____ Excessive acidity of body fluids. In the respiratory system it is caused by abnormally high levels of CO_2 in the body.

5. _____ A cold.

6. _____ Genetic disease of the exocrine glands with production of excessive mucus, causing severe congestion within the lungs and digestive systems.

7. _____ Pulmonary malignancy attributable to cigarette smoking.

8. _____ Abnormal presence of fluid in the pleural cavity.

9. _____ Accumulation of air in the pleural cavity.

10. _____ Crackling sound heard with stethoscope on inspiration.

11. _____ Collection of pus in the pleural space.

12. _____ A form of restrictive lung disease that follows severe infection or trauma in young and previously healthy individuals.

13. _____ Acute respiratory syndrome in children and infants, characterized by a resonant barking cough or stridor and severe dyspnea.

14. _____ Collapsed lung.

15. _____ Severe life-threatening infection of the epiglottis that occurs most often in children.

16. _____ Acute infectious disease characterized by an explosive cough; also called whooping cough.

17. _____ Whistling sound heard usually during expiration; caused by narrowing of an airway.

18 _____ Unexpected and unexplained death of an apparently well, or virtually well, infant.

19. _____ A deficiency of oxygen.

20. _____ Abnormal chest sounds resembling snoring, produced in obstructed airways.

VALIDATION FRAME: Check your answers in Appendix B, Answer Key. If you scored less than _____ %, review the vocabulary and retake the exercise.

To obtain a percentage score, multiply the number of correct answers times 5.

Number of Correct Answers: _____   **Percentage Score:** _____

Unit Summary

COMBINING FORMS RELATED TO THE RESPIRATORY SYSTEM

Combining Form	Pronunciation	Meaning
bronch/o bronchi/o	brŏng-kō brŏng-kē-ō	bronchus (plural: bronchi)
chondr/o	kŏn-drō	cartilage
epiglott/o	ĕp-ĭ-glŏt-ō	epiglottis
nas/o rhin/o	nā-zō rī-nō	nose
or/o	ōr-ō	mouth
pharyng/o	fă-rĭng-gō	pharynx (throat)
pleur/o	ploo-rō	pleura
pneum/o pneumon/o	nū-mō nū-mō-nō	lung, air
pulmon/o	pŭl-mō-nō	lung
sinus/o	sī-nŭs	sinus, cavity
thorac/o	thō-răk-ō	chest
tonsill/o	tŏn-sĭl-ō	tonsils
trache/o	trā-kē-ō	trachea (windpipe)

OTHER COMBINING FORMS IN UNIT 6

Combining Form	Pronunciation	Meaning
aer/o	ēr-ō	air
carcin/o	kăr-sĭn-ō	cancer
gastr/o	găs-trō	stomach
hem/o	hēm-ō	blood
hepat/o	hĕp-ă-tō	liver
hydr/o	hī-drō	water
melan/o	mĕl-ă-nō	black
muc/o	mū-kō	mucus
myc/o	mī-kō	fungus
my/o	mī-ō	muscle
odont/o	ō-dŏn-tō	teeth
or/o	ōr-ō	mouth
orth/o	ōr-thō	straight

SUFFIXES AND PREFIXES

Suffix (Prefix)	Pronunciation	Meaning
NOUN AND ADJECTIVE-ENDING SUFFIXES		
-ia	ē-ă	condition
-ist	ĭst	specialist
-ous	ŭs	pertaining to
SURGICAL SUFFIXES		
-centesis	sĕn-tē-sīs	surgical puncture
-ectomy	ĕk-tō-mē	excision, removal
-plasty	plăs-tē	surgical repair
-rrhaphy	ră-fē	suture
-tome	tōm	instrument to cut
-tomy	tō-mē	incision, cut into
OTHER SUFFIXES		
-algia -dynia	ăl-jē-ă dīn-ē-ă	pain
-cele	sēl	hernia, swelling
-ectasis	ĕk-tā-sĭs	expansion, dilation
-itis	ī-tĭs	inflammation
-logist	lō-jĭst	specialist in the study of
-malacia	mă-lā-shē-ă	softening
-oma	ō-mă	tumor
-osis	ō-sĭs	abnormal condition
-pathy	pă-thē	disease
-phagia	fă-jē-ă	swallow, eat
-phobia	fō-bē-ă	fear
-plasm	plăzm	formation, growth
-plegia	plē-jē-ă	paralysis
-pnea	nē-ă	breathing
-rrhagia	ră-jē-ă	bursting forth (of)
-scope	skōp	instrument to view
-scopy	skŏ-pē	visual examination
-spasm	spăzm	involuntary contraction, twitching
-stenosis	stĕ-nō-sĭs	stricture, narrowing
-therapy	thĕr-ă-pē	treatment

Suffix (Prefix)	Pronunciation	Meaning
PREFIXES		
epi-	ĕp-ĭ	above, upon
eu-	ū	good, normal
macro-	mă-krō	large
micro-	mī-krō	small
neo-	nē-ō	new
peri-	pĕr-ĭ	around

Endocrine and Nervous Systems

The endocrine and nervous systems work together like an interlocking supersystem to control many intricate activities of the body.

The ductless glands of the endocrine system produce specific effects on body functions by slowly releasing chemical substances called hormones into the bloodstream (Fig. 7–1).

In contrast, the nervous system is designed to act instantaneously through the transmission of electrical impulses to specific body locations (Figs. 7–2 to 7–4).

The combining forms related to the endocrine system are summarized here. Review this information before you begin to work the frames.

Endocrine System

COMBINING FORMS

Combining Form	Meaning	Example	Pronunciation
aden/o	gland	aden/oma tumor	ăd-ĕ-NŌ-mă
adrenal/o	adrenal gland	adrenal/ectomy excision	ăd-rē-năl-ĔK-tō-mē
adren/o		adren/al pertaining to	ăd-RĒ-năl
calc/o	calcium	calc/emia blood	kăl-SĒ-mē-ă
gluc/o	sugar, glucose	gluc/o/genesis producing, forming	gloo-kō-JĔN-ă-sĭs
glyc/o		hyper/glyc/emia excessive blood	hī-pĕr-glī-SĒ-mē-ă
pancreat/o	pancreas	pancreat/itis inflammation	păn-krē-ăt-Ī-tĭs
thym/o	thymus	thym/oma tumor	thī-MŌ-mă
thyroid/o	thyroid gland	thyroid/ectomy excision	thī-royd-ĔK-tō-mē

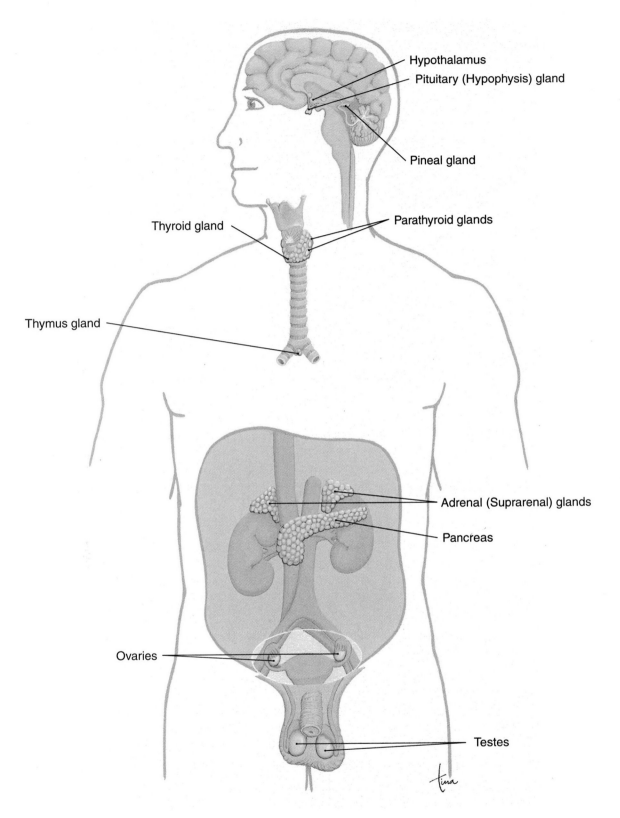

Figure 7–1. Locations of the many endocrine glands. Both male and female gonads (testes and ovaries) are shown. (From Scanlon, VC, and Sanders, T: Understanding Human Structure and Function. FA Davis, Philadelphia, 1997, p 178, with permission.)

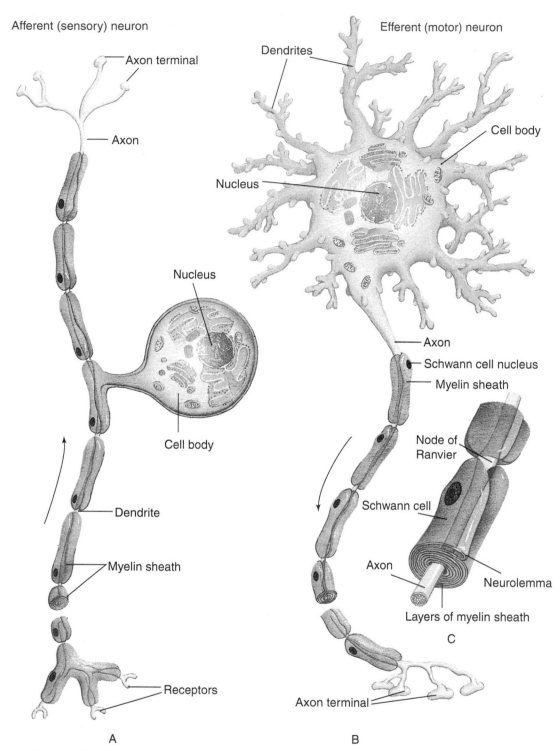

Afferent (sensory) neuron

Efferent (motor) neuron

Axon terminal

Axon

Nucleus

Cell body

Dendrites

Cell body

Nucleus

Axon

Schwann cell nucleus

Myelin sheath

Node of Ranvier

Dendrite

Schwann cell

Myelin sheath

Axon

Neurolemma

Layers of myelin sheath

Receptors

Axon terminal

A

B

C

Figure 7–2. (A) A typical sensory neuron. (B) A typical motor neuron. The arrows indicate the direction of impulse transmission. (C) Details of the myelin sheath and neurolemma formed by Schwann cells. (From Scanlon, VC, and Sanders, T: Understanding Human Structure and Function. FA Davis, Philadelphia, 1997, p 131, with permission.)

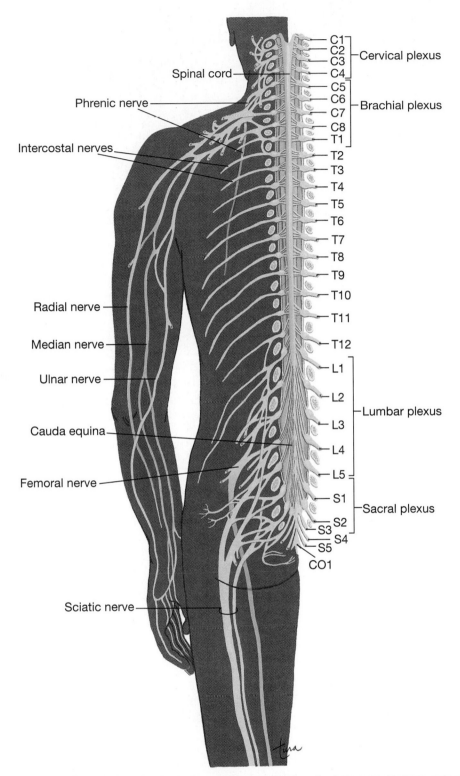

Figure 7–3. The spinal cord and spinal nerves. The distribution of spinal nerves is shown only on the left side. The nerve plexuses are labeled on the right side. A nerve plexus is a network of neurons from several segments of the spinal cord that combine to form nerves to specific parts of the body. For example, the radial and ulnar nerves to the arm emerge from the brachial plexus. (From Scanlon, VC, and Sanders, T: Understanding Human Structure and Function. FA Davis, Philadelphia, 1997, p 137, with permission.)

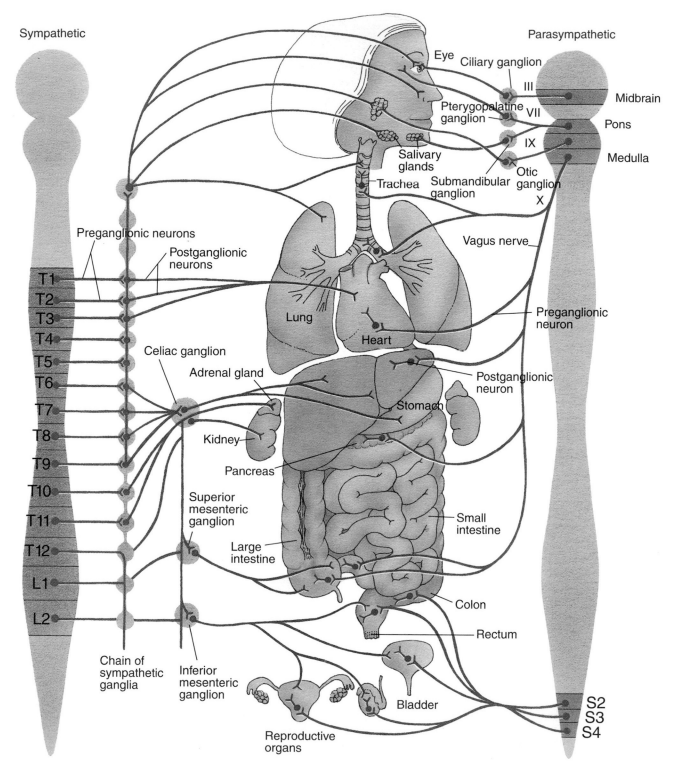

Sympathetic

Parasympathetic

Eye Ciliary ganglion

III

Midbrain

Pterygopalatine
ganglion VII

Pons

Salivary
glands

IX

Medulla

Trachea

Submandibular
ganglion

Otic
ganglion

X

Preganglionic neurons

Postganglionic
neurons

Vagus nerve

T1
T2
T3
T4
T5
T6
T7
T8
T9
T10
T11
T12
L1
L2

Lung

Heart

Preganglionic
neuron

Celiac ganglion

Adrenal gland

Stomach

Postganglionic
neuron

Kidney

Pancreas

Superior
mesenteric
ganglion

Large
intestine

Small
intestine

Chain of
sympathetic
ganglia

Inferior
mesenteric
ganglion

Colon

Rectum

S2
S3
S4

Bladder

Reproductive
organs

Figure 7–4. The autonomic nervous system. The sympathetic division is shown on the left and parasympathetic division is shown on the right (both divisions are bilateral). (From Scanlon, VC, and Sanders,
T: Understanding Human Structure and Function. FA Davis, Philadelphia, 1997, p 150, with permission.)

7-1 Use the Index of Medical Word Elements, Part A of Appendix A, to define the following elements.

Medical Word Element	Meaning
aden/o	_____
anter/o	_____
-gen , -genesis	_____
hyper-	_____
hypo-	_____
-megaly	_____
neur/o	_____

7-2 Although all major hormones circulate to virtually all tissues, each hormone exerts specific effects on a certain organ, referred to as its target organ.

If a hormone has a specific effect on the stomach, then that hormone's target organ is the stomach. If the hormone has a specific effect on the heart, then the

heart

target organ is the _____ .

7-3 Dys/function of an endocrine gland may result in either hypo/secretion or hyper/secretion of its hormone. Remember that the prefix hyper- denotes excessive. The prefix hypo-, on the other hand, denotes deficient, below, or under.

Identify the medical terms in this frame that mean

hyper/secretion
(hī-pĕr-sē-KRĒ-shŭn)
hypo/secretion
(hī-pō-sē-KRĒ-shŭn)

excessive secretion: _____ / _____

deficient secretion: _____ / _____

---

bad, painful

difficult

7-4 The prefix dys- means _____ , _____ , or

_____ .

7-5 Refer to Table 7-1 to complete Frames 7-5 and 7-6.
Define the term _hormone_.

_____

_____

_____

_____

7-6 List two common characteristics of hormones.

1. _____

_____

_____

2. _____

_____

_____

TABLE 7–1 **DEFINITION AND CHARACTERISTICS OF HORMONES**

♦ Hormones are chemical substances produced by specialized cells of the body.
♦ Hormones are released slowly in minute amounts directly into the bloodstream.
♦ Hormones are produced primarily by the endocrine glands.
♦ Most hormones are inactivated or excreted by the liver and kidneys.

Pituitary Gland

7–7   The **(1) pituitary gland** is the most important endocrine (hormone-secreting) gland. Located below the brain, it is no larger than a pea.

Label the pituitary gland in Figure 7–5.

---

hypo/secretion
(hī-pō-sē-KRĒ-shŭn)
hyper/secretion
(hī-pĕr-sē-KRĒ-shŭn)

7–8   Disorders of the endocrine glands are based on hypo/secretion or hyper/secretion of hormones.

Identify the words in this frame that are synonymous with

underproduction or deficiency: _____ / _____

overproduction or excessive: _____ / _____

---

posterior
(pŏs-TĒ-rē-or)

7–9   **Anter/o** and **poster/o** are combining forms. **Anter/o** means front or anterior; **poster/o** means back (of body), behind, or posterior.

Anterior is the opposite of _____ .

---

anterior
(ăn-TĒ-rē-or)
posterior
(pŏs-TĒ-rē-or)

7–10   The pituitary gland consists of two distinct portions—an anterior lobe and a posterior lobe.

The front lobe is called the _____ lobe.

The back lobe back is called the _____ lobe.

---

anter/o

poster/o

7–11   Identify the combining forms meaning

front or anterior: _____ / _____

back (of body), behind, or posterior: _____ / _____

---

back

7–12   The directional term anter/o/posterior means passing from the front to the _____ .

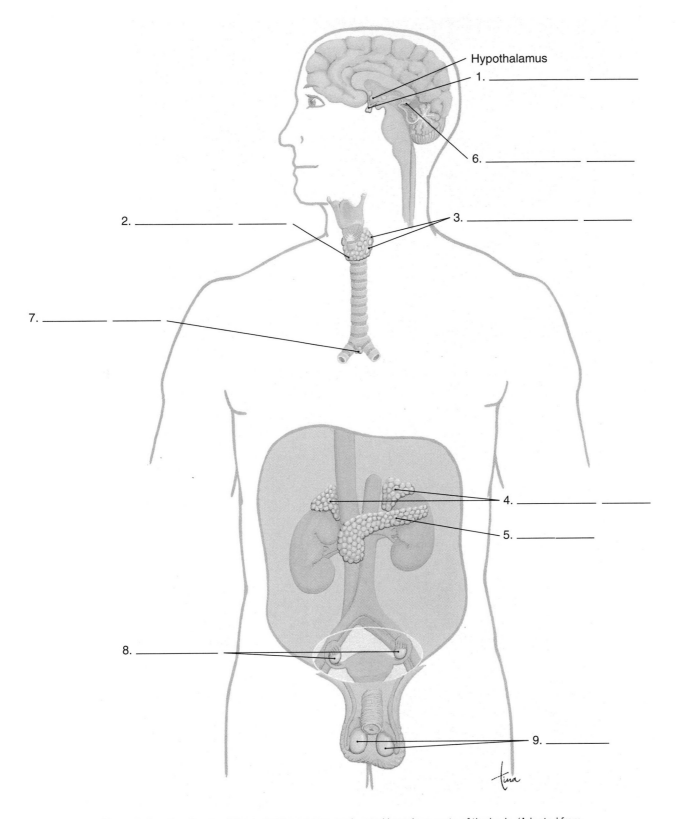

Hypothalamus

1. _____ _____

6. _____ _____

2. _____ _____

3. _____ _____

7. _____

4. _____ _____

5. _____

8. _____

9. _____

Figure 7–5. The glands of the endocrine system are located in various parts of the body. (Adapted from Scanlon, VC, and Sanders, T: Understanding Human Structure and Function. FA Davis, Philadelphia, 1997, p 178, with permission.)

radi/o	**7-13** Anter/o/posterior (AP) is used in radi/o/logy to describe the direction or path of an x-ray beam. From radi/o/logy, determine the combining form for x-ray or radiation: _____ / _____ .
posterior (pŏs-TĒ-rē-or)	**7-14** An AP view of the abdomen is a view from the anterior to the _____ part of the abdomen.
AP PA	**7-15** Poster/o/anterior (PA) means directed from the back toward the front (of the body). Identify the abbreviations that designate the path of an x-ray beam from the anterior to posterior of the body: _____ the posterior to the anterior of the body: _____
above below	**7-16** Use the words **above** or **below** to complete this frame. Poster/o/superior is a directional term meaning located behind and _____ a structure. Poster/o/inferior is a directional term meaning located behind and _____ a structure.
gland	**7-17** The pituitary gland is also known as the hypophysis. The anterior lobe of the pituitary gland is called the aden/o/hypophysis; the posterior lobe is called the neur/o/hypophysis. The combining form **neur/o** refers to nerve; the combining form **aden/o** refers to _____ .
anterior (ăn-TĒ-rē-or) posterior (pŏs-TĒ-rē-or) neur/o/hypophysis (nū-rō-hī-PŎF-ĭs-ĭs) aden/o/hypophysis (ăd-ĕ-nō-hī-PŎF-ĭ-sĭs)	**7-18** The anterior lobe, or aden/o/hypophysis, is composed of glandular tissue. The posterior lobe, or neur/o/hypophysis, is composed of nervous tissue. Both lobes secrete various hormones that regulate body functions. Identify the *words* in this frame that mean in front of: _____ behind, back (of body): _____ hypophysis composed or nervous tissue: _____ / _____ / _____ hypophysis composed of glandular tissue: _____ / _____ / _____

neur/o/hypophysis (nū-rō-hī-PŎF-ĭs-ĭs)	**7–19** The posterior lobe of the pituitary gland, composed primarily of nervous tissue, is called _____ / ____ / _____ .

aden/o/hypophysis (ăd-ē-nō-hī-PŎF-ĭ-sĭs)	**7–20** The anterior lobe of the pituitary gland, composed primarily of glandular tissue, is called _____ / ____ / _____ .

Hormones of the Pituitary Gland

7–21 Refer to Table 7–2 to complete Frames 7–21 through 7–26.

The two hormones produced by the neur/o/hypophysis are

_____ _____ and

_____ .

7–22 Define the following abbreviations:

GH _____

TSH _____

ADH _____

TABLE 7–2 HORMONES OF THE PITUITARY GLAND

Gland	Hormone	Function(s)
Adenohypophysis (anterior lobe)	Growth hormone (GH)	Stimulates bone and body growth
	Thyroid-stimulating hormone (TSH), or thyrotropin	Controls secretions of hormones from the thyroid gland
	Prolactin	Promotes growth of breast tissue Stimulates milk production after birth
	Adrenocorticotropic hormone (ACTH)	Stimulates secretions by the adrenal cortex, especially cortisol
	Follicle-stimulating hormone (FSH)	Stimulates development of eggs in the ovaries Stimulates secretion of estrogen in women Stimulates production of sperm cells in the testes
	Luteinizing hormone (LH), or interstitial cell-stimulating hormone (ICSH) in men	Promotes the secretion of sex hormones in both men and women Plays a role in the release of the egg cell in women
Neurohypophysis (posterior lobe)	Antidiuretic hormone (ADH)	Decreases volume of urine excreted Increases volume of water reabsorbed in kidney
	Oxytocin	Causes contraction of the uterus during labor and childbirth Stimulates milk secretion

Source: From Gylys, BA, and Wedding, ME: *Medical Terminology: A Systems Approach*, ed 3. FA Davis, Philadelphia, 1995, p 296, with permission.

7–23 Briefly state two functions of the ADH.

_____

_____

_____

_____

_____

_____

7–24 Briefly state two functions of the GH.

_____

_____

7–25 The hormone that causes contraction of the uterus during childbirth is

_____ .

7–26 Write the abbreviation of the hormone that initiates sperm production in men: _____

7–27 Overproduction of GH produces an exceptionally large person, a condition known as giant/ism. Underproduction of GH is likely to produce an exceptionally small person, a condition called dwarf/ism.

dwarf

giant

An abnormally short or undersized person is known as a _____ ; an abnormally tall or oversized person is known as a _____ .

enlargement

extremities

7–28 **Acr/o** is the combining form for extremities.

Acr/o/megaly is an _____ of the

_____ (Fig. 7–6).

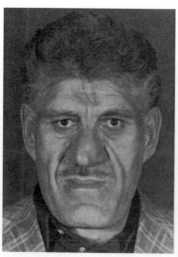 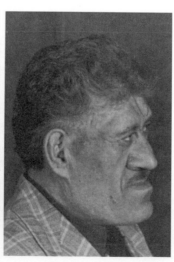

Figure 7–6. Acromegaly in a 56-year-old man. (From Martin, JB, Reichlin, S, and Brown, GM: Clinical Neuroendocrinology. FA Davis, Philadelphia, 1977, p 353, with permission.)

acr/o/megaly (ăk-rō-MĔG-ă-lē)	**7–29** Hyper/secretion of the aden/o/hypophysis after puberty results in an enlargement of the extremities or _____ / _____ / _____ .

acr/o/megaly (ăk-rō-MĔG-ă-lē)	**7–30** Acr/o/megaly is characterized by overgrowth of bones and soft tissue (see Fig. 7–6). A person with enlarged bones of the hands and feet, as well as some bones of the head, has an enlargement of the extremities. This is called _____ / _____ / _____ .

inflammation, skin extremities	**7–31** Acr/o/dermat/itis is an _____ of the _____ of the _____ .

extremities	**7–32** Acr/o/hyper/hidr/osis literally means an abnormal condition of excessive perspiration of the _____ .

acr/o/pathy (ăk-KRŎP-ă-thē)	**7–33** Form a word meaning any disease of the extremities: _____ / _____ / _____

7–34 Use the Index of Medical Word Elements, Part A of Appendix A, to define the following elements.

Medical Word Element	*Meaning*
-emia	_____
enter/o	_____
-ism	_____
neur/o	_____
toxic/o	_____

Thyroid Gland

7–35 The **(2) thyroid gland** is located on the front and sides of the trachea just below the larynx. Its two lobes are separated by a strip of tissue called the isthmus.

Label the thyroid gland in Figure 7–5.

thyroid/ectomy (thī-royd-ĔK-tō-mē)	**7–36** The combining forms for the thyroid gland are **thyr/o** and **thyroid/o**. Use thyroid/o to form a word meaning excision of the thyroid gland: _____ / _____ .

thyr/o/megaly
(thī-rō-MĔG-ă-lē)
thyr/o/pathy
(thī-RŎP-ă-thē)
thyr/o/tomy
(thī-RŎT-ō-mē)

7–37   Use **thyr/o** to construct words meaning

enlargement of the thyroid gland: _____ / _____ / _____

disease of the thyroid gland: _____ / _____ / _____

incision of the thyroid gland: _____ / _____ / _____

7–38   Refer to Table 7–3 to complete Frames 7–38 through 7–40. The thyroid gland produces two hormones that regulate the body's metabolism (rate at which food is converted into heat and energy).

These hormones are called _____ and

_____ .

7–39   Calcium and phosphate levels in the blood are controlled by the

hormone _____ .

7–40   The three hormones produced by the thyroid gland are:

_____ , _____ , and

_____ .

excessive

thyroid gland
(THĪ-royd GLĂND)

condition

7–41   Hyper/thyroid/ism is caused by excessive secretion of the thyroid gland, which increases the body's metabolism and intensifies the demand for food.

Analyze hyper/thyroid/ism by defining the elements.

Hyper- means _____ .

thyroid/o means _____ _____ .

-ism means _____ .

toxic
(TŎKS-ĭk)
thyr/o, thyroid

hyper-

7–42   Thyr/o/toxic/osis, also known as hyper/thyroid/ism, is a poisonous condition caused by hyper/activity of the thyroid gland.

Write the elements in this frame that mean

poison: _____

thyroid: _____ / _____ or _____

excessive: _____

TABLE 7–3   HORMONES OF THE THYROID GLAND

Hormone	Function(s)
Thyroxine and triiodothyronine	♦ Regulates metabolism of the body ♦ Increases energy production from all food types ♦ Increases rate of protein synthesis
Calcitonin	♦ Decreases reabsorption of calcium and phosphate from bones to blood

7–43   Toxic/o/logy is the scientific study of poisons, and the treatment of the conditions produced by them.

A specialist in the study of poisons is called a

_____ / _____ / _____ .

toxic/o/logist
(toks-i-KŎL-ō-jĭst)

---

poison

7–44   Toxic/o/pathy is any disease caused by _____ .

---

thyroid/o/tomy
(thī-royd-ŎT-ō-mē)
thyroid/o/tome
(thī-ROI-dō-tōm)

7–45   Use **thyroid/o** to formulate words meaning

incision of the thyroid gland: _____ / _____ / _____

instrument to incise the thyroid: _____ / _____ / _____

---

blood

7–46   The combining form for calcium is **calc/o**. The term calc/emia indicates

calcium in the _____ .

---

hyper/calc/emia
(hī-pĕr-kăl-SĒ-mē-ă)

7–47   Hypo/calc/emia is a condition of abnormally low blood calcium. A person with excessively high blood calcium has a condition called

_____ / _____ / _____ .

Review

Select the medical word element(s) that match(es) the meaning.

acr/o
aden/o
anter/o
calc/o
dermat/o
hidr/o
neur/o
poster/o
radi/o
thyr/o
thyroid/o
toxic/o

-ectomy
-emia
-logist
-logy
-megaly
-osis
-pathy
-tome
-tomy

dys-
hyper-
hypo-

a. _____ abnormal condition

b. _____ excessive

c. _____ back (of body), behind, posterior

d. _____ bad, painful, difficult

e. _____ blood

f. _____ calcium

g. _____ disease

h. _____ enlargement

i. _____ extremities

j. _____ front, anterior

k. _____ gland

l. _____ incision, cut into

m. _____ instrument to cut

n. _____ nerve

o. _____ poison

p. _____ radiation, x-ray

q. _____ skin

r. _____ specialist in the study of

s. _____ study of

t. _____ sweat

u. _____ thyroid gland

v. _____ under, below

Check your answers with the Review Answer Key on the following page.

Review Answer Key

a. -osis

b. hyper-

c. poster/o

d. dys-

e. -emia

f. calc/o

g. -pathy

h. -megaly

i. acr/o

j. anter/o

k. aden/o

l. -tomy

m. -tome

n. neur/o

o. toxic/o

p. radi/o

q. dermat/o

r. -logist

s. -logy

t. hidr/o

v. thyroid/o, thyr/o

v. hypo-

REINFORCEMENT FRAME: If you are not satisfied with your level of comprehension, go back to Frame 7–1 and rework the frames.

Parathyroid Glands

7-48 Four **(3) parathyroid glands** are located on the posterior surface of the thyroid gland. The parathyroid glands are so called because they are located around the thyroid gland.

Label the parathyroid glands in Figure 7–5.

---

para-

7-49 Identify the element in para/thyroid that means located near, beside, around: _____ .

---

inflammation

bladder

7-50 Para/cyst/itis is an _____ around the

_____ .

---

para/hepat/itis
(păr-ă-hĕp-ă-TĪ-tĭs)

7-51 Construct a medical word meaning inflammation around the liver:

_____ / _____ / _____ .

PTH

7-52 The hormone produced by the four para/thyroid glands is called para/thormone or para/thyroid hormone (PTH).

Write the abbreviation for para/thormone or parathyroid hormone: _____ .

7-53 Refer to Table 7–4 to complete this frame. The major function of PTH is to

regulate levels of _____ and _____ .

---

nephr/o, ren/o

enter/o

7-54 Recall the combining forms for the following

kidney: _____ / _____ or _____ / _____

intestine: _____ / _____

---

hyper/calc/emia
(hī-pĕr-kăl-SĒ-mē-ă)
hypo/calc/emia
(hī-pō-kăl-SĒ-mē-ă)

7-55 Calc/emia refers to calcium in the blood.

Use hypo- and hyper- to form words meaning

excessive calcium in the blood: _____ / _____ / _____

deficiency of calcium in the blood: _____ / _____ / _____

TABLE 7-4 HORMONE OF THE PARATHYROID GLANDS

Hormone	Function(s)
Parathyroid hormone (PTH)	♦ Increases the reabsorption of calcium and phosphate from bone to blood ♦ Increases the reabsorption of calcium and the excretion of phosphate by the kidneys ♦ Increases absorption of calcium and phosphate by the small intestine

Adapted from Scanlon, VC, and Sanders, T: *Essentials of Anatomy and Physiology*, ed 2. FA Davis, Philadelphia, 1995, p 227.

Adrenal Glands

7–56 The **(4) adrenal glands**, also known as the **suprarenal glands**, are paired structures located superior to the kidneys.

Label Figure 7–5 as you continue to learn about the endocrine system.

---

supra/ren/al

superior

7–57 Indicate the words in Frame 7–56 that mean

above a kidney: _____ / _____ / _____

above: _____

---

enlargement

7–58 **Adren/o** and **adrenal/o** are combining forms for the adrenal glands. Adren/o/megaly is an _____ of the adrenal glands.

---

adrenal/ectomy
(ăd-rē-năl-ĔK-tō-mē)

7–59 Each adrenal gland is composed of two parts: the outer adrenal cortex and the inner adrenal medulla. The hormones produced by each part have different functions.

Use **adrenal/o** to form a word meaning an excision of an adrenal gland:

_____ / _____

7–60 Refer to Tables 7–5 and 7–6 to complete Frames 7–60 through 7–65.

The three hormones produced by the adrenal cortex are

_____ , _____ , and

_____ .

7–61 Identify the hormone produced by the adrenal cortex that

maintains secondary sex characteristics: _____

regulates the amount of salts in the body: _____

7–62 One of the hormones produced by the adrenal medulla is epinephrine, also called _____ .

TABLE 7–5   HORMONES OF THE ADRENAL MEDULLA

Hormone	Function(s)
Epinephrine (adrenaline)	♦ Increases heart rate and force of contraction ♦ Dilates bronchial tubes ♦ Increases conversion of glycogen to glucose in the liver ♦ Increases use of fats for energy
Norepinephrine (noradrenaline)	♦ Raises blood pressure and constricts vessels

TABLE 7–6 **HORMONES OF THE ADRENAL CORTEX**

Hormone	Function(s)
Aldosterone	♦ Regulates the amount of salts in the body
Cortisol	♦ Regulates the metabolism of carbohydrates, proteins, and fats
Androgens	♦ Maintain secondary sex characteristics

7–63 Epinephrine (or adrenaline) helps the body to cope with dangerous situations. Nerves transmit the message of fear to the glands, which react by rushing adrenaline to all parts of the system. Epinephrine is also called

_____ .

7–64 When a person is experiencing a stressful situation, the adrenal medulla produces adrenaline, also called _____ .

7–65 The hormone produced by the adrenal medulla that raises blood pressure is called _____ or _____ .

Pancreas (Islets of Langerhans)

7–66 The **(5) pancreas** is located posterior to the stomach. The hormone-producing cells of the pancreas are called islets of Langerhans (islet cells of the pancreas); they produce two hormones called insulin and glucagon. These two hormones play a role in the proper metabolism of sugars and starches in the body.

Label the pancreas in Figure 7–5.

pancreat/oma
(păn-krē-ă-TŌ-mă)
pancreat/o/lith
(păn-krē-ĂT-ō-lĭth)

pancreat/o/lith/iasis
(păn-krē-ăt-ō-lĭ-THĪ-ă-sĭs)
pancreat/o/pathy
(păn-krē-ă-TŎP-ă-thē)

7–67 Use **pancreat/o** (pancreas) to build medical words meaning

tumor of the pancreas: _____ / _____

calculus or stone in the pancreas: _____ / ___ / _____

abnormal condition of a pancreatic stone:

_____ / ___ / _____ / _____

disease of the pancreas: _____ / ___ / _____

pancreas
(PĂN-krē-ăs)

7–68 The suffix -lysis is used in words to mean separation, destruction, loosening. Pancreat/o/lysis is a destruction of the _____ .

TABLE 7–7 **HORMONES OF THE PANCREAS**

Hormone	Function(s)
Insulin	♦ Lowers blood sugar by promoting the movement of glucose to the body cells
Glucagon	♦ Increases blood sugar by stimulating the liver to convert glycogen to glucose

7–69 Refer to Table 7–7 to complete Frames 7–69 through 7–71.

The two hormones produced by the pancreas are _____

and _____ .

7–70 Determine the pancreat/ic hormone that does the following:

lowers blood sugar: _____

increases blood sugar: _____

7–71 How does insulin lower blood sugar?

_____

_____

glyc/o/gen
(GLĪ-kō-jĕn)

7–72 Glucose is the chief source of energy for living organisms. **Gluc/o** and **glyc/o** are combining forms that refer to sugar and glucose.

The suffix -gen refers to producing or forming.

Combine **glyc/o** and -gen to form a word meaning producing or forming sugar.

_____ / _____ / _____

gluc/o/genesis
(gloo-kō-JĔN-ĕ-sĭs)
glyc/o/genesis
(glī-kō-JĔN-ĕ-sĭs)

7–73 Use -genesis to form words that mean producing or forming sugar or glucose: _____ / _____ / _____ and

_____ / _____ / _____

-emia

hyper-

hypo-

glyc

7–74 Hyper/glyc/emia is an excessive amount of glucose or sugar in the blood. A deficiency of glucose or sugar in the blood is known as hypo/glyc/emia.

Identify the elements in this frame that mean

blood: _____

above or excessive: _____

under, below, deficient: _____

sugar or glucose: _____

hyper/glyc/emia (hī-pĕr-glī-SĒ-mē-ă)	**7–75** Because glucose, or sugar, provides energy, a person that continuously feels sluggish may have hypo/glyc/emia. A person who is energetic may have an excessive amount of glucose in the blood or _____ / _____ / _____ .
discharge or **flow, sugar or glucose**	**7–76** Glyc/o/rrhea is a _____ of _____ from the body by way of the urine.
-gen, -genesis	**7–77** Glyc/o/gen and glyc/o/genesis both mean producing or forming sugar. Identify the elements that mean producing or forming: _____ , _____ .
insulin (ĬN-sū-lĭn)	**7–78** Hyper/glyc/emia is seen in diabetes. This can occur if the pancreas does not produce sufficient amounts of insulin. When the pancreas does not produce enough insulin, the diabetic person reduces the amount of glucose in the blood by injecting the hormone called _____ .
urine or **urination**	**7–79** Diabetes is a general term for diseases characterized by excessive urination and usually refers to the more common condition, diabetes mellitus. Recall that poly/uria means excessive _____ .
hypo/glyc/emia (hī-pō-glī-SĒ-mē-ă)	**7–80** People with diabetes who use too much insulin have abnormally low blood sugar, the condition called _____ / _____ / _____ .
hypo/glyc/emia (hī-pō-glī-SĒ-mē-ă)	**7–81** Hyper/glyc/emia increases susceptibility to infection and often precedes diabetic coma. The opposite of hyper/glyc/emia is _____ / _____ / _____ .
poly/dipsia (pŏl-ē-DĬP-sē-ă) **poly/uria** (pŏl-ē-Ū-rē-ă) **poly/phagia** (pŏl-ē-FĂ-jē-ă)	**7–82** The suffix -dipsia denotes a condition of thirst. Poly/dipsia, poly/uria, and poly/phagia are three cardinal signs of diabetes mellitus. Write the words used in this frame that mean excessive thirst: _____ / _____ too much or excessive urination: _____ / _____ excessive eating: _____ / _____

poly/uria (pŏl-ē-Ū-rē-ă)	**7–83** When a person drinks too much water, he or she may experience a condition of excessive urination or _____ / _____ .

Pineal and Thymus Glands

7–84 The **(6) pineal** and **(7) thymus glands** are classified as endocrine glands but little is known about their endocrine function.

Label these structures in Figure 7–5.

thym/ectomy (thī-MĔK-tō-mē) thym/oma (thī-MŌ-mă) thym/o/pathy (thī-MŎP-ă-thē) thym/o/lysis (thī-MŎL-ĭ-sĭs)	**7–85** **Thym/o** is the combining form for the thymus gland. Build medical words meaning excision of the thymus gland: _____ / _____ tumor of the thymus gland: _____ / _____ disease of the thymus gland: _____ / ____ / _____ destruction of the thymus gland: _____ / ____ / _____

Ovaries and Testes

7–86 The **(8) ovaries** are a pair of small almond-shaped glands positioned in the upper pelvic cavity, one on each side of the uterus. The **(9) testes** are paired oval glands surrounded by the scrotal sac. The functions of the ovaries and testes are covered in Unit 5, Reproductive System.

Label the ovaries and testes in Figure 7–5.

oophor/o (ō-ŎF-ō-rō) orchid/o, orchi/o (ŌR-kĭ-dō, ŌR-kē-ō)	**7–87** Recall the combining forms for ovaries: _____ / ____ testes: _____ / ____ or _____ / ____

oophor/o/pathy (ō-ŏf-or-ŎP-ă-thē) oophor/o/tomy (ō-ŏf-or-ŎT-ō-mē)	**7–88** Construct medical words meaning disease of the ovary: _____ / ____ / _____ incision of the ovary: _____ / ____ / _____

orchid/o/pexy (ŌR-kĭd-ō-pĕk-sē)	**7–89** Use **orchid/o** to form a word meaning surgical fixation of a testis: _____ / ____ / _____

VALIDATION FRAME: Check your labeling of Figure 7–5 in Appendix B, Answer Key.

Review

Select the medical word element(s) that match(es) the meaning.

adrenal/o	-dipsia	hypo-
adren/o	-gen	para-
enter/o	-genesis	poly-
gluc/o	-iasis	supra-
glyc/o	-lith	
orchid/o	-lysis	
orchi/o	-oma	
pancreat/o	-pathy	
thym/o	-pexy	
	-phagia	
	-rrhea	
	-uria	

a. _____ abnormal condition (produced by something specified)

b. _____ above

c. _____ adrenal glands

d. _____ disease

e. _____ fixation, suspension

f. _____ flow, discharge

g. _____ many, much

h. _____ near, beside, around

i. _____ pancreas

j. _____ producing, forming

k. _____ separation, destruction

l. _____ stone, calculus

m. _____ sugar, glucose

n. _____ swallowing, eating

o. _____ testes

p. _____ thirst

q. _____ thymus gland

r. _____ under, below

s. _____ urine, urination

Check your answers with the Review Answer Key on the following page.

Review Answer Key

a. -iasis

b. supra-

c. adrenal/o, adren/o

d. -pathy

e. -pexy

f. -rrhea

g. poly-

h. para-

i. pancreat/o

j. -gen, -genesis

k. -lysis

l. -lith

m. glyc/o, gluc/o

n. -phagia

o. orchid/o, orchi/o

p. -dipsia

q. thym/o

r. hypo-

s. -uria

REINFORCEMENT FRAME: If you are not satisfied with your level of comprehension, go back to Frame 7–48 and rework the frames.

NERVOUS SYSTEM

The nervous system is divided into the central nervous system (CNS), which includes the brain and spinal cord, and the peripheral nervous system (PNS), which includes the cranial nerves, arising from the brain, and the spinal nerves, rising from the spinal cord (see Figs. 7–2 to 7–4).

Neurons are the basic structural and functional units of the nervous system (see Fig. 7–2). They are specialized to respond to physical and chemical stimuli, conduct electrochemical impulses, and release specific chemical regulators. Through these activities, neurons perform such functions as the perception of sensory stimuli, learning, memory, and the control of muscles and glands.

Neuroglia, or **glial cells**, do not carry impulses but perform the functions of support and protection. Many neuroglial cells form a supporting network by twining around nerve cells or lining certain structures in the brain and spinal cord. Others bind nervous tissue to supporting structures and attach the neurons to their blood vessels. Certain small glial cells are phagocytic; they protect the CNS from disease by engulfing invading microbes and clearing away debris. Neuroglia are of clinical interest because they are a common source of tumors (gliomas) of the nervous system.

The combining forms related to the nervous system are summarized here. Review this information before you begin to work the frames.

COMBINING FORMS

Combining Form	Meaning	Example	Pronunciation
cerebr/o	cerebrum (brain)	cerebr/o/spin/al spine pertaining to	sĕr-ĕ-brō-SPĪ-năl
encephal/o	brain	encephal/itis inflammation	ĕn-sĕf-ă-LĪ-tĭs
gli/o	glue or gluelike; neuroglial tissue (binding, supportive tissue of nervous system)	gli/oma tumor	glē-Ō-mă
mening/o	meninges	mening/o/cele hernia, protrusion	mĕn-ĬN-gō-sēl
meningi/o		meningi/oma tumor	mĕn-ĭn-jē-Ō-mă
myel/o	spinal cord, bone marrow	myel/o/gram record	MĪ-ĕ-lō-grăm
neur/o	nerve	neur/algia pain	nū-RĂL-jē-ă

7–90 Examine the Index of Medical Word Elements, Part B of Appendix A. Use it to learn the medical word element for each of the following English terms that are used in this unit.

English	*Medical Word Elements*
bursting forth (of)	_____ or
	_____
glue	_____
speech	_____
meninges	_____ / _____ or
	_____ / _____
spinal cord, bone marrow	_____ / _____

brain	**7–91** The combining form for the brain is **encephal/o**. Encephal/itis is an inflammation of the _____ .

encephal/oma (ĕn-sĕf-ă-LŌ-mă)	**7–92** Build a word meaning a tumor of the brain: _____ / _____

myel/itis (mī-ĕ-LĪ-tĭs) myel/oma (mī-ĕ-LŌ-mă) myel/o/malacia (mī-ĕ-lō-mă-LĀ-shē-ă)	**7–93** The combining form **myel/o** refers to the spinal cord or bone marrow. Form medical words meaning inflammation of the spinal cord: _____ / _____ tumor of the spinal cord: _____ / _____ softening of the spinal cord: _____ / _____ / _____

myel/o neur/o encephal/o	**7–94** The nervous system consists of the brain, spinal cord, and peripheral nerves. Together with the endocrine system, the nervous system coordinates and controls many body activities. Identify the combining forms related to the nervous system. spinal cord, bone marrow: _____ / _____ nerve: _____ / _____ brain: _____ / _____

cell	**7–95** The combining form **thromb/o** refers to a blood clot. A thromb/o/cyte is a blood-clotting _____ .

thromb/o/cyte (THRŎM-bō-sīt)	**7–96** A thromb/o/cyte (platelet) promotes the formation of clots and prevents bleeding. Another name for platelet is _____ / _____ / _____ .

clot	**7–97** Thromb/o/lysis is the destruction or loosening of a blood _____ .

thromb/o/genesis (thrŏm-bō-JĔN-ĕ-sĭs)	**7–98** Use -genesis to form a word meaning producing or forming of a blood clot. _____ / _____ / _____

7–99 A cerebr/o/vascul/ar accident (CVA), or stroke, is damage to a blood vessel in the brain, resulting in lack of oxygen to that part of the brain. A more general term, such as hem/o/rrhage or thromb/us, indicates the nature of the disturbance.

Write the terms in this frame that mean

bursting forth (of) blood: _____ / ____ / _____

pertaining to the cerebrum and blood vessels:

_____ / ____ / _____ / _____

blood clot: _____

hem/o/rrhage
(HĔM-ĕ-rĭj)

cerebr/o/vascul/ar
(sĕr-ĕ-brō-VĂS-kū-lăr)
thrombus
(THRŎM-bŭs)

hardening
abnormal condition

7–100 Recall that **scler/o** means _____ and -osis

means _____ _____ .

cerebr/o/scler/osis
(sĕr-ĕ-brō-sklĕ-RŌ-sĭs)

7–101 An abnormal condition of hardening of the cerebrum is called

_____ / ____ / _____ / _____ .

cerebr/oid
(SĔR-ĕ-broyd)

7–102 Construct a medical term meaning resembling the cerebrum:

_____ / _____

cerebr/al
(sĕr-Ē-brăl)

7–103 Cerebr/al palsy is a nonprogressive partial paralysis and lack of muscular coordination caused by damage to the cerebrum prior to or during the birth process.

Form a word meaning pertaining to the cerebrum: _____ / _____

7–104 Define *palsy*, using your medical dictionary.

_____

_____

a/phasia
(ă-FĀ-zē-ă)
dys/phasia
(dĭs-FĀ-zē-ă)

7–105 After a stroke, a person may lose partial or all speech.

Form medical words meaning

without speech: ____ / _____

bad or difficult speech: _____ / _____

meninges
(mĕn-ĬN-jēz)

7-106 The three layers of membranes that cover the brain and spinal cord are the meninges. **Mening/o** and **meningi/o** are combining forms for the

_____ .

---

mening/itis
(mĕn-ĭn-JĪ-tĭs)
mening/o/pathy
(mĕn-ĭn-GŎP-ă-thē)

7-107 Use **mening/o** to construct a word meaning

inflammation of the meninges: _____ / _____

disease of the meninges: _____ / _____ / _____

---

meningi/oma
(mĕn-ĭn-jē-Ō-mă)

7-108 Use **meningi/o** to form a word meaning tumor of the meninges:

_____ / _____ .

---

mening/o

-cele

7-109 A mening/o/cele is a hernia in which the meninges protrude through the opening of the skull or spinal cord.

Identify the elements that mean

meninges: _____ / _____

hernia, swelling: _____

---

blood

7-110 Recall that a hem/o/rrhage is a bursting forth (of) _____ .

-rrhagia, -rrhage

7-111 A hem/o/rrhage of the cerebr/al or spin/al membrane is called mening/o/rrhagia.

Write the word elements meaning bursting forth (of):

_____ and _____ .

---

spin/al
(SPĪ-năl)
cerebr/al
(sĕr-Ē-brăl)
mening/o/rrhagia
(mĕn-ĭn-gō-RĂ-jē-ă)

7-112 Determine the words in Frame 7–111 that mean

pertaining to the spine: _____ / _____

pertaining to the cerebrum: _____ / _____

bursting forth of the meninges: _____ / _____ / _____

---

neur/o/glia
(nū-RŎG-lē-ă)

7-113 In spite of its complexity, the entire nervous system is composed of nerve cells interspersed with glia cells.

Combine **neur/o** and -glia to construct a word that literally means nerve glue:

_____ / _____ / _____

inflammation, nerves	**7-114** Neur/itis is an _____ of _____ .
nerve	**7-115** Neur/o/dynia and neur/algia refer to pain in a _____ .
inflammation, nerves	**7-116** Neur/o/myel/itis is an _____ of _____ and spinal cord.
nervous	**7-117** A neur/o/hormone is a hormone that affects the function of the _____ system.
cell	**7-118** A neur/o/cyte is a nerve _____ .

Review

Select the combining form(s) that match(es) the meaning of each of the following terms.

encephal/o	-glia	a-
hem/o	-itis	dys-
mening/o	-malacia	
meningi/o	-oid	
myel/o	-oma	
neur/o	-osis	
scler/o	-phasia	
thromb/o	-rrhage	
vascul/o	-rrhagia	

a. _____ abnormal condition

b. _____ bad, painful, difficult

c. _____ blood

d. _____ blood clot

e. _____ blood vessel

f. _____ brain

g. _____ bursting forth (of)

h. _____ glue or gluelike

i. _____ hardening

j. _____ inflammation

k. _____ meninges

l. _____ nerve

m. _____ resembling

n. _____ softening

o. _____ speech

p. _____ spinal cord, bone marrow

q. _____ tumor

r. _____ without, not

Check your answers with the Review Answer Key on the following page.

Review Answer Key

a. -osis

b. dys-

c. hem/o

d. thromb/o

e. vascul/o

f. encephal/o

g. -rrhage, -rrhagia

h. -glia

i. scler/o

j. -itis

k. mening/o, meningi/o

l. neur/o

m. -oid

n. -malacia

o. -phasia

p. myel/o

q. -oma

r. a-

REINFORCEMENT FRAME: If you are not satisfied with your level of comprehension, go back to Frame 7–90 and rework the frames.

Additional Pathological Conditions

ENDOCRINE SYSTEM

Addison's disease (Ă-dĭ-sŭnz dĭ-ZĒZ) results from a deficiency in the secretion of adrenocortical (adrenal cortex) hormones.

Cushing's syndrome (KOOSH-ĭngz SĬN-drōm) excessive production of glucocorticoids caused by hypersecretion of the adrenal cortex.

exophthalmos (ĕks-ŏf-THĂL-mŏs) abnormal protrusion of eyeball. May be due to thyrotoxicosis, tumor of the orbit, orbital cellulitis, leukemia, or aneurysm.

Graves' disease (GRĀVZ dĭ-ZĒZ) hyperthyroidism, also called toxic goiter, involves growth of the thyroid associated with hypersecretion of thyroxine; characterized by exophthalmos (bulging of the eyes), which develops because of edema in the tissues of the eye sockets and swelling of the extrinsic eye muscles.

insulinoma (ĭn-sū-lĭn-Ō-mă) tumor of the islets of Langerhans of the pancreas.

myxedema (mĭks-ĕ-DĒ-mă) advanced hypothyroidism in adults resulting from hypofunction of the thyroid gland. This disorder affects body fluids, causing edema and increasing blood volume, thereby increasing blood pressure.

panhypopituitarism (păn-hī-pō-pĭ-TŪ-ĭ-tăr-ĭzm) total pituitary impairment that brings about a progressive and general loss of hormonal activity.

pheochromocytoma (fē-ō-krō-mō-sī-TŌ-mă) small chromaffin cell tumor, usually located in the adrenal medulla.

pituitarism (pĭ-TŪ-ĭ-tăr-ĭzm) any disorder of the pituitary gland and its function.

NERVOUS SYSTEM

Alzheimer's disease (ĂLTS-hī-mĕrz dĭ-ZĒZ) a chronic, organic mental disorder; a form of presenile dementia caused by atrophy of frontal and occipital lobes. Onset is usually between ages 40 and 60. Involves progressive irreversible loss of memory, deterioration of intellectual functions, apathy, speech and gait disturbances, and disorientation. Course may take from a few months to 4 or 5 years to progress to complete loss of intellectual function.

Bell's palsy (bĕlz pawl-ZĒ) facial paralysis caused by a functional disorder of the seventh cranial nerve and any or all of its branches. It may be unilateral, bilateral, transient, or permanent.

cerebrovascular accident (CVA) (sĕr-ĕ-brō-VĂS-kū-lăr ĂKS-ĭ-dĕnt) brain tissue damage caused by a disorder within the blood vessels; usually due to the formation of a clot or a ruptured blood vessel; the resulting functional deficit depends on the area of the brain affected; also called apoplexy, stroke, or CVA.

epilepsy (ĔP-ĭ-lĕp-sē) disorder affecting the central nervous system, characterized by recurrent seizures.

Huntington's chorea (HŬN-tĭng-tŭnz kō-RĒ-ă) hereditary nervous disorder caused by the progressive loss of brain cells, leading to bizarre, involuntary, dance-like movements.

hydrocephalus (hī-drō-SĔF-ă-lŭs) cranial enlargement caused by accumulation of fluid within the ventricles of the brain.

multiple sclerosis (MS) (MŬL-tĭ-pl sklĕ-RŌ-sĭs) a progressive degenerative disease of the CNS characterized by inflammation, hardening, and finally, loss of myelin throughout the spinal cord and brain, which produces weakness and other muscular symptoms.

neuroblastoma (nū-rō-blăs-TŌ-mă) a malignant tumor composed principally of cells resembling neuroblasts; occurs chiefly in infants and children.

palsy (PAWL-zē) partial or complete loss of motor function; paralysis.

Parkinson's disease (PĂR-kĭn-sŭnz dĭ-ZĒZ) a progressive, degenerative neurological disorder affecting the portion of the brain responsible for controlling movement. The unnecessary skeletal muscle movements often interfere with voluntary movement, causing the hand to shake. This shaking is called tremor, the most common symptom of Parkinson's disease.

poliomyelitis (pō-lē-ō-mī-ĕl-Ī-tĭs) inflammation of the gray matter of the spinal cord caused by a virus, often resulting in spinal and muscle deformity and paralysis.

sciatica (sī-ĂT-ĭ-kă) severe pain in the leg along the course of the sciatic nerve, which travels from the hip to the foot.

shingles (SHĬNG-lz) eruption of acute, inflammatory, herpetic vesicles on the trunk of the body along a peripheral nerve caused by herpes zoster virus.

spina bifida (SPĪ-nă BĬF-ĭ-dă) congenital defect characterized by incomplete closure of the spinal canal through which the spinal cord and meninges may or may not protrude. It usually occurs in the lumbosacral area and has several forms. **Spina bifida occulta** is the most common and least severe form of this defect; no protrusion of the spinal cord or meninges occurs in this form. **Spina bifida cystica** is a more severe type, involving protrusion of the meninges (**meningocele**), spinal cord (**myelocele**), or both (**meningomyelocele**).

transient ischemic attack (TRĂN-zhĕnt ĭs-KĒ-mĭk ă-TĂK) temporary interference with blood supply to the brain, lasting from a few minutes to a few hours.

Medical Record

The following medical reports are related to the medical specialties called endocrinology and neurology. An endocrinologist treats diseases and malfunctions of the endocrine glands (i.e., diabetes, thyroid disorders, obesity). A neurologist specializes in diagnosing and treating diseases and disorders of the central nervous system (CNS).

MEDICAL RECORD 7–1. Cerebrovascular Accident

Dictionary Exercise

This exercise will help you master the terminology in the medical record. Underline the following terms in the reading exercise and use a medical dictionary to define the words. The pronunciations of medical terms in this report are included in the Audiocassette Exercise on pages 317–319.

adenocarcinoma _____

anorexia _____

aphasia _____

biliary _____

cardiovascular _____

cholecystojejunostomy _____

CVA _____

deglutition _____

diagnosed _____

diplopia _____

Dx _____

jaundice _____

jejunojejunostomy _____

lesion _____

metastasis _____

metastatic _____

paralysis _____

pruritus _____

vertigo _____

Word Elements Exercise

Break down the following words into their basic elements:

adenocarcinoma
cardiovascular

cholecystojejunostomy
jejunojejunostomy

VALIDATION FRAME: Check your answers in Appendix B, Answer Key.

Reading Exercise

Read the case study out loud.

The patient is a moderately obese white woman who was admitted to Riverside Hospital because of a sudden episode of CVA. She recalls an episode of vertigo 3 days ago. The patient is being nursed at home by her daughter because of terminal adenocarcinoma of the head of the pancreas with metastasis to the liver, which was diagnosed in December. About 5 hours before the CVA, the patient fell to the floor with paralysis of the right arm and left leg and aphasia. She has not noticed any difficulty with deglutition. Apparently with the onset of the CVA attack she also experienced diplopia. She denies any difficulty with her cardiovascular system in the past. The patient was in the hospital 5 years ago because of generalized biliary type disease with jaundice, pruritus, weight loss, and anorexia. Subsequently, she was seen in consultation and cholecystojejunostomy and jejunojejunostomy was performed.

Dx: 1. CVA, probably secondary to metastatic lesion of the brain or **cerebrovascular** disease.

2. Evidence of the previously described deterioration secondary to carcinoma of the pancreas with metastases of the liver.

MEDICAL RECORD EVALUATION 7–1. Cerebrovascular Accident

1. What is a CVA?

2. Did the patient have a history of cardiovascular problems prior to her CVA?

3. What symptoms did the patient experience just prior to her CVA?

4. What is the primary site of this patient's cancer?

5. What is cerebrovascular disease?

6. What is the probable cause of the patient's CVA?

MEDICAL RECORD 7–2. Diabetes Mellitus

Dictionary Exercise

This exercise will help you master the terminology in the medical record. Underline the following terms in the reading exercise and use a medical dictionary to define the words. The pronunciations of medical terms in this report are included in the Audiocassette Exercise on pages 317–319.

diabetes mellitus _____

insulin-dependent diabetes mellitus _____

polydipsia _____

polyuria _____

glycosuria _____

electrolytes _____

WNL _____

ketones _____

BS _____

acidosis _____

insulin _____

fingersticks _____

Humulin L _____

Humulin R _____

glycemic _____

ADA _____

Reading Exercise

Read the case study out loud.

Admitting Diagnosis: Diabetes mellitus, new onset.

Discharge Diagnosis: Insulin-dependent diabetes mellitus, new onset.

History of Present Illness: This patient is a 15-year-old white boy who presented in the office complaining of increased appetite, polydipsia, and polyuria and was found to have elevated blood sugar of 400 and glycosuria. He was sent to the hospital for further evaluation and treatment.

Hospital Course: Upon admission, lab tests showed electrolytes WNL and ketones were negative. Urinalysis showed a trace of sugar, BS was 380, and there was no evidence of acidosis. Metabolically the patient was quite stable. Patient was started on split-mixed insulin dosing. The patient and his family received full diabetic instruction during his hospitalization and seemed to understand this very well. The patient picked up on all of this information quickly, asked appropriate questions, and appeared to be coping well with his new condition. By the 5th day his polyuria and polydipsia resolved. Once the patient was able to draw up and give his own insulin and perform his own fingersticks, he was discharged.

Discharge Instructions: The patient was discharged to home with parents, on a mixture of Humulin L 12 units and Humulin R 6 units each morning, with Humulin L 5 units and Humulin R 6 units each afternoon. He will continue with fingerstick BS four times daily at home until seen in the office for follow-up. I warned him of all glycemic symptoms to watch for, and he is to call the office with any problems that may occur. He is to follow an ADA 2000-calorie diet.

Discharge Condition: The patient's overall condition was much improved, and at the time of discharge BS levels were stabilized and he was doing well.

MEDICAL RECORD EVALUATION 7–2. Diabetes Mellitus

1. What symptoms of DM did the patient experience before his office visit?

2. What confirmed the patient's new diagnosis of DM?

3. What conditions had to be met before the patient could be discharged from the hospital?

4. How many times a day does the patient have to take insulin?

5. Why does the patient have to perform fingersticks four times a day?

6. What is an ADA 2000-calorie diet? Why is it important?

Abbreviations

Endocrine System

ADH	antidiuretic hormone	IDDM	insulin-dependent diabetes mellitus
AP	anteroposterior	LH	luteinizing hormone
BS	blood sugar	PA	posteroanterior
DM	diabetes mellitus	PGH	pituitary growth hormone
GH	growth hormone	PTH	parathyroid hormone
ICSH	interstitial cell-stimulating hormone	TSH	thyroid-stimulating hormone

Nervous System

CNS	central nervous system	EEG	electroencephalogram
CSF	cerebospinal fluid	EMG	electromyogram
CVA	cerebral vascular accident	LP	lumbar puncture
CVD	cerebrovascular disease	MRI	magnetic resonance imaging

Audiocassette Exercise

The audiocassette tape helps you master the pronunciation of medical words. Listen to the tape for instructions to complete this exercise. You may also use this list without the audiotape to practice correct pronunciation and spelling of the terms.

Frame	Word	Pronunciation	Spelling Exercise
7–31	[] acrodermatitis	(ăk-rō-děr-mă-TĪ-tĭs)	_____
7–32	[] acrohyperhidrosis	(ăk-rō-hī-pěr-hī-DRŌ-sĭs)	_____
7–28	[] acromegaly	(ăk-rō-MĔG-ă-lē)	_____
Reading Exercise	[] adenocarcinoma	(ăd-ĕ-nō-kăr-sĭn-Ō-mă)	_____
7–33	[] acropathy	(ă-KRŎP-ă-thē)	_____
7–17	[] adenohypophysis	(ăd-ĕ-nō-hī-PŎF-ĭ-sĭs)	_____
7–59	[] adrenalectomy	(ăd-rě-năl-ĔK-tō-mē)	_____
7–58	[] adrenomegaly	(ăd-rĕn-ō-MĔG-ă-lē)	_____
Reading Exercise	[] anorexia	(ăn-ō-RĔK-sē-ă)	_____
7–12	[] anteroposterior	(ăn-těr-ō-pŏs-TĒ-rē-ŏr)	_____
7–105	[] aphasia	(ă-FĀ-zē-ă)	_____
Reading Exercise	[] biliary	(BĬL-ē-ār-ē)	_____
Reading Exercise	[] carcinoma	(kăr-sĭn-Ō-mă)	_____
Reading Exercise	[] cardiovascular	(kăr-dē-ō-VĂS-kū-lăr)	_____
7–103	[] cerebral palsy	(SĔR-ĕ-brăl pawl-zē)	_____
7–102	[] cerebroid	(SĔR-ĕ-broyd)	_____
7–101	[] cerebrosclerosis	(sěr-ĕ-brō-sklĕ-RŌ-sĭs)	_____
Combining Forms	[] cerebrospinal	(sěr-ĕ-brō-SPĪ-năl)	_____
7–99	[] cerebrovascular accident	(sěr-ĕ-brō-VĂS-cū-lăr ĂKS-ĭ-děnt)	_____
Reading Exercise	[] cholecystojejunostomy	(kō-lē-sĭs-tō-jě-jū-NŎS-tō-mē)	_____
Reading Exercise	[] deglutition	(dē-gloo-TĬSH-ŭn)	_____
7–79	[] diabetes mellitus	(dī-ă-BĒ-tēz mě-LĪ-tŭs)	_____
Reading Exercise	[] diabetic	(dī-ă-BĔT-ĭk)	_____
Reading Exercise	[] diplopia	(dĭp-LŌ-pē-ă)	_____
7–105	[] dysphasia	(dĭs-FĀ-zē-ă)	_____
7–92	[] encephaloma	(ĕn-sĕf-ă-LŌ-mă)	_____
7–7	[] endocrine	(ĔN-dō-krĭn)	_____
7–72	[] glucose	(GLOO-kōs)	_____
7–72	[] glycogen	(GLĪ-kō-jěn)	_____
7–73	[] glycogenesis	(glī-kō-JĔN-ě-sĭs)	_____
7–76	[] glycorrhea	(glī-kō-RĒ-ă)	_____
Reading Exercise	[] glycosuria	(glī-kō-sū-RĒ-ă)	_____
7–99	[] hemorrhage	(HĔM-ě-rĭj)	_____
7–55	[] hypercalcemia	(hī-pěr-kăl-SĒ-mē-ă)	_____
7–78	[] hyperglycemia	(hī-pěr-glī-SĒ-mē-ă)	_____
7–41	[] hyperthyroidism	(hī-pěr-THĪ-royd-ĭzm)	_____
7–47	[] hypocalcemia	(hī-pō-kăl-SĒ-mē-ă)	_____
7–74	[] hypoglycemia	(hī-pō-glī-SĒ-mē-ă)	_____

Frame	Word	Pronunciation	Spelling Exercise
7–66	[] insulin	(ĬN-sū-lĭn)	_____
7–35	[] isthmus	(ĬS-mŭs)	_____
Reading Exercise	[] jaundice	(JAWN-dĭs)	_____
Reading Exercise	[] lesion	(LĒ-zhŭn)	_____
7–106	[] meninges	(mĕn-ĬN-jēz)	_____
7–108	[] meningioma	(mĕn-ĭn-jē-Ō-mă)	_____
7–107	[] meningitis	(mĕn-ĭn-JĪ-tĭs)	_____
7–109	[] meningocele	(mĕn-ĬN-gō-sēl)	_____
7–107	[] meningopathy	(mĕn-ĭn-GŎP-ă-thē)	_____
7–111	[] meningorrhagia	(mĕn-ĭn-gō-RĂ-jē-ă)	_____
7–38	[] metabolism	(mĕ-TĂB-ō-lĭzm)	_____
Reading Exercise	[] metastasis	(mĕ-TĂS-tă-sĭs)	_____
7–93	[] myelitis	(mī-ĕ-LĪ-tĭs)	_____
7–93	[] myeloma	(mī-ĕ-LŌ-mă)	_____
7–93	[] myelomalacia	(mī-ĕ-lō-mă-LĀ-sē-ă)	_____
7–115	[] neuralgia	(nū-RĂL-jē-ă)	_____
7–118	[] neurocyte	(NŪ-rō-sīt)	_____
7–115	[] neurodynia	(nū-rō-DĬN-ē-ă)	_____
7–113	[] neuroglia	(nū-RŎG-lē-ă)	_____
7–117	[] neurohormone	(NŪ-rō-hōr-mōn)	_____
7–17	[] neurohypophysis	(nū-rō-hī-PŎF-ĭs-ĭs)	_____
7–116	[] neuromyelitis	(nū-rō-mī-ĕ-LĪ-tĭs)	_____
7–89	[] orchidopexy	(ŌR-kĭd-ō-pĕk-sē)	_____
7–88	[] oophoropathy	(ō-ŏf-ōr-ŎP-ă-thē)	_____
7–88	[] oophorotomy	(ō-ŏf-ō-RŎT-ō-mē)	_____
7–21	[] oxytocin	(ŏk-sē-TŌ-sĭn)	_____
7–50	[] paracystitis	(păr-ă-sĭs-TĪ-tĭs)	_____
7–51	[] parahepatitis	(păr-ă-hĕp-ă-TĪ-tĭs)	_____
7–48	[] parathyroid	(păr-ă-THĪ-royd)	_____
7–82	[] polydipsia	(pŏl-ē-DĬP-sē-ă)	_____
7–82	[] polyphagia	(pŏl-ē-FĂ-jē-ă)	_____
7–79	[] polyuria	(pŏl-ē-Ū-rē-ă)	_____
7–16	[] posteroinferior	(pŏs-tĕr-ō-ĭn-FĒ-rē-ōr)	_____
7–16	[] posterosuperior	(pŏs-tĕr-ō-soo-PĒ-rē-ōr)	_____
Reading Exercise	[] pruritus	(proo-RĪ-tĭs)	_____
7–13	[] radiology	(rā-dē-ŎL-ō-jē)	_____
7–56	[] suprarenal	(soo-pră-RĒ-năl)	_____
7–85	[] thymectomy	(thī-MĔK-tō-mē)	_____
7–85	[] thymolysis	(thī-MŎL-ĭ-sĭs)	_____
7–85	[] thymoma	(thī-MŌ-mă)	_____
7–85	[] thymopathy	(thī-MŎP-ă-thē)	_____
7–36	[] thyroidectomy	(thī-royd-ĔK-tō-mē)	_____
7–45	[] thryoidotome	(thī-ROY-dō-tōm)	_____

Frame	Word	Pronunciation	Spelling Exercise
7–45	[] thyroidotomy	(thī-royd-ŎT-ō-mē)	_____
7–37	[] thyromegaly	(thī-rō-MĔG-ă-lē)	_____
7–37	[] thyropathy	(thī-RŎP-ă-thē)	_____
7–37	[] thyrotomy	(thī-RŎT-ō-mē)	_____
7–42	[] thryotoxicosis	(thī-rō-tŏks-ĭ-KŌ-sĭs)	_____
7–42	[] toxic	(TŎKS-ĭk)	_____
7–43	[] toxicologist	(tŏks-ĭ-KŎL-ō-jĭst)	_____
7–43	[] toxicology	(tŏks-ĭ-KŎL-ō-jē)	_____
Reading Exercise	[] vertigo	(VĔR-tĭ-gō)	_____

Unit Exercises

DEFINITIONS

Review Unit 7 Endocrine and Nervous System Summary (pages 327–329) before completing this exercise.
Write the meaning for each element.

SUFFIXES, PREFIXES, AND ABBREVIATIONS

Element	Meaning

SURGICAL SUFFIXES

1. -lysis _____
2. -pexy _____
3. -tome _____
4. -tomy _____

OTHER SUFFIXES

5. -dipsia _____
6. -emia _____
7. -genesis _____
8. -iasis _____
9. -malacia _____
10. -megaly _____
11. -oid _____
12. -oma _____
13. -osis _____
15. -phagia _____
16. -phasia _____
17. -rrhagia _____
18. -rrhea _____

PREFIXES

19. a- _____
20. para- _____

COMBINING FORMS RELATED TO ENDOCRINE AND NERVOUS SYSTEMS

21. aden/o _____
22. adrenal/o, adren/o _____
23. anter/o _____
24. calc/o _____
25. cerebr/o _____
26. encephal/o _____
27. gluc/o, glyc/o _____
28. mening/o, meningi/o _____
29. myel/o _____
30. neur/o _____

Element	Meaning
31. thryoid/o	_____

OTHER COMBINING FORMS IN UNIT 7

Element	Meaning
32. acr/o	_____
33. carcin/o	_____
34. hem/o	_____
35. scler/o	_____
36. toxic/o	_____

VALIDATION FRAME: Check your answers in the Index of Medical Word Elements, Part A of Appendix A.

If you scored less than _____ %,* review Unit Summary (pages 327–329).
To obtain a percentage score, multiply the number of correct answers times 2.78.

Number of Correct Answers: _____   **Percentage Score:** _____

*Enter the percentage required by your instructor to complete this course.

Vocabulary

Match the medical term(s) below with the definitions in the numbered list.

acromegaly
adenohypophysis
adrenalectomy
adrenaline
cerebral palsy
deglutition
diabetes mellitus
glycogenesis
hormone

hypercalcemia
hyperglycemia
insulin
jaundice
meningorrhagia
metastasis
neurohypophysis
neuromalacia

pancreatolith
pancreatolysis
pancreatopathy
polydipsia
polyphagia
pruritus
thyrotoxicosis
vertigo

1. _____ Enlargement of the extremities.

2. _____ Destruction of the pancreatic substance by pancreatic enzymes.

3. _____ Anterior lobe of the pituitary, composed of glandular tissue.

4. _____ Partial paralysis and lack of muscular coordination caused by damage to the cerebrum prior to or during the birth process.

5. _____ Excessive amounts of calcium in the blood.

6. _____ Pancreatic hormone that decreases blood sugar level.

7. _____ Posterior lobe of the pituitary, composed primarily of nerve tissue.

8. _____ Any disease of the pancreas.

9. _____ Excessive consumption of food.

10. _____ Pathology arising from hyposecretion or hypoactivity of insulin.

11. _____ Increase of blood sugar, as in diabetics.

12. _____ Calculus or stone in the pancreas.

13. _____ Excessive thirst.

14. _____ Toxic condition due to hyperactivity of the thyroid gland; exophthalmic goiter.

15. _____ Excision of an adrenal gland.

16. _____ Hormone secreted by the adrenal medulla that causes some of the physiological expressions of fear and anxiety; epinephrine.

17. _____ Production or formation of sugar.

18. _____ Hemorrhage of the cerebral or spinal membrane.

19. _____ Softening of nerve tissue.

20. _____ Severe itching.

21. _____ Act of swallowing.

22. _____ Illusion of movement.

23. _____ Yellowish discoloration of the skin and eyes.

24. _____ Spread of a malignant tumor beyond its primary site to a secondary organ or location.

25. _____ Chemical substance produced by specialized cells of the body and released slowly into the bloodstream.

VALIDATION FRAME: Check your answers Appendix B, Answer Key.

If you scored less than _____ %, review the vocabulary and retake the exercise.
To obtain a percentage score, multiply the number of correct answers times 4.

Number of Correct Answers: _____   **Percentage Score:** _____

Additional Pathological Changes

Match the medical term(s) below with the definitions in the numbered list.

Alzheimer's disease
Bell's palsy
cerebrovascular accident (CVA)
Cushing's syndrome
epilepsy
exophthalmos
Graves' disease

Huntington's chorea
hydrocephalus
insulinoma
myxedema
neuroblastoma
panhypopituitarism
Parkinson's disease

pheochromocytoma
pituitarism
poliomyelitis
sciatica
shingles
spina bifida

1. _____ Facial paralysis caused by a functional disorder of the seventh cranial nerve and any or all of its branches. It may be unilateral, bilateral, transient, or permanent.

2. _____ Brain tissue damage caused by a disorder within the blood vessels; usually due to the formation of a clot or a ruptured blood vessel; also called apoplexy, stroke, or CVA.

3. _____ Central nervous system disorder characterized by recurrent seizures.

4. _____ Abnormal protrusion of eyeball that may be due to thyrotoxicosis.

5. _____ Hyperthyroidism, also called toxic goiter; involves growth of the thyroid associated with hypersecretion of thyroxine; characterized by exophthalmos.

6. _____ Tumor of the islets of Langerhans of the pancreas.

7. _____ Advanced hypothyroidism in adults, resulting from hypofunction of the thyroid gland, causing edema and increasing blood pressure.

8. _____ Small chromaffin cell tumor, usually located in the adrenal medulla.

9. _____ Progressive degenerative neurological disorder affecting the portion of the brain responsible for controlling movement, causing hand tremors.

10. _____ Inflammation of the gray matter of the spinal cord caused by a virus, often resulting in spinal and muscle deformity and paralysis.

11. _____ Severe pain in the leg along the course of the sciatic nerve, which travels from the hip to the foot.

12. _____ Congenital defect characterized by incomplete closure of the spinal canal through which the spinal cord and meninges may or may not protrude. It usually occurs in the lumbosacral area and has several forms.

13. _____ Cranial enlargement caused by accumulation of fluid within the ventricles of the brain.

14. _____ Malignant tumor composed principally of cells resembling neuroblasts; occurs chiefly in infants and children.

15. _____ Brain disorder marked by deterioration of mental capacity (dementia), beginning in middle age, and leading to total disability and death.

16. _____ Eruption of acute, inflammatory, herpetic vesicles on the trunk of the body along a peripheral nerve caused by herpes zoster virus.

17. _____ Any disorder of the pituitary gland and its function.

18. _____ Total pituitary impairment that brings about a progressive and general loss of hormonal activity.

19. _____ Hereditary nervous disorder caused by the progressive loss of brain cells that leads to bizarre, involuntary, dancelike movements.

20. _____ Results from hypersecretion of the adrenal cortex in which there is excessive production of glucocorticoids.

VALIDATION FRAME: Check your answers in Appendix B, Answer Key. If you scored less than _____%, review the vocabulary and retake the exercise.

To obtain a percentage score, multiply the number of correct answers times 5.

Number of Correct Answers: _____   **Percentage Score:** _____

Unit Summary

COMBINING FORMS RELATED TO THE ENDOCRINE AND NERVOUS SYSTEMS

Combining Form	Pronunciation	Meaning
aden/o	ăd-ĕ-nō	gland
adren/o adrenal/o	ăd-rē-nō ă-drĕn-ă-lō	adrenal glands
anter/o	ăn-tĕr-ō	front, anterior
calc/o	kăl-kō	calcium
cerebr/o	sĕr-ĕ-brō	cerebrum (brain)
encephal/o	ĕn-sĕf-ă-lō	brain
gli/o	glē-ō	glue or gluelike; neuroglial tissue (supportive tissue of nervous system)
gluc/o glyc/o	gloo-kō glī-kō	sugar, glucose
mening/o meningi/o	mĕn-ĭn-gō mĕn-ĭn-jē-ō	meninges
myel/o	mī-ĕ-lō	spinal cord, bone marrow
neur/o	nū-rō	nerve
orchid/o orchi/o	or-kŭ-dō or-kē-ō	testes
pancreat/o	păn-krē-ă-tō	pancreas
thym/o	thī-mō	thymus gland
thyroid/o	thī-royd-ō	thyroid gland
vascul/o	văs-kū-lō	blood vessel

OTHER COMBINING FORMS IN UNIT 7

Combining Form	Pronunciation	Meaning
acr/o	ăk-ro	extremities
carcin/o	kăr-sĭn-ō	cancer
cyst/o	sĭs-tō	bladder, sac
cyt/o	sī-tō	cell
dermat/o	dĕr-mă-tō	skin
enter/o	ĕn-tĕr-ō	intestines (usually small)
gastr/o	găs-trō	stomach
hem/o	hēm-ō	blood
hepat/o	hĕp-ă-tō	liver
hidr/o	hī-drō	sweat
nephr/o ren/o	nĕf-rō rĕ-nō	kidney

Combining Form	Pronunciation	Meaning
poster/o	pŏs-tĕr-ō	back (of body), behind, posterior
scler/o	sklĕr-rō	hardening
spin/o	spī-nō	spine
thromb/o	thrŏm-bō	blood clot
toxic/o	tŏks-ĭ-kō	poison

SUFFIXES AND PREFIXES

Suffix (Prefix)	Pronunciation	Meaning
SURGICAL SUFFIXES		
-ectomy	ĕk-tō-mē	excision, removal
-lysis	lī-sĭs	separation, destruction, loosening
-pexy	pĕk-sē	surgical fixation
-tome	tōm	instrument to cut
-tomy	tō-mē	incision, cut into
OTHER SUFFIXES		
-dipsia	dĭp-sē-ă	thirst
-dynia	dīn-ē-ă	pain
-emia	ē-mē-ă	blood
-gen -genesis	jĕn jĕn-ĕ-sĭs	producing, forming
-glia	glē-a	glue or gluelike; neuroglial tissue (supportive tissue of nervous system)
-iasis	ī-ă-sĭs	abnormal condition (produced by something specified)
-ism	ĭzm	condition (of)
-itis	ī-tĭs	inflammation
-lith	lĭth	stone, calculus
-logist	lō-jĭst	specialist in the study of
-logy	lō-jē	study of
-megaly	mĕg-ă-lē	enlargement
-malacia	mă-lā-shē-ă	softening
-oid	oyd	resemble
-oma	ō-mă	tumor
-osis	ō-sĭs	abnormal condition
-pathy	pă-thē	disease
-penia	pē-nē-ă	decrease
-phagia	fă-jē-ă	swallow, eat

Suffix (Prefix)	Pronunciation	Meaning
-phasia	fā-zē-ă	speech
-plegia	plē-jē-ă	paralysis
-rrhagia	ră-jē-ă	bursting forth (of)
-rrhea	rē-ă	flow, discharge
-uria	ū-rē-ă	urine
PREFIXES		
a-	ă	without
dys-	dĭs	bad, painful, difficult
endo-	ĕn-dō	within
hyper-	hī-pĕr	above, excessive
hypo-	hī-pō	under, below
para-	păr-ă	near, beside, around
poly-	pŏl-ē	many, much
supra-	soo-pră	above

Musculoskeletal System

The musculoskeletal system is composed of bones, joints, and muscles. Bones form a skeleton to support and protect the body, and serve as storage areas for mineral salts, especially calcium and phosphorus (Fig. 8–1). Joints are the places where two bones articulate, or connect. Because bones cannot move without the help of muscles, contraction must be provided by muscular tissue (Fig. 8–2).

The combining forms related to the skeletal system are summarized here. Review this information before you begin to work the frames.

Skeletal System

COMBINING FORMS OF SPECIFIC BONES

Combining Form	Meaning	Example	Pronunciation
BONES OF UPPER EXTREMITIES			
crani/o	cranium (skull)	crani/o/tomy incision	krā-nē-ŎT-ō-mē
stern/o	sternum (breastbone)	stern/o/cost/al ribs pertaining to	stĕr-nō-KŎS-tăl
cost/o	ribs	sub/cost/al under pertaining to	sŭb-KŎS-tăl
spondyl/o (used to form words about the condition of the structure)	vertebrae (backbone)	spondyl/itis inflammation	spŏn-dĭl-Ī-tĭs
vertebr/o(used to form words that describe the structure)		vertebr/al pertaining to	VĔR-tĕ-brăl
humer/o	humerus (upper arm bone)	humer/al pertaining to	HŪ-mĕr-ăl
carp/o	carpus (wrist bones)	carp/o/ptosis dropping, falling	kăr-pŏp-TŌ-sĭs
metacarp/o	metacarpus (bones of the hand)	metacarp/ectomy excision	mĕt-ă-kăr-PĔK-tō-mē
phalang/o	phalanges (finger bones)	phalang/itis inflammation	făl-ăn-JĪ-tĭs
BONES OF LOWER EXTREMITIES			
pelv/i	pelvis (hip bone)	pelv/i/metry process of measuring	pĕl-VĬM-ĕ-trē

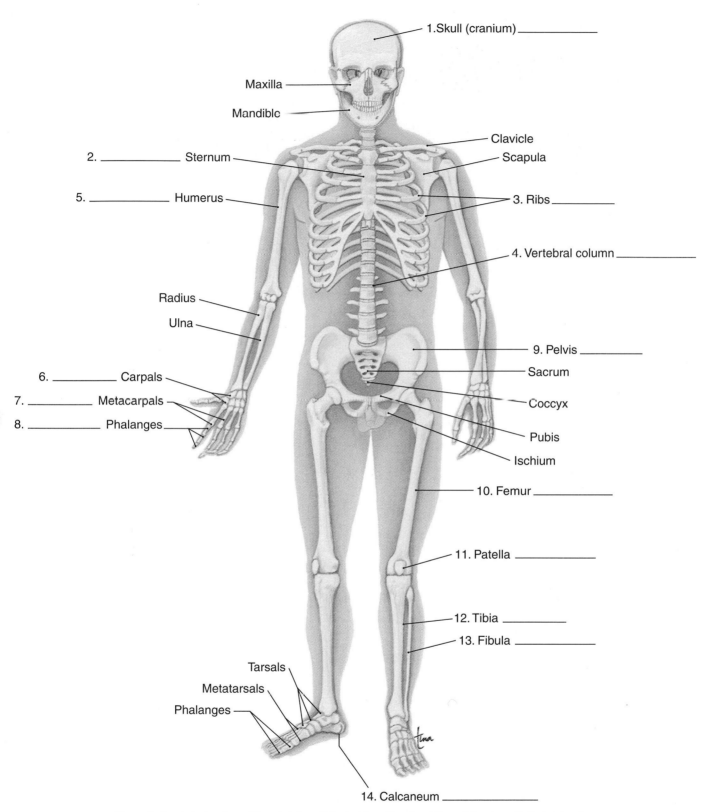

1.Skull (cranium)_____

Maxilla

Mandible

Clavicle

Scapula

2._____ Sternum

5._____ Humerus

3. Ribs_____

4. Vertebral column_____

Radius

Ulna

9. Pelvis_____

Sacrum

6._____ Carpals

7._____ Metacarpals

Coccyx

8._____ Phalanges

Pubis

Ischium

10. Femur_____

11. Patella_____

12. Tibia_____

13. Fibula_____

Tarsals

Metatarsals

Phalanges

14. Calcaneum_____

Figure 8–1.   Anterior view of the skeleton. (Adapted from Scanlon, VC, and Sanders, T: Understanding Human Structure and Function. FA Davis, Philadelphia, 1997, p 89, with permission.)

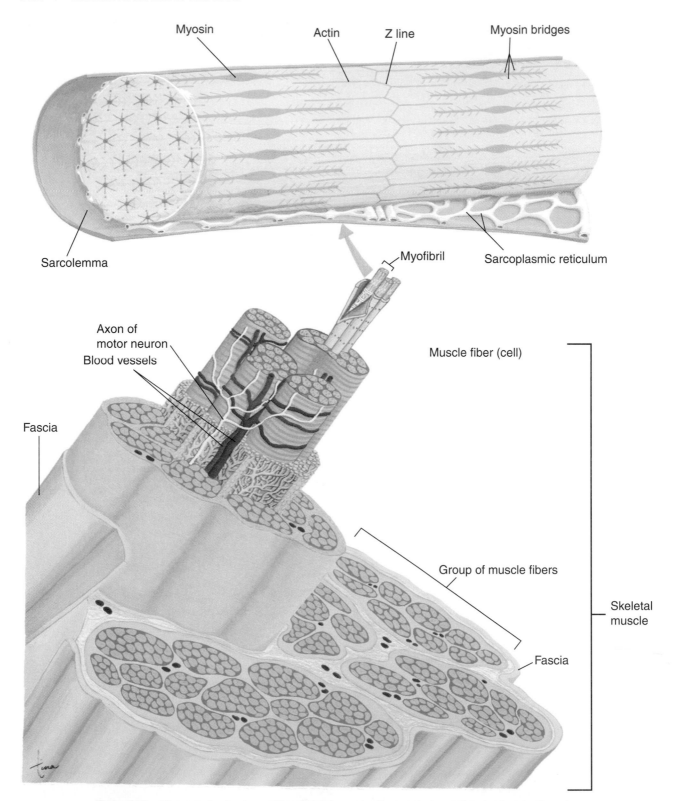

Figure 8–2. Microscopic structure of the skeletal muscle. Progressively smaller structure is shown in the expanded portions. The arrow indicates a highly magnified view of the structure of sarcomeres. (From Scanlon, VC, and Sanders, T: Understanding Human Structure and Function. FA Davis, Philadelphia, 1997, p 115, with permission.)

Combining Form	Meaning	Example	Pronunciation
femor/o	femur (thigh bone)	femor/al pertaining to	FĔM-ŏr-ăl
patell/o	patella (kneecap)	patell/o/pexy fixation	pă-TĔL-ō-pĕk-sē
tibi/o	tibia (shin bone)	tibi/al pertaining to	TĬB-ē-ăl
fibul/o	fibula (smaller bone of lower leg)	fibul/ar pertaining to	FĬB-ū-lă
calcane/o	calcaneum (heel bone)	calcane/o/dynia pain	kăl-kăn-ē-ō-DĬN-ē-ă

OTHER RELATED COMBINING FORMS

ankyl/o	stiff, bent, crooked	ankyl/osis abnormal condition	ăng-kĭ-LŌ-sĭs
arthr/o	joint	arthr/itis inflammation	ăr-THRĪ-tĭs
cervic/o	neck	cervic/al pertaining to	SĔR-vĭ-kăl
lamin/o	lamina (part of the vertebral arch)	lamin/ectomy excision	lăm-ĭ-NĔK-tō-mē
myel/o	spinal cord, bone marrow	myel/o/cele herniation	MĪ-ĕ-lō-sēl
orth/o	straight	orth/o/ped/ic child pertaining to	ŏr-thō-PĒ-dĭk
oste/o	bone	oste/itis inflammation	ŏs-tē-Ī-tĭs

8–1 Use the Index of Medical Word Elements, Part A of Appendix A, to define the following elements.

Medical Word Element	*Meaning*
calc/o	_____
chondr/o	_____
-cyte	_____
-genesis	_____
-gram	_____
myel/o	_____
my/o	_____
-plegia	_____
spin/o	_____

oste/o/dynia
(ŏs-tē-ō-DĬN-ē-ă)

8–2 The combining form **oste/o** refers to bone or bony. Oste/algia refers to pain in a bone.

Construct another word meaning pain in a bone:

_____ / _____ / _____ .

---

oste/o/cytes
(ŎS-tē-ō-sītz)

8–3 Bone is living tissue composed of oste/o/cytes, blood vessels, and nerves.

Determine the medical term for bone cells:

_____ / _____ / _____ .

---

oste/itis
(ŏs-tē-Ī-tĭs)
oste/o/pathy
(ŏs-tē-ŎP-ă-thē)
oste/o/tomy
(ŏs-tē-ŎT-ō-mē)

oste/o/rrhaphy
(ŏs-tē-ŎR-ă-fē)

oste/o/scler/osis
(ŏs-tē-ō-sklĕ-RŌ-sĭs)

8–4 Practice developing medical words meaning

inflammation of bone: _____ / _____

disease of bone: _____ / _____ / _____

incision or cutting into bone: _____ / _____ / _____

suture of bone (wiring of bone fragments):

_____ / _____ / _____

abnormal condition of bone hardening:

_____ / _____ / _____ / _____

---

oste/o

8–5 Bones are constructed of various shapes and sizes. Regardless of whether the bone is short, flat, or irregular, the combining form for bone(s) is still

_____ / _____ .

-genesis

oste/o

8–6 Oste/o/genesis is the formation or development of bones.

Identify the elements in this frame that mean

production or formation: _____

bone: _____ / _____

---

oste/o/malacia
(ŏs-tē-ō-mă-LĀ-shē-ă)
oste/o/genesis
(ŏs-tē-ō-JĔN-ĕ-sĭs)

8–7 Milk is a good source of vitamin D. A deficiency of this vitamin results in a softening and weakening of the skeleton, causing pain and bowing of the bones.

Construct medical terms meaning

softening of bones: _____ / _____ / _____

producing or forming bone: _____ / _____ / _____

oste/o/malacia (ŏs-tē-ō-mă-LĀ-shē-ă)	**8–8** Oste/o/malacia is a disease in which there is an inefficient mineralization of the bone-forming tissue. The bones become flexible and brittle, causing deformities. When the disease occurs in children, it is called rickets. Rickets is another name for _____ / _____ / _____ .
oste/o/malacia (ŏs-tē-ō-mă-LĀ-shē-ă)	**8–9** Rickets is marked by an abnormality in the shapes of bones and is a form of _____ / _____ / _____ .
rickets (RĬK-ĕts)	**8–10** Calcium provides bone the strength that is needed for its supportive functions. Many children in underdeveloped countries suffer from rickets because of inadequate milk supplies. When oste/o/malacia occurs in children, it is called _____ .
calc/emia (kăl-SĒ-mē-ă)	**8–11** Combine **calc/o** and -emia to form a word meaning calcium in the blood. _____ / _____
below, under deficient	**8–12** Recall that hypo- means _____ , _____ , _____ .
hyper/calc/emia (hī-pĕr-kăl-SĒ-mē-ă)	**8–13** Hypo/calc/emia is a deficiency of calcium in the blood. An excessive amount of calcium in the blood is called _____ / _____ / _____ .

Structure of Bones

8–14 Typically, long bones are found in the extremities of the body. The **(1) diaphysis** is the shaft or main portion of the bone. The **(2) bone marrow** is the soft tissue that fills the **(3) medullary cavities** of long bones.

Label the parts of a long bone in Figure 8–3.

muscle bone marrow, spinal cord	**8–15** Even though **my/o** and **myel/o** sound somewhat alike, you know they have different meanings. **My/o** refers to _____ ; **myel/o** refers to _____ _____ or _____ _____ .

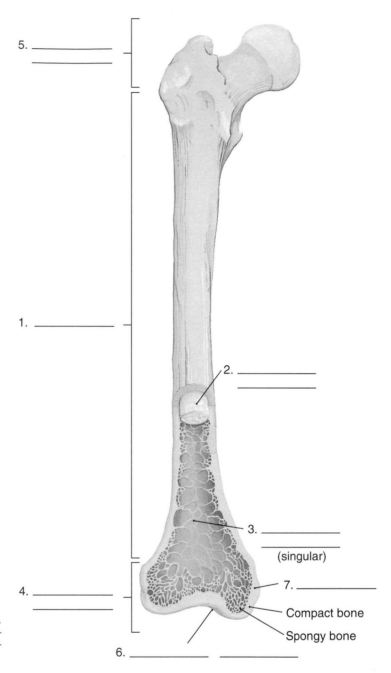

5. _____

1. _____

2. _____

3. _____
(singular)

7. _____
Compact bone

Spongy bone

4. _____

6. _____

Figure 8–3. A longitudinal section of the femur bone. (Adapted from Scanlon, VC, and Sanders, T: Understanding Human Structure and Function. FA Davis, Philadelphia, 1997, p 84, with permission.)

8–16 To acquaint yourself with words that contain **myel/o**, find three such words in your medical dictionary and write brief definitions in the space provided.

Word	*Definition*
_____	_____
	_____
_____	_____
	_____
_____	_____
	_____

8–17   **Radi/o** is the combining form that refers to x-rays or radiation.

Form medical words meaning

radi/o/logy
(rā-dē-ŎL-ō-jē)
radi/o/logist
rā-dē-ŎL-ō-jĭst)

    The study of x-rays: _____ / _____ / _____

    A specialist in the study of x-rays: _____ / _____ / _____

8–18   Use -graphy to form a word meaning the process of recording an x-ray:

radi/o/graphy
(rā-dē-ŎG-rä-fē)

_____ / _____ / _____

---

x-ray

8–19   A radi/o/gram is a picture record or image of an _____ .

8–20   Radi/o/logy, the study of x-rays and radioactive substances, is used for diagnosing and treating diseases.

A physician who specializes in the study of x-rays is called a

radi/o/logist
(rā-dē-ŎL-ō-jĭst)

_____ / _____ / _____ .

8–21   Radi/o/logy, also called roentgen/o/logy, was developed after the discovery of an unknown ray in 1895 by Wilhelm Roentgen, who called his discovery an x-ray.

x-rays

Roentgen/o/logy is also known as the study of _____ .

8–22   You will find that radi/o/logy is the preferred term in the medical field, but occasionally you may see words with the combining form **roentgen/o**. Both **radi/o** and **roentgen/o** refer to x-rays.

Use **roentgen/o** to form words that mean

roentgen/o/gram
(rĕnt-GĔN-ō-grăm)

roentgen/o/graphy
(rĕnt-gĕn-ŎG-rä-fē)

    record of an x-ray: _____ / _____ / _____

    process of recording an x-ray:

    _____ / _____ / _____

8–23   A roentgen/o/logist is a physician who specializes in the use of x-rays for diagnosis and treatment of disease.

Identify the elements in this frame meaning

roentgen/o

-logist

    x-rays: _____ / _____

    specialist in the study of: _____

8–24   A myel/o/gram is an x-ray of the spinal cord after injection of a dye. The

myel/o

combining form for bone marrow and spinal cord is _____ / _____ .

myel / o / genesis (mī-ĕ-lō-JĔN-ĕ-sĭs)	**8–25** Use -genesis to build a word meaning formation of bone marrow. _____ / _____ / _____
myel / o / malacia (mī-ĕl-ō-mă-LĀ-shē-ă) myel / o / gram (mī-ĔL-ō-grăm)	**8–26** Develop medical words meaning softening of the spinal cord: _____ / _____ / _____ record of the spinal cord: _____ / _____ / _____
mening / o	**8–27** **Mening / o** is the combining form for the meninges, which are the three membranes that line the brain and spinal cord. From mening / itis, construct the combining form that denotes the meninges: _____ / _____
mening / o / cele (mĕn-ĬN-gō-sēl)	**8–28** Use -cele to form a word meaning hernia or swelling of the meninges: _____ / _____ / _____
-cele mening / o myel / o	**8–29** A mening / o / myel / o / cele (Fig. 8–4) is a herniation of the meninges and spinal cord through a defect in the spin / al column. Identify the elements in mening / o / myel / o / cele that mean hernia, swelling: _____ meninges: _____ / _____ spinal cord: _____ / _____
mening / o / pathy mĕn-ĭn-GŎP-ă-thē) mening / o / cele (mĕn-ĬN-gō-sēl) mening / itis (mĕn-ĭn-JĪ-tĭs) mening / o / myel / itis (mĕn-ĭn-gō-mī-ĕl-Ī-tĭs) mening / o / myel / o / cele or myel / o / mening / o / cele (mĕ-nĭng-gō-MĪ-ĕ-lō-sēl) (mī-ĕ-lō-mĕn-ĬN-gō-sēl)	**8–30** Spina bifida usually occurs in the lumbar region and has several forms. Mening / o / myel / o / cele is a form of spina bifida (see Fig. 8–4). Use elements in this frame to develop words meaning disease of the meninges: _____ / _____ / _____ hernia or swelling of the meninges: _____ / _____ / _____ inflammation of the meninges: _____ / _____ inflammation of the meninges and spinal cord: _____ / _____ / _____ / _____ hernia of the meninges and spinal cord: _____ / _____ / _____ / _____ / _____

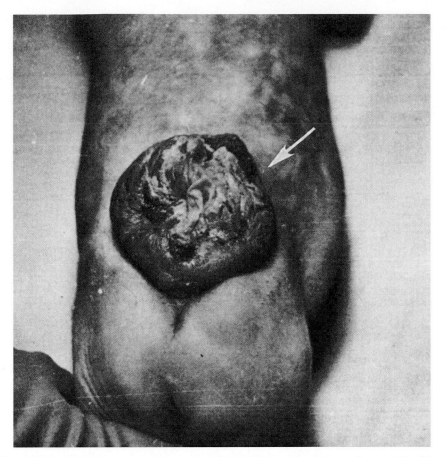

Figure 8–4. Lumbar myelomeningocele in an infant with hydrocephalus and paraplegia. (From Adams, JF, and Duchen, LW: Greenfield's Neuropathy, ed 5. Oxford University Press, New York, 1992, p 542, with permission.)

8–31 The **(4) distal epiphysis** and **(5) proximal epiphysis** are the two ends of bone. Both have a somewhat bulbous shape to provide space for muscle and ligament attachments near the joints.

Label these structures in Figure 8–3.

---

dist / o

8–32 Dist / al is a directional word meaning farthest from the point of attachment to the trunk, or far from the beginning of a structure.

From dist / al, construct the combining form that means far or farthest:

_____ / _____ .

---

proxim / o

8–33 Proxim / al is a directional word meaning near the point of attachment to the trunk, or near the beginning of a structure.

From proxim / al, construct the combining form that means near or nearest:

_____ / _____ .

---

farthest

nearest

8–34 Use the words "farthest" or "nearest" to complete this frame.

The dist / al epiphysis is located _____ from the trunk.

The proxim / al epiphysis is located _____ the trunk.

8–35 A thin layer of **(6) articular cartilage** provides the joints with a cushion against jars and blows.

Label the articular cartilage in Figure 8–3.

---

chondr/itis
(kŏn-DRĪ-tĭs)
chondr/oma
(kŏn-DRŌ-mă)
chondr/o/genesis
(kŏn-drō-JĔN-ĕ-sĭs)

8–36 Cartilage, which is more elastic than bone, makes up parts of the skeleton such as the tip of the nose.

Use **chondr/o** (cartilage) to form words meaning

inflammation of cartilage: _____ / _____

tumor composed of cartilage: _____ / _____

producing or forming cartilage: _____ / _____ / _____

---

chondr/o/cyte
(KŎN-drō-sīt)

8–37 Use -cyte to build a word meaning cartilage cell:

_____ / _____ / _____ .

8–38 The **(7) periosteum** is the tough and fibrous outermost covering of bone. It contains many blood and lymph vessels, and nerves.

Label the periosteum in Figure 8–3.

---

around

bone

8–39 Analyze peri/oste/um by defining the elements.

peri- means _____ .

oste means _____ .

-um is a noun ending.

VALIDATION FRAME: Check your labeling of Figure 8–3 in Appendix B, Answer Key.

Review

Select the medical word element(s) that match(es) the meaning.

calc/o
chondr/o
cyt/o
dist/o
mening/o
myel/o
my/o
oste/o
radi/o
roentgen/o
scler/o

-algia
-cele
-dynia
-emia
-genesis
-gram
-graphy
-itis
-logist
-malacia
-oma
-rrhaphy
-tomy

hyper-
hypo-
peri-

a. _____ excessive

b. _____ around

c. _____ blood

d. _____ bone

e. _____ cartilage

f. _____ calcium

g. _____ cell

h. _____ far, farthest

i. _____ hardening

j. _____ hernia, swelling

k. _____ incision, cut into

l. _____ inflammation

m. _____ meninges

n. _____ muscle

o. _____ pain

p. _____ process of recording

q. _____ producing, forming

r. _____ record

s. _____ softening

t. _____ specialist in the study of

u. _____ spinal cord, bone marrow

v. _____ suture

w. _____ tumor

x. _____ under, below

y. _____ x-rays

Check your answers with the Review Answer Key on the following page.

Review Answer Key

a. hyper-

b. peri-

c. -emia

d. oste/o

e. chondr/o

f. calc/o

g. -cyte

h. dist/o

i. scler/o

j. -cele

k. -tomy

l. -itis

m. mening/o

n. my/o

o. -algia, -dynia

p. -graphy

q. -genesis

r. -gram

s. -malacia

t. -logist

u. -myel/o

v. -rrhaphy

w. -oma

x. hypo-

y. radi/o, roentgen/o

REINFORCEMENT FRAME: If you are not satisfied with your level of comprehension, go back to Frame 8–1 and rework the frames.

Joints

8-40   A joint is the place where two bones articulate, or connect, to allow motion between the parts.

Use your medical dictionary to define *articulation*.

_____

_____

---

arthr/o/pathy
(ăr-THRŎP-ă-thē)
arthr/itis
(ăr-THRĪ-tĭs)
arthr/o/centesis
(ăr-thrō-sĕn-TĒ-sĭs)

8-41   Use **arthr/o**, which is the combining form for joint, to develop medical words meaning

disease of a joint: _____ / _____ / _____

inflammation of a joint: _____ / _____

surgical puncture of a joint: _____ / _____ / _____

---

joints

8-42   Just as a piece of machinery is lubricated by oil, joints are lubricated by synovial fluid, which is secreted within the synovial membranes.

Synovial fluid allows free movement of the _____ .

---

arthr/o/centesis
(ăr-thrō-sĕn-TĒ-sĭs)

8-43   To remove accumulated fluid from a joint, a surgical puncture of a joint is performed. This surgical procedure is called

_____ / _____ / _____ .

---

arthr/o/dynia
(ăr-thrō-DĬN-ē-ă)

8-44   A person with arthr/itis suffers not only from an inflammation of the joints but also from arthr/algia.

Construct another medical word meaning pain in a joint:

_____ / _____ / _____

---

arthr/itis
(ăr-THRĪ-tĭs)

oste/o/arthr/itis
(ŏs-tē-ō-ăr-THRĪ-tĭs)

8-45   Although there are various forms of arthr/itis, all of them result in an inflammation of the joints that is usually accompanied by pain and swelling.

Form medical words meaning

inflammation of joints: _____ / _____ .

inflammation of bones and joints:

_____ / _____ / _____ / _____

---

oste/o/arthr/o/pathy
(ŏs-tē-ō-ăr-THRŎP-ă-thē)

8-46   A disease of the bones and joints is called

_____ / _____ / _____ / _____ / _____ .

8-47 Select element(s) from oste/o/arthr/o/pathy to build a word meaning an abnormal condition of the bones and joints.

_____ / _____ / _____ / _____ .

oste/o/arthr/osis
(ŏs-tē-ō-ăr-THRŌ-sĭs)

Reinforcement of Combining Forms Related to Specific Bones

8-48 The word roots/combining forms of bones are derived from the names of the bones. Learn the combining forms for the bones as you label them in Figure 8–1.

1. **crani/o** refers to the cranium or skull.
2. **stern/o** refers to the sternum or chest plate.
3. **cost/o** refers to the ribs, which are attached to the sternum.
4. **vertebr/o** refers to the vertebrae or the backbone. The vertebral column is also called the spinal column and is composed of 26 bones called vertebr/ae (plural).
5. **humer/o** refers to the humerus or upper arm bone. It articulates with the scapula at the shoulder and with the radius and ulna at the elbow.
6. **carp/o** refers to the carpals, which are the eight wrist bones.
7. **metacarp/o** refers to the metacarpals, which radiate from the wrist like spokes and form the palm of the hand.
8. **phalang/o** refers to the phalanges or bones of the fingers and toes.
9. **pelv/i** and **pelv/o** refer to the pelvis. The pelvis provides attachment for the legs and also supports the soft organs of the abdominal cavity.
10. **femor/o** refers to the femur or thigh bone. The femur is the longest and strongest bone in the body. It articulates with the hip bone and the bones of the lower leg.
11. **patell/o** refers to the patella, or kneecap. It articulates with the femur, but essentially is a "floating bone." The main function of this bone is to protect the knee joint, but its exposed position makes it vulnerable to dislocation and fracture.
12. **tibi/o** refers to the tibia. It is the weight-bearing bone of the lower leg.
13. **fibul/o** refers to the fibula. The fibula is not a weight-bearing bone but is important because muscles are attached and anchored to it.
14. **calcane/o** refers to the calcaneum or heel bone.

VALIDATION FRAME: Check your labeling of Figure 8–1 in Appendix B, Answer Key.

REMINDER FRAME: You are not expected to know the combining forms and the names of the bones from memory. You can always refer to Figure 8–1, the Index of Medical Terms, Part A of Appendix A, or a medical dictionary to obtain information about a bone or its combining form.

8-49 Words containing **cephal/o** refer to the head. Cephal/o/dynia is a
_____ in the _____ .

pain, head

8-50 Cephal/o/dynia is the medical term for a headache.
Construct another word meaning pain in the head:
_____ / _____ .

cephal/algia
(sĕf-ă-LĂL-gē-ă)

head -meter	**8–51** A meter is an instrument to measure. A cephal/o/meter is an instrument to measure the _____ . In cephal/o/meter, the element meaning an instrument to measure is _____ .
brain brain brain	**8–52** When the prefix en-, meaning "in," is combined with **cephal/o**, meaning head, the new combining form **encephal/o** is created. This refers to the brain. Encephal/oma is a tumor of the _____ . Encephal/itis is an inflammation of the _____ . Encephal/o/malacia is a softening of the _____ .
inflammation, brain	**8–53** Mosquitoes can transmit viruses that cause encephal/itis, which is an _____ of the _____ .
disease, brain	**8–54** Encephal/o/pathy is a _____ of the _____ .
brain	**8–55** An encephal/o/cele is a protrusion of _____ substance through an opening of the skull.
inter- cost -al	**8–56** Inter/cost/al muscles, located between the ribs, move the ribs during the breathing process. Write the elements in this frame that mean between: _____ ribs: _____ pertaining to: _____
under or below, ribs	**8–57** Sub/cost/al refers to the area _____ the _____ .
pain, rib	**8–58** Cost/algia is a _____ in a _____ .

Fractures and Repairs

8–59 A fracture is a break in the continuity of bone. Fractures are defined according to the type and extent of the break. Label and examine the fractures in Figure 8–5 as you read the following information.

With a **(1) simple**, or **closed, fracture**, the bone is broken, but there is no external wound. The surrounding tissue damage is minimal.

With an **(2) open**, or **compound, fracture**, the broken end of a bone has been moved and it pierces the skin. There may be extensive damage to surrounding blood vessels, nerves, and muscles. In a **(3) greenstick fracture**, the bone is partially bent and partially broken. These fractures occur in children, because their bones tend to splinter rather than break completely. In a **(4) comminuted fracture**, the bone is broken into pieces.

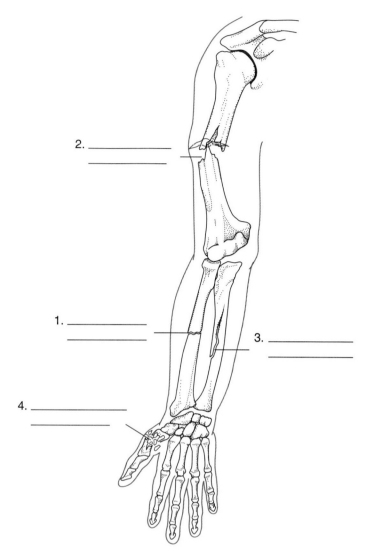

2. _____
   _____

1. _____
   _____

3. _____
   _____

4. _____
   _____

Figure 8–5. Types of fractures. (Adapted from Scanlon, VC, and Sanders, T: Essentials of Anatomy and Physiology. FA Davis, 1995, p 107, with permission.)

VALIDATION FRAME: Check your labeling of Figure 8–5 in Appendix B, Answer Key.

8–60 Refer to Figure 8–5 to complete this frame.

Identify the following fractures

Bone pierces the skin and causes extensive damage to surrounding blood

open, compound   vessels: _____ or _____ .

simple, closed   Bone is broken with no external wound present: _____ or

_____ .

Bone is partially bent and partially broken; found more commonly in

greenstick   children: _____ .

Broken ends of a bone segments are wedged into one another:

impacted   _____ .
(ĭm-PĂK-tĕd)

Vertebral Column

spin/al column (SPĪ-năl KŎL-ŭm) spin/o	**8–61** The vertebr/al or spin/al column (Fig. 8–6) supports the body and provides a protective bony canal for the spinal cord. Another name for the vertebr/al column is _____ / _____ _____ . From the word spin/al, construct the combining form for the spine: _____ / _____
vertebra (VĔR-tĕ-bră) vertebra (VĔR-tĕ-bră)	**8–62** **Spondyl/o** and **vertebr/o** are combining forms that refer to the vertebrae (singular, vertebra), or backbone. Vertebr/ectomy is an excision of a _____ . Spondyl/o/dynia is a painful condition of a _____ .

8–63 Vertebr/ae is the plural form of vertebr/a. Change the following words from singular to plural form by retaining the **a** and adding an **e**.

	Singular	Plural
vertebrae (VĔR-tĕ-brē)	vertebra	_____
bursae (BĔR-sē)	bursa	_____
pleurae (PLOO-rē)	pleura	_____

spondyl/itis (spŏn-dĭl-Ī-tĭs) spondyl/o/pathy (spŏn-dĭl-ŎP-ă-thē) spondyl/o/malacia (spŏn-dĭl-ō-mă-LĀ-shē-ă)	**8–64** **Spondyl/o** is used to form words about the condition of the structure. Build medical words meaning inflammation of the vertebrae: _____ / _____ disease of the vertebrae: _____ / _____ / _____ softening of the vertebrae: _____ / _____ / _____
vertebra vertebra (VĔR-tĕ-bră)	**8–65** **Vertebr/o** is used to form words that describe the structure. For example, vertebr/o/cost/al means pertaining to a _____ and a rib; vertebr/o/stern/al means pertaining to a _____ and the sternum or chest plate.

8–66 Vertebrae are separate and cushioned from each other by **(1) intervertebral disks** made up of cartilage.

Label Figure 8–6 as you learn about the vertebr/al or spin/al column.

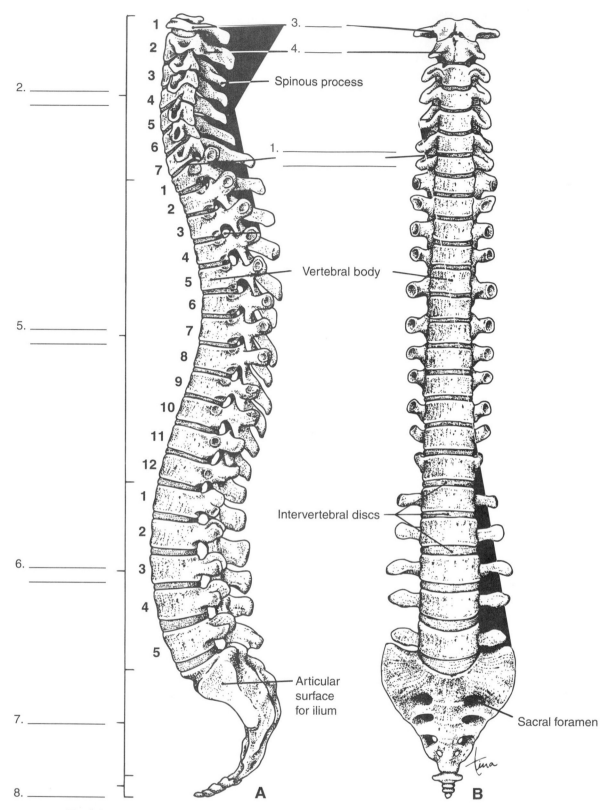

Figure 8–6. Vertebral column. (**A**) Lateral view of the left side. (**B**) Anterior view. (Adapted from Scanlon, VC, and Sanders, T: Understanding Human Structure and Function. FA Davis, Philadelphia, 1997, p 95, with permission.)

inter- vertebr -al	**8–67** Determine the elements in inter/vertebr/al that mean between: _____ vertebrae: _____ pertaining to: _____

8–68 The vertebr/al column is divided into five groups of bones. Each group derives its name from its location within the spinal column. The seven **(2) cervical vertebrae** form the skeletal framework of the neck. The first cervical vertebra is called the **(3) atlas** and supports the skull. The second cervical vertebra, the **(4) axis**, makes possible rotation of the skull on the neck.

Label these structures in Figure 8–6.

neck	**8–69** Recall that **cervic/o** is the combining form for both the neck and the cervic uteri (neck of the uterus). Cervic/o/facial refers to the face and _____ .

atlas (ĂT-lăs) cervic/al (SĔR-vi-kăl)	**8–70** The first cervic/al vertebra is the _____ . Write a word meaning pertaining to the neck: _____ / _____ .

C5 or C₅	**8–71** In medical reports, the first cervical vertebra is designated as C1. The fifth cervical vertebra is designated as _____ .

C5 or C₅	**8–72** When the radi/o/logist interprets an x-ray film and indicates a herniation or rupture at C3 to C4 disk in a report, he or she is referring to a herniation or rupture of the inter/vertebr/al disk between C3 and C4. When the radi/o/logist indicates a herniation at C4 to C5 disk in a report, he or she is referring to a herniation of the inter/vertebr/al disk between C4 and _____ .

C2 or C₂	**8–73** The second vertebra is identified as _____ .

seven	**8–74** There are a total of _____ cervic/al vertebrae.

8–75 Twelve **(5) thoracic vertebrae** support the chest and serve as a point of articulation for the ribs. The next five vertebrae are the **(6) lumbar vertebrae**. These are situated in the lower back and carry most of the weight of the torso.

Label these structures in Figure 8–6.

articulation (ăr-tĭk-ū-LĀ-shŭn) thorac/ic (thō-RĂS-ĭk)	**8–76** Identify the terms in Frame 8–75 that mean a place where two bones meet: _____ pertaining to the chest: _____ / _____
pertaining to, back	**8–77** The combining form **lumb/o** refers to the lower back or loin. Lumb/ar means _____ _____ the loin or lower _____ .
pain	**8–78** Lumb/o/dynia is a _____ in the lower back.
lumbar, five (LŬM-băr)	**8–79** Examine the position of the five lumbar vertebrae in Figure 8–6. These are designated as L1 to L5 on medical reports. An obese person with weak abdominal muscles tends to experience pain in the lower back area or L1 to L5. L5 refers to _____ vertebra _____ .
	8–80 Below the lumbar vertebrae are five **sacral vertebrae** that are fused into a single bone in the adult and are referred to as the **(7) sacrum** and the tail of the vertebral column, the **(8) coccyx**. Label the sacrum and coccyx in Figure 8–6.
pain sacrum, spine (SĀ-krŭm)	**8–81** **Sacr/o** is the combining form for the sacrum. Sacr/o/dynia is a _____ in the sacrum. Sacr/o/spin/al refers to the _____ and _____ .

VALIDATION FRAME: Check your labeling of Figure 8–6 in Appendix B, Answer Key.

S5 or S$_5$	**8–82** To designate the exact position of abnormalities on the sacrum, the label S1 to S5 is used. The first vertebra of the sacrum is designated as S1. The fifth vertebra of the sacrum is designated as _____ .
lumbar, sacrum (LŬM-băr), (SĀ-krŭm)	**8–83** A ruptured disk can cause severe pain, muscle weakness, or numbness in either leg. The disk that most often ruptures is the L5 to S1 disk. L5 refers to _____ five; S1 refers to _____ one.

Review

Select the medical word element(s) that match(es) the meaning.

arthr/o	-centesis	inter-
cephal/o	-ectomy	
cervic/o	-osis	
cost/o	-pathy	
encephal/o	-al	
lumb/o		
oste/o		
sacr/o		
spondyl/o		
thorac/o		
vertebr/o		

a. _____ abnormal condition

b. _____ between

c. _____ bone

d. _____ brain

e. _____ chest

f. _____ disease

g. _____ excision, removal

h. _____ head

i. _____ joint

j. _____ lower back, loin

k. _____ neck, cervix uteri

l. _____ pertaining to

m. _____ ribs

n. _____ sacrum

o. _____ surgical puncture

p. _____ vertebrae (backbone)

Check your answers with the Review Answer Key on the following page.

Review Answer Key

a. -osis

b. inter-

c. oste/o

d. encephal/o

e. thorac/o

f. -pathy

g. -ectomy

h. cephal/o

i. arthr/o

j. lumb/o

k. cervic/o

l. -al

m. cost/o

n. sacr/o

o. -centesis

p. spondyl/o, vertebr/o

REINFORCEMENT FRAME: If you are not satisfied with your level of comprehension, go back to Frame 8–40 and rework the frames.

MUSCULAR SYSTEM

All muscles, through contraction, provide the body with motion or body posture. The less-apparent motions provided by muscles include the passage and elimination of food through the digestive system, propulsion of blood through the arteries, and contraction of the bladder to eliminate urine.

The combining forms related to the muscular system are summarized here. Review this information before you begin to work the frames.

COMBINING FORMS

Combining Form	Meaning	Example	Pronunciation
chondr/o	cartilage	chondr/o/pathy disease	kŏn-DRŎP-ă-thē
lumb/o	lower back, loins	lumb/o/dynia pain	lŭm-bō-DĬN-ē-ă
my/o	muscle	my/algia pain	mī-ĂL-jē-ă
ten/o	tendon	ten/o/tomy incision	tĕn-ŎT-ō-mē
tend/o		tend/o/lysis separation, loosening	tĕn-DŎL-ĭ-sĭs
tendin/o		tendin/itis inflammation	tĕn-dĭn-Ī-tĭs

8-84 Use the Index of Medical Word Elements, Part A of the Appendix A, to define the following elements.

Medical Word Element	*Meaning*
-cyte	_____
enter/o	_____
my/o	_____
-plegia	_____
-rrhexis	_____
scler/o	_____
tend/o	_____

---

muscle(s)

8-85 Muscles are responsible for movement. They lie between the skin and the skeleton. Remember, the combining form for muscle is **my/o**. My/o/genesis is the formation of _____ .

---

my/o/plasty
(MĪ-ō-plăs-tē)
my/o/rrhaphy
(mī-ŌR-ă-fē)
my/o/tomy
(mī-ŎT-ō-mē)

8-86 Build medical words meaning

surgical repair of muscle: _____ / _____ / _____

suture of muscle: _____ / _____ / _____

incision of muscle: _____ / _____ / _____

---

rupture, muscle

8-87 The suffix -rrhexis means rupture.

My/o/rrhexis is a _____ of _____ .

8-88 Using your dictionary, define *rupture*.

_____

_____

hepat/o/rrhexis
(hĕp-ă-tō-RĔKS-ĭs)
cyst/o/rrhexis
(sĭs-tō-RĔKS-ĭs)
enter/o/rrhexis
(ĕn-tĕr-ō-RĔKS-ĭs)

8-89 Practice building words with the following organs

rupture of the liver: _____ / _____ / _____

rupture of the bladder: _____ / _____ / _____

rupture of the intestine: _____ / _____ / _____

my/algia
(mī-ĂL-jē-ă)

8-90 My/o/dynia is a muscle pain. Formulate another word that means muscle pain: _____ / _____

my/o/pathy
(mī-ŎP-ă-thē)

8-91 The medical word meaning disease of muscle is _____ / _____ / _____ .

muscle

8-92 My/o/genesis is the formation of _____ .

hardening

8-93 The combining form **scler/o** refers to a _____ .

scler/osis
(sklĕ-RŌ-sĭs)

8-94 An abnormal condition of hardening is called _____ / _____ .

my/o/scler/osis
(mī-ō-sklĕr-Ō-sĭs)

8-95 Form a word that means an abnormal condition of muscle hardening: _____ / _____ / _____ / _____ .

anterior

posterior

8-96 To become familiar with the names of the major muscles of the body, study Figure 8–7.

Write the word in the Figure 8–7 legend that means

in front of: _____

back (of body), behind: _____

tendon

8-97 **Tend/o** is a combining form for tendon, which is the fibrous connective tissue that attaches muscles to bone.

Tend/o/plasty is a surgical repair of a _____ .

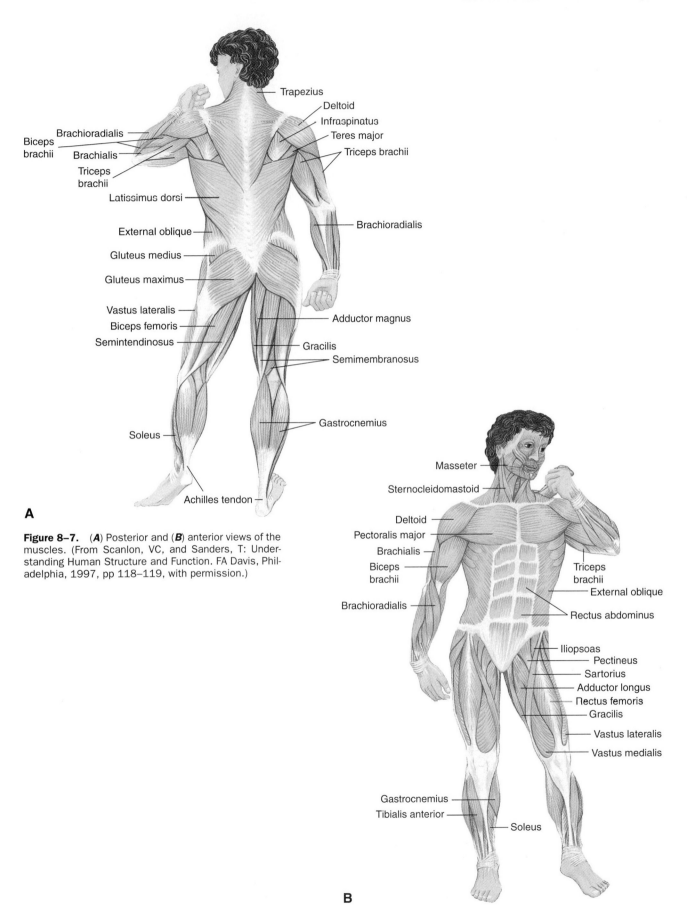

Figure 8–7. (**A**) Posterior and (**B**) anterior views of the muscles. (From Scanlon, VC, and Sanders, T: Understanding Human Structure and Function. FA Davis, Philadelphia, 1997, pp 118–119, with permission.)

A

B

tend/o/tome
(TĔN-dō-tōm)
tend/o/tomy
(tĕn-DŎT-ō-mē)
tend/o/plasty
(TĔN-dō-plăs-tē)

8–98   Use **tend/o** to form words meaning

instrument to cut a tendon: _____ / _____ / _____

incision of a tendon: _____ / _____ / _____

surgical repair of a tendon: _____ / _____ / _____

---

inferior

8–99   The **Achilles tendon** connects to a muscle in the lower leg. Locate the Achilles tendon in Figure 8–7. It is (superior, inferior) _____ to the gastrocnemius muscle.

---

paralysis
(pă-RĂL-ĭ-sĭs)

8–100   The prefix quadri- refers to four. Quadri/plegia is a
_____ of all four extremities.

---

quadri/plegia
(kwŏd-rĭ-PLĒ-jē-ă)

8–101   A paralysis of all four limbs is also called
_____ / _____ .

---

paralysis
(pă-RĂL-ĭ-sĭs)

8–102   The prefix hemi- refers to half or partly. Hemi/plegia is a
_____ of half the body.

Review

Select the medical word element(s) that match(es) the meaning.

cyst / o   -cyte   hemi-
enter / o   -genesis   quadri-
hepat / o   -osis
my / o   -plasty
scler / o   -plegia
tend / o   -rrhaphy
                 -rrhexis
                 -tomy

a. _____ abnormal condition

b. _____ bladder

c. _____ cell

d. _____ four

e. _____ half, partly

f. _____ hardening

g. _____ incision, cut into

h. _____ intestines

i. _____ liver

j. _____ muscle

k. _____ paralysis

l. _____ producing, forming

m. _____ rupture

n. _____ surgical repair

o. _____ suture

p. _____ tendon

Check your answers with the Review Answer Key on the following page.

Review Answer Key

a. -osis

b. cyst/o

c. -cyte

d. quadri-

e. hemi-

f. scler/o

g. -tomy

h. enter/o

i. hepat/o

j. my/o

k. -plegia

l. -genesis

m. -rrhexis

n. -plasty

o. -rrhaphy

p. tend/o

REINFORCEMENT FRAME: If you are not satisfied with your level of comprehension, go back to Frame 8–84 to rework the frames.

Additional Pathological Conditions

ankylosis (ăng-kĭ-LŌ-sĭs): immobility of a joint.

carpal tunnel syndrome (CTS) (KĂR-păl TŬN-ĕl SĬN-drōm): pain or numbness resulting from compression of the median nerve within the carpal tunnel (wrist canal through which the flexor tendons and median nerve pass).

contracture (kŏn-TRAK-chŭr): fibrosis of connective tissue in skin, fascia, muscle or joint capsule that prevents normal mobility of the related tissue or joint.

crepitation (krĕp-ĭ-TĀ-shŭn): grating sound made by movement of bone ends rubbing together, indicating a fracture or joint destruction.

Ewing's sarcoma (Ū-wĭngz săr-KŌ-mă): malignant growth found in the shaft of long bones that spreads to the periosteum.

gout (GOWT): hereditary metabolic disease that is a form of acute arthritis characterized by excessive uric acid in the blood and around the joints.

herniated disk (HĔR-nē-ā-tĕd dĭsk): herniation or rupture of the nucleus pulposus (center gelatinous material within an intervertebral disk) between two vertebrae. Occurs most often in the lumbar region (Fig. 8–8).

kyphosis (kī-FŌ-sĭs): increased convexity in the curvature of the thoracic section of the vertebral column; hunchback or humpback.

lordosis (lōr-DŌ-sĭs): forward curvature of the lumbar spine; swayback.

muscular dystrophy (MŬS-kū-lăr DĬS-trō-fē): group of hereditary diseases characterized by gradual atrophy and weakness of muscle tissue. There is no cure, and most individuals die before the age of 20 years. Duchenne's dystrophy is the most common form.

musculotendinous (mŭs-kū-lō-TĔN-dĭ-nŭs) or rotator cuff injuries: four of the nine muscles that cross the shoulder joint, the supraspinatus, infraspinatus, teres minor, and subscapularis (see Fig. 8-7A), are commonly called the musculotendinous cuff, or rotator cuff muscles. The type of injury to this structure is a compete abduction of the shoulder, followed by a rapid and forceful rotation and flexion of the shoulder, which may strain the musculotendinous cuff. These are common injuries in baseball players when they throw a baseball; it also occurs, but less frequently, in tennis players when they are serving or completing an overhead stroke.

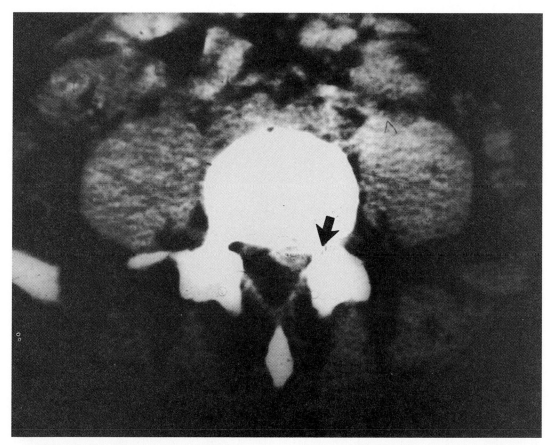

Figure 8–8. Herniated disk in the lateral recess, shown on MRI. (Photo courtesy of Dr. M. Patel, Long Island Jewish Medical Center.)

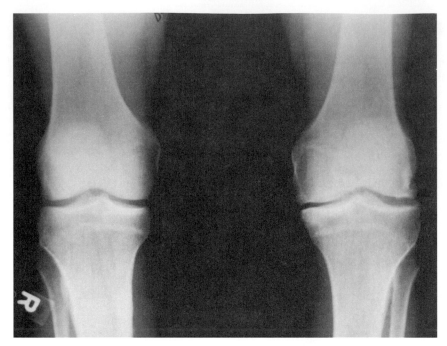

Figure 8–9. X-ray of an arthritic joint. Note the loss of definition in the joint space of the left knee. (From Starkey, C, and Ryan, J: Evaluation of Orthopedic and Athletic Injuries. FA Davis, Philadelphia, 1996, p 35, with permission.)

myasthenia gravis (mī-ăs-THĒ-nē-ă GRĂV-ĭs): autoimmune neuromuscular disorder characterized by severe muscular weakness and progressive fatigue.

osteoporosis (ŏs-tē-ō-pōr-Ō-sĭs): decrease in bone density and an increase in porosity, causing bones to become brittle and increasing the risk of fractures.

Paget's disease (PĂJ-ĕtz dĭs-ZĒZ): skeletal disease of the elderly with chronic inflammation of bones, resulting in thickening and softening of bones and bowing of long bones; osteitis deformans.

rheumatoid arthritis (ROO-mă-toyd ăr-THRĪ-tĭs): chronic, systemic disease characterized by inflammatory changes in joints and related structures that result in crippling deformities (Fig. 8–9).

sequestrum (sē-KWĔS-trŭm): fragment of a necrosed bone that has become separated from surrounding tissue.

sprain (SPRĀN): trauma to a joint that causes injury to the surrounding ligament, accompanied by pain and disability.

strain (STRĀN): trauma to a muscle from overuse or excessive forcible stretch.

talipes (TĂL-ĭ-pĕz): congenital deformity of the foot; clubfoot.

tendinitis (tĕn-dĭn-Ī-tĭs): inflammation of a tendon usually caused by injury or overuse.

torticollis (tŏr-tĭ-KŎL-ĭs): spasmodic contraction of the neck muscles causing stiffness and twisting of the neck that may be congenital or acquired; wryneck.

Medical Report

The reports that follow are related to the medical specialty called Orthopedics. An orthopedist specializes in diagnosing and treating diseases and disorders of the bones, joints, and muscles. An orthopedist is also known as an orthopedic surgeon.

MEDICAL RECORD 8–1. Degenerative, Intervertebral Disk Disease

Dictionary Exercise

This exercise will help you master the terminology in the medical record. Underline the following terms in the reading exercise, and use a medical dictionary to define the words. The pronunciations of medical terms in this report are included in the Audiocassette Exercise on pages 365–367.

AP _____

anteroposterior _____

degenerative _____

flexion _____

bilateral _____

hypertrophic _____

intervertebral _____

L3 to L4 _____

L5 to S1 _____

L5 on S1 _____

laminectomy _____

lateral _____

lipping _____

lumbar _____

lumbosacral _____

sacroiliac _____

spine _____

vertebral _____

Word Element Exercise

Break down the following words into their basic elements.

anteroposterior
bilateral
hypertrophic
intervertebral

lateral
lumbosacral
sacroiliac
vertebral

VALIDATION FRAME: Check your answers in Appendix B, Answer Key.

Reading Exercise

Read the medical report out loud.

Anteroposterior and lateral views of the lumbar spine and an AP view of the sacrum show a placement of L5 on S1. The L5 to S1 intervertebral disk space contains a slight shadow of decreased density. There is now slight narrowing of the L3 to L4 and L4 to L5 spaces. Bilateral laminectomies appear to have been done at L5 to S1. Slight hypertrophic lipping of the upper lumbar vertebral bodies is now seen, as is slight lipping of the upper margin of the body of L4. The sacroiliac joint spaces are well preserved. Lateral views of the lumbosacral spine taken with the spine in flexion and extension demonstrate slight motion at all of the lumbar and lumbosacral levels.

Impression

1. Degenerative, intervertebral disk disease at L5 to S1, now also accompanied by slight narrowing of the L3 to L4 and L4 to L5 disk spaces.

2. Slight motion at all of the lumbar and lumbosacral levels.

MEDICAL RECORD EVALUATION 8–1. Degenerative, Intervertebral Disk Disease

1. Why does the x-ray show a decreased density at L5 to S1?

2. What is the most common cause of degenerative intervertebral disk disease?

3. What happens to the gelatinous material of the disk as aging occurs?

4. What is the probable cause of the narrowing of the L3 to L4 and L4 to L5 spaces?

MEDICAL RECORD 8–2. Rotator Cuff Tear, Right Shoulder

Dictionary Exercise

This exercise will help you master the terminology in the medical record. Underline the following terms in the reading exercise, and use a medical dictionary to define the words. The pronunciations of medical terms in this report are included in the Audiocassette Exercise on pages 365–367.

AC joint _____

acromial _____

acromioclavicular _____

anterior _____

arthritis _____

arthroscopy _____

biceps _____

bursectomy _____

calcification _____

degenerative _____

glenohumeral _____

glenoid _____

gouty _____

intra-articular _____

labra _____

osteoarthritis _____

osteophyte _____

posterior _____

spur _____

subacromial _____

superior _____

tendinitis _____

tuberosity _____

Word Elements Exercise

Break down the following words into their basic elements.

arthritis   subacromial
arthroscopy   tendinitis
osteoarthritis

VALIDATION FRAME: Check your answers in Appendix B, Answer Key.

Reading Exercise

Read the medical report out loud.

Preoperative and Postoperative Diagnosis: Rotator cuff tear, right shoulder. Degenerative arthritis right acromioclavicular joint. Calcific tendinitis at the level of the superior glenoid tuberosity, right shoulder. Early degenerative osteoarthritis of the right shoulder. History of gouty arthritis (see Fig. 8–9).

Operation: Open repair of rotator cuff, open incision outer end of clavicle, anterior acromioplasty, glenohumeral and subacromial arthroscopy with arthroscopic bursectomy.

Findings: A glenohumeral arthroscopy revealed the superior, anterior, inferior, and posterior glenoid labra were intact. There was some fraying of the anterior glenoid labrum. The long head of the biceps was intact. We were unable to visualize any intra-articular calcification. We observed the takeoff of the long head of the biceps from the posterior superior edge of the glenoid labrum and the glenoid tuberosity. There was an osteophyte inferiorly on the humeral head. There was a deep surface tear of the rotator cuff at the posterior superior corner of the greater tuberosity of the humerus at the infraspinatus insertion. There was an extremely dense subacromial bursal scar. There was prominence of the inferior edge of the AC joint, with inferior AC joint and anterior acromial spurs.

MEDICAL RECORD EVALUATION 8–2. Rotator Cuff Tear, Right Shoulder

1. Locate the area and structures that make up the rotator cuff. Use the following references: Figure 8–7, anatomy and physiology textbook, or medical dictionary.

2. What type of arthritis did the patient have?

3. Did the patient have calcium deposits in the right shoulder?

4. Refer to Figure 8–1, and observe the location of the clavicle. Now feel the outer end of your clavicle. What does it feel like?

5. What type of instrument did the physician use to visualize the glenoid labra?

6. What are labra?

7. Did the patient have any outgrowths of bone? If so, where?

8. Did they find any deposits of calcium salts within the shoulder joint?

Abbreviations

Abbreviation	Meaning	Abbreviation	Meaning
AE	above the elbow	HNP	herniated nucleus pulposus (herniated disk)
AK	above the knee		
AP	anteroposterior	IM	intramuscular
BE	below the elbow	L1, L2 to L5	first lumbar vertebra, second lumbar vertebra, and so on
BK	below the knee		
C1, C2 to C7	first cervical vertebra, second cervical vertebra, and so on	Ortho, ORTH	orthopedics
		RA	rheumatoid arthritis
CT	computed tomography	S1, S2 to S5	first sacral vertebra, second sacral vertebra, and so on
CTS	carpal tunnel syndrome		
Fx	fracture	T1, T2 to T12	first thoracic vertebra, second thoracic vertebra, and so on
HD	hip disarticulation; hemodialysis; hearing distance	TKR	total knee replacement

Audiocassette Exercise

The audiocassette tape helps you master the pronunciation of medical words. Listen to the tape for instructions to complete this exercise. You may also use this list without the audiotape to practice correct pronunciation and spelling of the terms.

Frame	Word	Pronunciation	Spelling Exercise
Reading Exercise	[] acromioclavicular	(ă-krō-mē-ŏ-klă-VĬK-ū-lăr)	_____
Reading Exercise	[] anteroposterior	(ăn-tĕr-ō-pŏs-TĒ-rē-ŏr)	_____
8–44	[] arthralgia	(ăr-THRĂL-jē-ă)	_____
8–41	[] arthritis	(ăr-THRĪ-tĭs)	_____
8–41	[] arthrocentesis	(ăr-thrō-sĕn-TĒ-sĭs)	_____
8–44	[] arthrodynia	(ăr-thrō-DĬN-ē-ă)	_____
8–41	[] arthropathy	(ăr-THRŎP-ă-thē)	_____
Reading Exercise	[] arthroscopy	(ăr-THRŎS-kō-pē)	_____
8–76	[] articulation	(ăr-tĭk-ū-LĀ-shŭn)	_____
Reading Exercise	[] biceps	(BĪ-sĕps)	_____
Reading Exercise	[] bilateral	(bī-LĂT-ĕr-ăl)	_____
8–48	[] calcaneum	(kăl-KĀ-nē-ŭm)	_____
8–11	[] calcemia	(kăl-SĒ-mē-ă)	_____
Reading Exercise	[] calcification	(kăl-sĭ-fĭ-KĀ-shŭn)	_____
8–50	[] cephalalgia	(sĕf-ă-LĂL-jē-ă)	_____
8–49	[] cephalodynia	(sĕf-ă-lō-DĬN-ē-ă)	_____
8–51	[] cephalometer	(sĕf-ă-LŎM-ĕ-ter)	_____
8–69	[] cervicofacial	(sĕr-vĭ-kō-FĀ-shē-ăl)	_____
8–36	[] chondritis	(kŏn-DRĪ-tĭs)	_____
8–37	[] chondrocyte	(KŎN-drō-sīt)	_____
8–36	[] chondrogenesis	(kŏn-drō-JĔN-ĕ-sĭs)	_____
8–36	[] chondroma	(kŏn-DRŌ-mă)	_____
8–89	[] cystorrhexis	(sĭs-tō-RĔK-sĭs)	_____
Reading Exercise	[] degenerative	(dē-JĔN-ĕr-ă-tĭv)	_____
8–32	[] distal	(DĬS-tăl)	_____
8–52	[] encephalitis	(ĕn-sĕf-ā-LĪ-tĭs)	_____
8–55	[] encephalocele	(ĕn-SĔF-ă-lō-sēl)	_____
8–52	[] encephaloma	(ĕn-sĕf-ă-LŌ-mă)	_____
8–54	[] encephalopathy	(en-sĕf-ă-LŎP-ă-thē)	_____
8–89	[] enterorrhexis	(ĕn-tĕr-ō-RĔK-sĭs)	_____
Reading Exercise	[] flexion	(FLĔK-shŭn)	_____
Reading Exercise	[] glenohumeral	(glĕ-nō-HŪ-mĕr-ăl)	_____
8–102	[] hemiplegia	(hĕm-ē-PLĒ-jē-ă)	_____
8–89	[] hepatorrhexis	(hĕp-ă-tō-RĔK-sĭs)	_____
8–13	[] hypocalcemia	(hī-pō-kăl-SĒ-mē-ă)	_____
8–60	[] impacted	(ĭm-PĂK-tĕd)	_____
8–56	[] intercostal	(ĭn-tĕr-KŎS-tăl)	_____
8–66	[] intervertebral	(ĭn-tĕr-VĔR-tĕ-brăl)	_____

Frame	Word	Pronunciation	Spelling Exercise
Reading Exercise	[] labra	(LĀ-bră)	_____
Reading Exercise	[] laminectomies	(lăm-ĭ-NĔK-tō-mēz)	_____
Reading Exercise	[] lateral	(LĂT-ĕr-ăl)	_____
8–77	[] lumbar	(LŬM-băr)	_____
8–78	[] lumbodynia	(lŭm-bō-DĬN-ē-ă)	_____
Reading Exercise	[] lumbosacral	(lŭm-bō-SĀ-krăl)	_____
8–27	[] meningitis	(mĕn-ĭn-JĪ-tĭs)	_____
8–28	[] meningocele	(mĕn-ĬN-gō-sēl)	_____
8–30	[] meningomyelitis	(mĕn-ĭn-gō-mī-ĕl-Ī-tĭs)	_____
8–29	[] meningomyelocele	(mĕ-nĭng-gō-MĪ-ĕl-ō-sēl)	_____
8–90	[] myalgia	(mī-ĂL-jē-ă)	_____
8–25	[] myelogenesis	(mī-ĕl-ō-JĔN-ĕ-sĭs)	_____
8–24	[] myelogram	(MĪ-ĕl-ō-grăm)	_____
8–26	[] myelomalacia	(mī-ĕl-ō-mă-LĀ-shē-ă)	_____
8–90	[] myodynia	(mī-ō-DĬN-ē-ă)	_____
8–85	[] myogenesis	(mī-ō-JĔN-ĕ-sĭs)	_____
8–91	[] myopathy	(mī-ŎP-ă-thē)	_____
8–86	[] myoplasty	(MĪ-ō-plăs-tē)	_____
8–86	[] myorrhaphy	(mī-ŌR-ă-fē)	_____
8–95	[] myosclerosis	(mī-ō-sklĕr-Ō-sĭs)	_____
8–86	[] myotomy	(mī-ŎT-ō-mē)	_____
8–2	[] ostealgia	(ŏs-tē-ĂL-jē-ă)	_____
8–4	[] osteitis	(ŏs-tē-Ī-tĭs)	_____
8–45	[] osteoarthritis	(ŏs-tē-ō-ăr-THRĪ-tĭs)	_____
8–46	[] osteoarthropathy	(ŏs-tē-ō-ăr-THRŎP-ă-thē)	_____
8–3	[] osteocytes	(ŎS-tē-ō-sīts)	_____
8–2	[] osteodynia	(ŏs-tē-ō-DĬN-ē-ă)	_____
8–6	[] osteogenesis	(ŏs-tē-ō-JĔN-ĕ-sĭs)	_____
8–7	[] osteomalacia	(ŏs-tē-ō-mă-LĀ-shē-ă)	_____
8–4	[] osteopathy	(ŏs-tē-ŎP-ă-thē)	_____
Reading Exercise	[] osteophyte	(ŎS-tē-ō-fīt)	_____
8–4	[] osteorrhaphy	(ŏs-tē-ŎR-ă-fē)	_____
8–4	[] osteosclerosis	(ŏs-tē-ō-sklĕ-RŌ-sĭs)	_____
8–4	[] osteotomy	(ŏs-tē-ŎT-ō-mē)	_____
8–38	[] periosteum	(pĕr-ē-ŎS-tē-ŭm)	_____
8–33	[] proximal	(PRŎK-sĭm-ăl)	_____
8–100	[] quadriplegia	(kwŏd-rĭ-PLĒ-jē-ă)	_____
8–19	[] radiogram	(RĀ-dē-ō-grăm)	_____
8–18	[] radiography	(rā-dē-ŎG-ră-fē)	_____
8–17	[] radiologist	(rā-dē-ŎL-ō-jĭst)	_____
8–17	[] radiology	(rā-dē-ŎL-ō-jē)	_____
8–10	[] rickets	(RĬK-ĭts)	_____
8–22	[] roentgenogram	(rĕnt-GĔN-ō-grăm)	_____

Frame	Word	Pronunciation	Spelling Exercise
8–22	[] roentgenography	(rĕnt-gĕn-ŎG-ră-fē)	_____
8–21	[] roentgenology	(rĕnt-gĕn-ŎL-ō-jē)	_____
8–81	[] sacrodynia	(sā-krō-DĬN-ē-ă)	_____
Reading Exercise	[] sacroiliac	(sā-krō-ĬL-ē-ăk)	_____
8–81	[] sacrospinal	(sā-krō-SPĪ-năl)	_____
8–83	[] sacrum	(SĀ-krŭm)	_____
8–94	[] sclerosis	(sklĕ-RŌ-sĭs)	_____
8–64	[] spondylitis	(spŏn-dĭ-LĪ-tĭs)	_____
8–62	[] spondylodynia	(spŏn-dĭ-lō-DĬN-ē-ă)	_____
8–64	[] spondylomalacia	(spŏn-dĭ-lō-mă-LĀ-shē-ă)	_____
8–64	[] spondylopathy	(spŏn-dĭl-ŎP-ă-thē)	_____
Reading Exercise	[] spur	(SPŬR)	_____
8–57	[] subcostal	(sŭb-KŎS-tăl)	_____
Reading Exercise	[] tendinitis	(tĕn-dĭn-Ī-tĭs)	_____
8–97	[] tendoplasty	(TĔN-dō-plăs-tē)	_____
8–98	[] tendotome	(TĔN-dō-tōm)	_____
8–98	[] tendotomy	(tĕn-DŎT-ō-mē)	_____
Reading Exercise	[] tuberosity	(tū-bĕr-ŎS-ĭ-tē)	_____
8–63	[] vertebrae	(VĔR-tĕ-brē)	_____
8–61	[] vertebral	(VĔR-tĕ-brăl)	_____
8–62	[] vertebrectomy	(vĕr-tĕ-BRĔK-tō-mē)	_____
8–65	[] vertebrocostal	(vĕr-tĕ-brō-KŎS-tăl)	_____
8–65	[] vertebrosternal	(vĕr-tĕ-brō-STĔR-năl)	_____

Unit Exercises

DEFINITIONS

Review Unit Summary (pages 375–377) before completing this exercise. Write the definition for each word part.

SUFFIXES AND PREFIXES

ELEMENT	MEANING
Surgical Suffixes	
1. -centesis	_____ \
2. -plasty	_____
3. -rrhaphy	_____
4. -tomy	_____
Other Suffixes	
5. -algia	_____
6. -cyte	_____
7. -dynia	_____
8. -emia	_____
9. -gram	_____
10. -graphy	_____
11. -malacia	_____
12. -meter	_____
13. -oma	_____
14. -osis	_____
15. -pathy	_____
16. -rrhexis	_____
Prefixes	
17. hemi-	_____
18. hypo-	_____
19. inter-	_____
20. peri-	_____
21. quadri-	_____
Combining Forms	
22. arthr/o	_____
23. calc/o	_____
24. cephal/o	_____
25. chondr/o	_____
26. dist/o	_____
27. encephal/o	_____
28. lumb/o	_____
29. myel/o	_____
30. my/o	_____

ELEMENT	MEANING
31. oste/o	_____
32. roentgen/o	_____
33. scler/o	_____
34. spondyl/o	_____
35. tend/o	_____

VALIDATION FRAME: Check your answers in the Index of Medical Word Elements, Part A of Appendix A. If you scored less than _____ %,* review Unit Summary (pages 375–377).

To obtain a percentage score, multiply the number of correct answers times 2.86.

Number of Correct Answers: _____   **Percentage Score:** _____

*Enter the percentage required by your instructor to complete this course.

Vocabulary

Match these medical word(s) with the definitions in the numbered list.

AP
arthrocentesis
atlas
articulation
bilateral
bone marrow
cephalometer
cervical vertebrae

compound or open fracture
diaphysis
distal
intervertebral
myelogram
myorrhexis

proximal
quadriplegia
radiology
roentgenologist
simple or closed fracture
spondylomalacia

1. _____ Study of x-rays and radioactive substances used for diagnosing and treating diseases.

2. _____ Shaft or main part of the bone.

3. _____ Passing from the front to the rear.

4. _____ A fracture in which the bone is broken but there is no external wound. The surrounding tissue damage is minimal.

5. _____ Pertaining to or affecting two sides.

6. _____ Near the point of attachment to the trunk.

7. _____ The place of union between two or more bones; a joint.

8. _____ A fracture in which the broken end of a bone has been moved, so that it pierces the skin. There may be extensive damage to surrounding blood vessels, nerves, and muscles.

9. _____ First cervical vertebra, which supports the skull.

10. _____ Surgical puncture of a joint to remove fluid.

11. _____ Soft tissue that fills the medullary cavities of long bones.

12. _____ Instrument used to measure the head.

13. _____ A roentgenogram of the spinal canal after injection of a radiopaque dye.

14. _____ Rupture of a muscle.

15. _____ Softening of vertebrae.

16. _____ Directional term that means farthest from the point of attachment to the trunk.

17. _____ A physician who specializes in the use of x-rays for diagnosis and the treatment of disease.

18. _____ Bones that form the skeletal framework of the neck.

19. _____ Situated between two adjacent vertebrae.

20. _____ Paralysis of all four extremities.

VALIDATION FRAME: Check your answers in Appendix B, Answer Key. If you scored less than _____ %, review the vocabulary and retake the exercise.

To obtain a percentage score, multiply the number of correct answers times 5.

Number of Correct Answers: _____   **Percentage Score:** _____

Additional Pathological Conditions

Match the medical word(s) that follow with the definitions in the numbered list.

ankylosis	kyphosis	sequestrum
carpal tunnel syndrome	lordosis	sprain
contracture	muscular dystrophy	strain
crepitation	myasthenia gravis	talipes
Ewing's sarcoma	osteoporosis	tendinitis
gout	Paget's disease	torticollis
herniated disk	rheumatoid arthritis	

1. _____ Decrease in bone density and an increase in porosity, which increases the risk of fractures.

2. _____ Inflammation of a tendon.

3. _____ Trauma to a joint, causing causes injury to the surrounding ligament.

4. _____ Trauma to a muscle that results from overuse or excessive, forcible stretch.

5. _____ Hunchback or humpback.

6. _____ Malignant growth found in the shaft of long bones that spreads to the periosteum.

7. _____ Wryneck.

8. _____ Disease characterized by excessive uric acid in the blood and around the joints.

9. _____ Disease characterized by inflammatory changes in joints and related structures that result in crippling deformities.

10. _____ Skeletal disease of the elderly with chronic inflammation of bones, resulting in thickening and softening of bones and bowing of long bones; osteitis deformans.

11. _____ Fragment of necrosed bone that has become separated from surrounding tissue.

12. _____ Clubfoot.

13. _____ Grating sound made by the ends of bone rubbing together.

14. _____ A neuromuscular disorder characterized by muscular weakness and progressive fatigue.

15. _____ Forward curvature of the lumbar spine; swayback.

16. _____ Group of hereditary diseases characterized by gradual atrophy and weakness of muscle (i.e., Duchenne's dystrophy).

17. _____ Connective tissue fibrosis that prevents normal mobility of the related tissue or joint.

18. _____ Immobility of a joint.

19. _____ Rupture of the nucleus pulposus between two vertebrae.

20. _____ Pain or numbness resulting from compression of the median nerve within the carpal tunnel.

VALIDATION FRAME: Check your answers in Appendix B, Answer Key. If you scored less than _____ %, review the vocabulary and retake the exercise.

To obtain a percentage score, multiply the number of correct answers times 5.

Unit Summary

COMBINING FORMS RELATED TO THE MUSCULOSKELETAL SYSTEM

Combining Form	Pronunciation	Meaning
arthr/o	ăr-thrō	joint
calc/o	kăl-kō	calcium
calcane/o	kăl-kā-nē-ō	calcaneum (heel bone)
carp/o	kăr-pō	carpus (wrist bones)
cephal/o	sĕf-ăl-ō	head
cervic/o	sĕr-vĭ-kō	neck
chondr/o	kŏn-drō	cartilage
cost/o	kŏs-tō	ribs
crani/o	krā-nē-ō	cranium (skull)
encephal/o	ĕn-sĕf-ă-lō	brain
femor/o	fĕm-ō-rō	femur (thigh bone)
fibul/o	fĭb-ū-lō	fibula
humer/o	hū-mĕr-ō	humerus
lumb/o	lŭm-bō	lower back, loin
metacarp/o	mĕt-ă-kăr-pō	metacarpus (bones of the hand)
myel/o	mī-ĕl-ō	spinal cord, bone marrow
my/o	mī-ō	muscle
oste/o	ŏs-tē-ō	bone
patell/o	pă-tĕl-ō	knee cap
radi/o	rā-dē-ō	x-rays, radiation
roentgen/o	rĕnt-gĕn-ō	x-rays
sacr/o	sā-krō	sacrum
spin/o	spī-nō	spine
spondyl/o (used to construct words about the condition of the structure) vertebr/o (used to construct words that describe the structure)	spŏn-dĭ-lō ver-tĕ-brō	vertebra (backbone)
stern/o	stĕr-nō	sternum (breastbone)
tend/o	tĕn-dō	tendon
tibi/o	tĭb-ē-ō	tibia

OTHER COMBINING FORMS IN UNIT 8

Combining Form	Pronunciation	Meaning
cyt/o	sī-tō	cell
cyst/o	sĭs-tō	bladder, sac
dist/o	dĭs-tō	far, farthest
enter/o	ĕn-tĕr-ō	intestine (usually small)
hepat/o	hĕp-ă-tō	liver
proxim/o	prŏk-sĭm-ō	near
scler/o	sklĕ-rō	hardening, sclera (white of the eye)

SUFFIXES AND PREFIXES

Suffix (Prefix)	Pronunciation	Meaning
SURGICAL SUFFIXES		
-centesis	sĕn-tē-sĭs	surgical puncture
-ectomy	ĕk-tō-mē	excision, removal
-plasty	plăs-tē	surgical repair
-rrhaphy	ră-fē	suture
-tomy	tō-mē	incision, cut into
OTHER SUFFIXES		
-al	ăl	pertaining to
-algia dynia	ăl-jē-ă dĭn-ē-ă	pain
-cele	sēl	hernia, swelling
-cyte	sīt	cell
-emia	ē-mē-ă	blood
-genesis	jĕn-ĕ-sĭs	producing, forming
-gram	grăm	record
-graphy	gră-fē	process of recording
-ist	ĭst	specialist
-itis	ī-tĭs	inflammation
-logist	lō-jĭst	specialist in the study of
-malacia	mă-lā-shē-ă	softening
-meter	mē-tĕr	measure, instrument for measuring
-oma	ō-mă	tumor
-osis	ō-sĭs	abnormal condition
-pathy	pă-thē	disease
-plegia	plē-jē-ă	paralysis
-rrhexis	rĕk-sĭs	rupture

Suffix (Prefix)	Pronunciation	Meaning
PREFIXES		
en-	ĕn	in
hemi-	hĕm-ē	half, partly
hypo-	hī-pō	under, below, deficient
inter-	ĭn-tĕr	between
peri-	pĕr-ē	around
quadri-	kwŏd-rī	four

CARDIOVASCULAR AND LYMPHATIC SYSTEMS

The heart and blood vessels compose the cardiovascular system, which circulates blood throughout the body.

The lymphatic system is composed of lymph nodes, lymph vessels, and lymph fluid. It is responsible for draining fluid from the tissues and returning it to the bloodstream.

The relationship of the lymphatic vessels to the cardiovascular system is illustrated in Figure 9–1.

CARDIOVASCULAR SYSTEM

The combining forms related to the cardiovascular system are summarized here. Review this information before you begin to work the frames.

COMBINING FORMS

Combining Form	Meaning	Example	Pronunciation
angi/o	vessel	angi/o/gram record	ĂN-jē-ō-grăm
vas/o		vas/o/spasm twitching, involuntary contraction	VĂS-ō-spăzm
aort/o	aorta	aort/o/stenosis stricture, narrowing	ā-ōr-tō-stĕn-Ō-sĭs
arteri/o	artery	arteri/o/scler/ osis hardening abnormal condition	ăr-tē-rē-ō-sklĕ-RŌ-sĭs
ather/o	fatty plaque	ather/oma tumor	ăth-ĕr-Ō-mă
atri/o	atrium	atri/o/ventricul/ar ventrical pertaining to	ā-trē-ō-vĕn-TRĬK-ū-lăr
cardi/o	heart	cardi/o/megaly enlargement	kăr-dē-ō-MĔG-ă-lē
electr/o	electric	electr/o/cardi/o/gram heart record	ē-lĕk-trō-KĂR-dē-ō-grăm
phleb/o	vein	phleb/itis inflammation	flĕb-Ī-tĭs
ven/o		ven/ous pertaining to	VĒ-nŭs

Combining Form	Meaning	Example	Pronunciation
thromb/o	blood clot	thromb/o/lysis destruction, loosening, separation	thrŏm-BŎL-ĭ-sĭs
ventricul/o	ventricle (of brain or heart)	inter/ventricul/ar between pertaining to	ĭn-tĕr-vĕn-TRĬK-ū-lăr

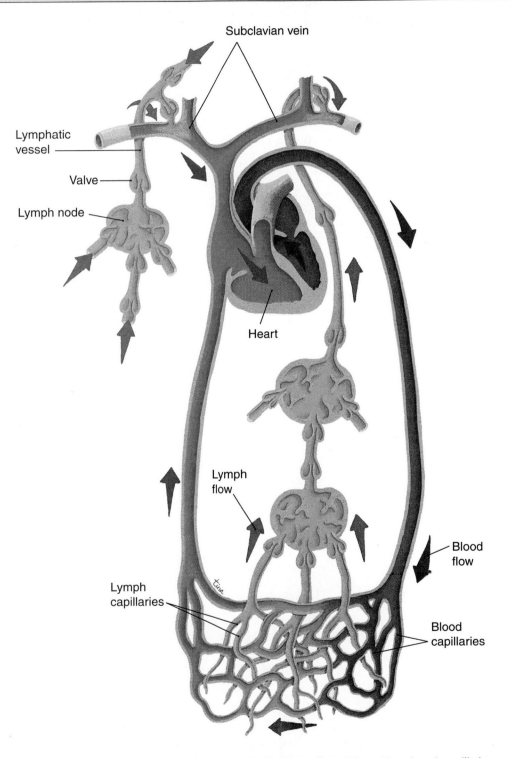

Figure 9–1. Relationship of the lymphatic system with the cardiovascular system. Lymph capillaries collect tissue fluid, which is returned to the blood. The arrows indicate direction of flow of the blood and lymph. (From Scanlon, VC, and Sanders, T: Understanding Human Structure and Function. FA Davis, Philadelphia, 1997, p 248, with permission.)

9–1 Use the Index of Medical Word Elements, Part A of Appendix A, to define the following elements.

Word Element	Meaning
brady-	_____
epi-	_____
cardi/o	_____
peri-	_____
-phagia	_____
tachy-	_____
-um	_____

9–2 The heart has three distinct layers of tissue: the **(1) endocardium**, the **(2) myocardium**, and the **(3) epicardium**.

---

my/o/cardi/um
(mī-ō-KĂR-dē-ŭm)
epi/cardi/um
(ĕp-ĭ-KĂR-dē-ŭm)
endo/cardi/um
(ĕn-dō-KĂR-dē-ŭm)

9–3 The combining form **cardi/o** means heart. Refer to Figure 9–2 to identify the layers of the heart.

The middle layer of the heart, composed of muscular tissue, is the

_____ / _____ / _____ / _____ .

The external layer of the heart is the _____ / _____ / _____ .

The inner layer of the heart is the _____ / _____ / _____ .

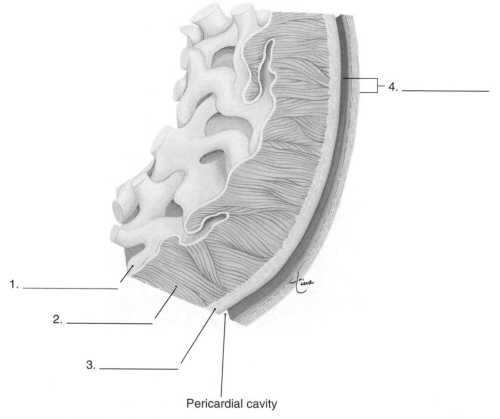

1. _____

2. _____

3. _____

4. _____

Pericardial cavity

Figure 9–2. The layers of the heart wall. (Adapted from Scanlon, VC, and Sanders, T: Understanding Human Structure and Function. FA Davis, Philadelphia, 1997, p 211, with permission.)

9-4   The heart is a muscular organ that pumps blood and is enclosed in a membranous sac called the **(4) pericardium**.

Label the pericardium in Figure 9–2.

---

peri/card/itis
(pĕr-ĭ-kăr-DĪ-tis)
peri/cardi/um
(pĕr-ĭ-KĂR-dē-ŭm)

9-5   Remember that the prefix peri- means around. Peri/card/itis is an inflammation of the peri/cardi/um. This condition causes an accumulation of fluid around the heart and decreases the heart's ability to pump blood.

Write the words in this frame that mean

   inflammation around the heart: _____ / _____ / _____

   around the heart: _____ / _____ / _____

---

peri/cardi/ectomy
(pĕr-ĭ-kăr-dē-ĔK-tō-mē)

9-6   The surgical procedure in which all or part of the peri/cardi/um is excised is called _____ / _____ / _____ .

---

peri/cardi/o/rrhaphy
(pĕr-ĭ-kăr-dē-OR-ă-fē)

9-7   A suture of a wound in the peri/cardi/um is called

_____ / _____ / _____ / _____ .

---

my/o/cardi/um
(mī-ō-KĂR-dē-ŭm)

9-8   The muscular layer of the heart is called the

_____ / _____ / _____ / _____ .

VALIDATION FRAME: Check your labeling of Figure 9–2 in Appendix B, Answer Key.

Structures of the Heart

9-9   There are two sides to the heart. Each side is subdivided into two chambers, for a total of four chambers. The upper chambers of the heart consist of the **(1) right atrium (RA)** and **(2) left atrium (LA)**.

Label the structures in Figure 9–3.

---

atri/al
(Ă-trē-ăl)

9-10   The combining form **atri/o** refers to the atrium, which is the upper chamber of each half of the heart.

Build a word that means pertaining to the atrium: _____ / _____ .

---

atrium, left
(Ā-trē-ŭm)

9-11   The heart consists of two upper chambers. These include the right _____ and the _____ atrium.

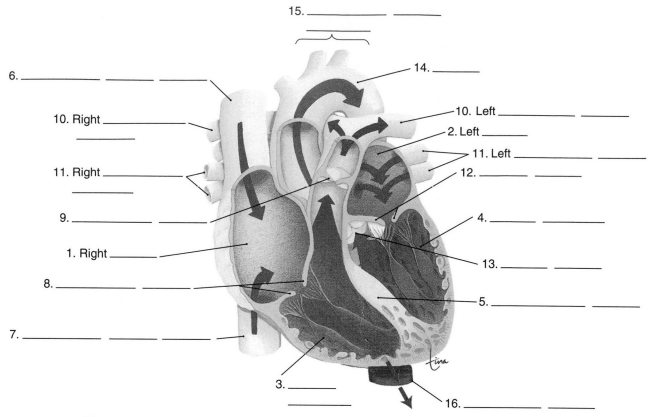

15. _____ _____

6. _____ _____ _____

10. Right _____ _____

14. _____

10. Left _____ _____

2. Left _____

11. Left _____ _____

11. Right _____ _____

12. _____ _____

9. _____ _____

4. _____ _____

1. Right _____

13. _____ _____

8. _____ _____

5. _____ _____

7. _____ _____ _____

3. _____ _____

16. _____ _____

Figure 9–3. Frontal section of the heart in anterior view, showing internal structures. (Adapted from Scanlon, VC, and Sanders, T: Understanding Human Structure and Function. FA Davis, Philadelphia, 1997, p 213, with permission.)

RA LA	**9–12** Write the abbreviation for right atrium: _____ left atrium: _____

9–13 The two lower chambers of the heart consist of the **(3) right ventricle (RV)** and **(4) left ventricle (LV)**.

Label the ventricles in Figure 9–3.

ventricul/o/tomy (vĕn-trĭk-ū-LŎT-ō-mē)	**9–14** The combining form **ventricul/o** refers to both the ventricles of the heart and the ventricles of the brain. An incision of a ventricle is known as a _____ / _____ / _____ .

ventricle (VĔN-trĭk-l)	**9–15** Remember that both -ar and -al are adjective-ending suffixes that mean "pertaining to." Atri/o/ventricul/ar (AV) refers to both the atrium and _____ .

ventricul/ar (vĕn-TRĬK-ū-lăr)	**9–16** A flutter is a rapid contraction of the atrium or ventricle. When the flutter occurs in the atrium, it is called an atri/al flutter. When the flutter occurs in the ventricle, it is called a _____ / _____ flutter.
right atrium (Ā-trē-ŭm) **left atrium** (Ā-trē-ŭm)	**9–17** An atri/al flutter can cause chest pain and shortness of breath (SOB), which is not uncommon in the elderly population. An atri/al flutter originates in the upper chambers of the heart, which are the right atrium and the left atrium. An RA flutter originates in the _____ _____ . An LA flutter originates in the _____ _____ .
RV **LV**	**9–18** Write the abbreviations for the two lower chambers of the heart. right ventricle: _____ left ventricle: _____

9–19 The rule for forming plural words from singular words that end in -um is to drop -um and add -a .

	Singular	*Plural*
atria (Ā-trē-ă)	atrium	_____
cardia (KĂR-dē-ă)	cardium	_____
septa (SĔP-tă)	septum	_____
bacteria (băk-TĒ-rē-ă)	bacterium	_____

9–20 The **(5) interventricular septum** (IVS) separates the LV from the RV. Label the structure in Figure 9–3.

LA	**9–21** A wall or partition dividing a body space or cavity is known as a septum (septa, plural). Some septa are membranous, some are composed of bone, and some are composed of cartilage. Each is named according to its location. For example, the interatrial septum (IAS) separates the RA from the _____ .

9–22 Form singular words from the following plural words. Apply the rule that was covered in Frame 9–19.

	Plural	*Singular*
bacterium (băk-TĒ-rē-ŭm)	bacteria	_____
septum (SĔP-tŭm)	septa	_____
atrium (Ā-trē-ŭm)	atria	_____
cardium (KĂR-dē-ŭm)	cardia	_____

rapid	**9–23** The prefix tachy- is used in words to mean rapid. Tachy/cardia is a heart rate that is _____ .
rapid eating	**9–24** Tachy/pnea refers to rapid breathing; tachy/phagia refers to rapid swallowing or _____ _____ .
brady/cardia (brād-ē-KĂR-dē-ă)	**9–25** The prefix brady- is used in words to mean slow. Combine brady- and -cardia to form a word meaning slow heart rate. _____ / _____ .
brady/cardia (brād-ē-KĂR-dē-ă)	**9–26** People with brady/cardia often have difficulty pumping enough blood to body tissues. A person with a slow heart rate has a condition called _____ / _____ .
brady/pnea (brād-ĭp-NĒ-ă) brady/phagia (brād-ē-FĂ-jē-ă)	**9–27** Form medical words that literally mean slow breathing: _____ / _____ slow eating: _____ / _____
tachy/pnea (tăk-ĭp-NĒ-ă) tachy/phagia (tăk-ē-FĂ-jē-ă)	**9–28** Construct medical words that mean rapid breathing: _____ / _____ rapid eating: _____ / _____
RA LA RV LV IVS IAS	**9–29** Review the chambers and structures of the heart (Fig. 9–3) by writing the abbreviation for the right atrium: _____ left atrium: _____ right ventricle: _____ left ventricle: _____ inter/ventricul/ar septum: _____ inter/atri/al septum: _____

Blood Flow Through The Heart

9–30 The right atrium receives oxygen-poor blood from all tissues except those of the lungs. The blood from the head and arms is delivered to the RA through the **(6) superior vena cava (SVC)**. The blood from the legs and torso is delivered to the RA through the **(7) inferior vena cava (IVC)**.

Label the structures in Figure 9–3.

inferior

superior

9-31 Determine the directional words in Frame 9–30 that mean

below (another structure): _____

above (another structure): ___ _____

---

superior

inferior

9-32 Refer to Figure 9–3 and use the words "superior" or "inferior" to complete this frame.

The left atrium is _____ to the left ventricle.

The right ventricle is _____ to the right atrium.

9-33 Blood flows from the right atrium through the **(8) tricuspid valve** and into the right ventricle. The leaflets (cusps) are shaped so that they form a one-way passage, which keeps the blood flowing in only one direction.

Label the tricuspid valve in Figure 9–3.

---

tri / cuspid valve
(trī-KŬS-pĭd)

9-34 The prefix `tri-` means three. The valve that has three leaflets or flaps is known as the _____ / _____ _____ .

---

three

9-35 In the English language, a tri / angle is a figure that has _____ sides.

---

two

9-36 The prefix `bi-` refers to two or double. A bi / cuspid valve has _____ leaflets or flaps.

---

three

9-37 In the English language, a bi / cycle has two wheels; a tri / cycle has _____ wheels.

---

two, three

9-38 By relating `bi-` and `tri-` to words in the English language, these prefixes should not be difficult to recall.

`bi-` means _____; `tri-` means _____ .

9-39 The ventricles are the pumping chambers of the heart. As the right ventricle contracts to pump oxygen-deficient blood through the **(9) pulmonary valve** into the pulmonary artery, the tri / cuspid valve remains closed, preventing a backflow of blood into the right atrium.

Once the blood passes through the main pulmonary artery, it branches into the **(10) right pulmonary artery** and **(10) left pulmonary arteries**. The pulmonary arteries carry the oxygen-deficient blood to the lungs.

Label the structures introduced in this frame in Figure 9–3.

---

artery
(ĂR-tĕr-ē)

9-40 The combining form **arteri / o** refers to an artery.

Arteri / al bleeding is bleeding from an _____ .

arteries (ĂR-tĕr-ēs)	**9–41** Arteri/al circulation is movement of blood through the _____ .
arteri/o/scler/osis (ăr-tē-rē-ō-sklĕr-Ō-sĭs)	**9–42** Arteri/o/scler/osis is a disease characterized by thickening and loss of elasticity of arteri/al walls. A person with a disease or abnormal condition of arteri/al hardening suffers from _____ / _____ / _____ / _____ .
stone, artery (ĂR-tĕr-ē)	**9–43** An arteri/o/lith, also called an arteri/al calculus, is a calculus or _____ in an _____ .
artery (ĂR-tĕr-ē)	**9–44** An arteri/al spasm is a spasm of an _____ .
arteri/o/rrhexis (ăr-tē-rē-ō-RĔK-sĭs) **arteri/o/rrhaphy** (ăr-tē-rē-ŌR-ă-fē) **arteri/o/pathy** (ăr-tē-rē-ŎP-ă-thē) **arteri/o/spasm** (ăr-TĒ-rē-ō-spăzm)	**9–45** Develop medical words that mean rupture of an artery: _____ / _____ / _____ suture of an artery: _____ / _____ / _____ disease of an artery: _____ / _____ / _____ spasm of an artery: _____ / _____ / _____
ten (10)	**9–46** The right and left pulmonary arteries leading to the lungs branch and subdivide until ultimately they form capillaries around the alveoli. Carbon dioxide is passed from the blood into the alveoli to be breathed out of the lungs. Oxygen breathed in by the lungs is passed from the alveoli into the blood. (Refer to Unit 6, Frame 6–58 to review the alveolar structure). The left and right pulmonary arteries are identified in Figure 9–3 as number _____ .
	9–47 The oxygenated blood leaves the lungs and returns to the heart via the **(11) right pulmonary veins** and **(11) left pulmonary veins**. The four pulmonary veins empty into the LA. The LA contracts to force blood through the **(12) mitral valve** into the LV. Label the structures in Figure 9–3.
two	**9–48** The mitral valve, located between the LA and LV, is a bi/cuspid or bi/leaflet valve. This means that the number of leaflets or flaps that the mitral valve has is _____ .

9–49 Write the meaning for the following abbreviations.

left atrium
(Ā-trē-ŭm)

LA: _____ _____

left ventricle
(VĔN-trik-l)

LV: _____ _____

inter/ventricul/ar
   septum
(ĭn-tĕr-vĕn-TRĬK-ū-lăr
SĔP-tum)

IVS: _____ / _____ / _____ _____

inter/atri/al septum
(ĭn-tĕr-Ā-trē-ăl SĔP-tŭm)

IAS: _____ / _____ / _____ _____

---

vein
(VĀN)

9–50 Recall that **ven/o** is a combining form meaning _____ .

---

vein
(VĀN)

9–51 **Phleb/o** is another combining form for vein. Phleb/o/tomy is a procedure used to draw blood from a _____ .

9–52 Use **phleb/o** to construct words meaning

phleb/o/rrhaphy
(flĕb-ŌR-ă-fē)

suture of a vein: _____ / ____ / _____

phleb/o/rrhexis
(flĕb-ō-RĔK-sĭs)

rupture of a vein: _____ / ____ / _____

phleb/o/stenosis
(flĕb-ō-stĕ-NŌ-sĭs)

stricture or narrowing of a vein:

_____ / ____ / _____

9–53 Use **ven/o** to form words meaning

ven/o/scler/osis
(vĕn-ō-sklĕ-RŌ-sĭs)

hardening of a vein: _____ / ____ / _____ / _____

ven/o/tomy
(vĕ-NŎT-ō-mē)

incision of a vein: _____ / ____ / _____

ven/o/spasm
(VĔ-nō-spăzm)

contraction or twitching of a vein: _____ / ____ / _____

9–54 To classify a heart abnormality, it is important to identify the part of the organ in which the abnormality occurs.
   For example, a mitral valve murmur is a murmur caused by an incompetent or faulty valve. The murmur occurs in the _____ _____ .

mitral valve
(MĪ-trăl)

9–55 Replacement surgery can be performed to replace a damaged heart valve. Figure 9–4 is an illustration of a heart valve replacement at the level of the

tri/cuspid valve
(trī-KŬS-pĭd)

_____ / _____ _____ .

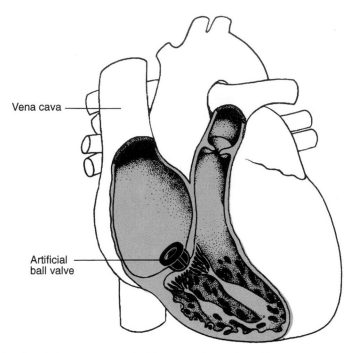

Vena cava

Artificial
ball valve

Figure 9–4. Heart valve replacement at the level of the tricuspid valve. (From Gylys, BA, and Wedding, ME: Medical Terminology: A Systems Approach, ed 3. FA Davis, Philadelphia, 1995, p 155 with permission.)

blood	**9–56** Recall that **hemat/o** and **hem/o** mean _____ .
hemat/o/logy (hē-mă-TŎL-ō-jē) hemat/o/logist (hē-mă-TŎL-ō-jĭst)	**9–57** Use **hemat/o** to form words meaning study of blood: _____ / _____ _____ specialist in the study of blood: _____ / _____ / _____
vessels	**9–58** **Angi/o** is a combining form for vessel, usually blood or lymph vessels. An angi/o/ma is a tumor consisting primarily of blood or lymph _____ .
hemangi/oma (hē-măn-jē-Ō-mă)	**9–59** You can combine **hem/o** and **angi/o** into a new element that also means blood vessel. Use **hemangi/o** (blood vessel) to develop a word meaning tumor of blood vessels: _____ / _____
expansion	**9–60** Hemangi/ectasis is a dilation or _____ of a blood vessel.

9–61 Contractions of the LV send oxygenated blood through the **(13) aortic valve** and into the **(14) aorta**. The three ascending **(15) branches of the aorta**

transport blood to the head and arms. The **(16) descending aorta** transports the blood to the legs and torso.

Label the structures in Figure 9–3 as you continue to learn about the heart.

VALIDATION FRAME: Check your labeling of Figure 9–3 in Appendix B, Answer Key.

aort / o / pathy (ā-ŏr-TŎP-ă-thē)	**9–62** The aorta is the largest artery of the body and originates at the LV of the heart. The combining form **aort / o** refers to the aorta. Any disease of the aorta is called _____ / _____ / _____ .
aort / o / malacia (ā-ŏr-tō-mă-LĀ-shē-ă)	**9–63** A softening of the aorta is known as _____ / _____ / _____ .
artery small vein	**9–64** The suffixes -ole and -ule refer to small. An arteri / ole is a small _____ ; a ven / ule is a _____ _____ .
arteries arteri / oles (ăr-TĒ-rē-ōls)	**9–65** Arteries are large vessels that convey blood away from the heart; they branch into smaller vessels called arteri / oles (see Fig. 9–1). The arteri / oles deliver blood to adjoining minute vessels called capillaries. Large vessels that transport blood away from the heart are called _____ . Smaller vessels that are formed from arteries are called _____ / _____ .
arteri / oles (ăr-TĒ-rē-ōls)	**9–66** Arteries convey blood to adjacent smaller vessels called _____ / _____ .
capillaries (KĂP-ĭ-lă-rēz)	**9–67** Arteri / oles are thinner than arteries and carry blood to minute vessels called _____ (see Fig. 9–1).
arteri / o / scler / osis (ăr-tē-rē-ō-sklĕ-RŌ-sĭs)	**9–68** Arteries carry blood under high pressure, so deterioration of their walls is part of the aging process. As a person ages, the arteries lose their elasticity, thicken, and become weakened. This process of deterioration is also known as an abnormal condition of artery hardening, or _____ / _____ / _____ / _____ .

arteri/o/scler/osis
(ăr-tē-rē-ō-sklĕ-RŌ-sĭs)

9–69 High blood pressure and high-fat diets contribute greatly to early arteri/o/scler/osis. A healthy diet can decrease the risk for hardening of the arteries, also called _____ / ____ / _____ / _____ .

superior vena cava
(VĒ-nă) (KĂ-vă)
inferior vena cava
(VĒ-nă) (KĂ-vă)

9–70 Capillaries carry blood from arteri/oles to ven/ules. Ven/ules form a collecting system to return oxygen-deficient blood to the heart through two large veins, the SVC and the IVC.

Define the following abbreviations

SVC: _____ _____ _____

IVC: _____ _____ _____

6, 7

9–71 In Figure 9–3, the SVC is number ____ ; the IVC is number ____ .

arteri/o/spasm
(ăr-TĒ-rē-ō-spăzm)

9–72 Combine **arteri/o** and -spasm to form a word meaning arterial spasm. _____ / ____ / _____

Review

Select the element(s) that match(es) the meaning.

aort/o	-ectasis	bi-
arteri/o	-malacia	brady-
atri/o	-ole	endo-
cardi/o	-osis	epi-
hem/o	-pathy	peri-
hemat/o	-phagia	tachy-
my/o	-pnea	tri-
phleb/o	-rrhexis	
scler/o	-spasm	
ven/o	-stenosis	
ventricul/o	-ule	

a. _____ abnormal condition

b. _____ above, upon

c. _____ aorta

d. _____ around

e. _____ artery

f. _____ atrium

g. _____ blood

h. _____ breathing

i. _____ disease

j. _____ expansion, dilation

k. _____ hardening

l. _____ heart

m. _____ involuntary contraction, twitching

n. _____ muscle

o. _____ rapid

p. _____ rupture

q. _____ slow

r. _____ small

s. _____ softening

t. _____ stricture, narrowing

u. _____ swallowing, eating

v. _____ three

w. _____ two, double

x. _____ vein

y. _____ ventricle (of brain or heart)

Check your answers with the Review Answer Key on the following page.

Review Answer Key

a. -osis

b. epi-

c. aort/o

d. peri-

e. arteri/o

f. atri/o

g. hem/o, hemat/o

h. -pnea

i. -pathy

j. -ectasis

k. scler/o

l. cardi/o

m. -spasm

n. my/o

o. tachy-

p. -rrhexis

q. brady-

r. -ole, -ule

s. -malacia

t. -stenosis

u. -phagia

v. tri-

w. bi-

x. phleb/o, ven/o

y. ventricul/o

REINFORCEMENT FRAME: If you are not satisfied with your level of comprehension, go back to Frame 9–1 and rework the frames.

The Conduction Pathway of the Heart

9–73 The primary responsibility for initiating the heartbeat rests with the pacemaker of the heart or the **(1) sinoatrial (SA) node**. The SA node is a small region of specialized cardiac muscle tissue located on the posterior wall of the **(2) RA**.

Label the two structures in Figure 9–5.

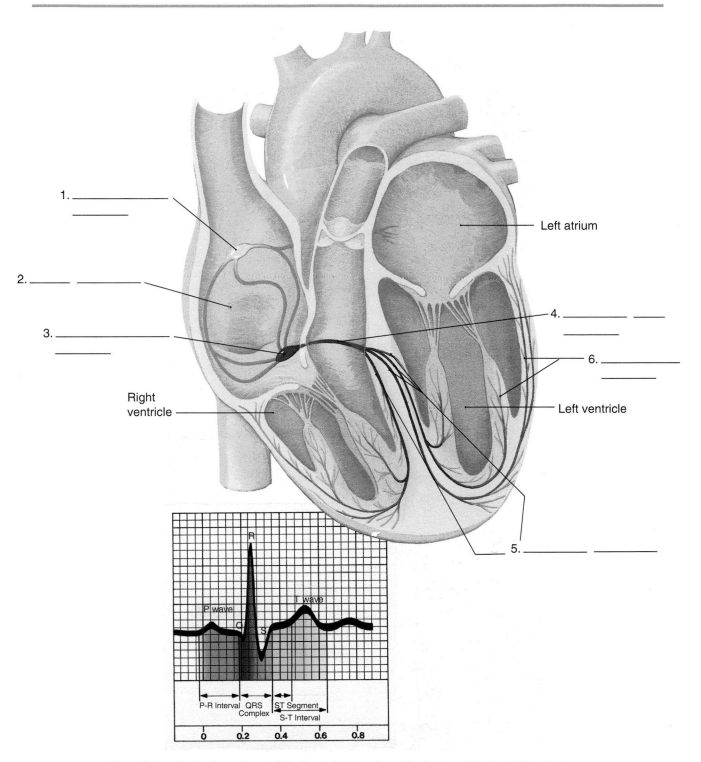

Figure 9–5. Conduction pathway of the heart. Anterior view of the interior of the heart. The electrocardiogram tracing is one normal heartbeat. (Adapted from Scanlon, VC, and Sanders, T: Understanding Human Structure and Function. FA Davis, Philadelphia, 1997, p 217, with permission.)

SA
RA

9–74 Write the abbreviations for

sinoatrial: _____

right atrium: _____

electricity

9–75 The combining form **electr/o** refers to electricity.

Electric/al and electr/ic both mean pertaining to _____ .

9–76 The electrical current generated by the heart's pacemaker causes the atrial walls to contract and forces the flow of blood into the ventricles. The wave of electricity moves to another region of the myo/cardi/um called the **(3) atrioventricular (AV) node**.

Label the structure in Figure 9–5 as you learn about the conduction pathway of the heart.

atri/o/ventricul/ar
(ā-trē-ō-věn-TRĬK-ū-lăr)
electric/al

atri/al
(Ā-trē-ăl)

9–77 Identify the words in Frame 9–76 that mean pertaining to the atrium and ventricles:

_____ / ____ / _____ / _____

pertaining to electricity: _____ / _____

pertaining to the atrium: _____ / _____

AV
SA

9–78 Write the abbreviations for

atri/o/ventricul/ar: _____

sino/atri/al: _____

9–79 The AV node instantaneously sends impulses to a bundle of specialized muscle fibers called the **(4) bundle of His**, which transmits them down the right and left **(5) bundle branches**.

Label the structures in Figure 9–5.

9–80 From the right and left bundle branches, impulses travel through the **(6) Purkinje fibers** to the rest of the ventricul/ar my/o/cardi/um, and bring about ventricul/ar contraction.

Label the Purkinje fibers in Figure 9–5.

9–81 Use your dictionary to define *contraction*.

_____

_____

VALIDATION FRAME: Check your labeling of Figure 9–5 in Appendix B, Answer Key.

The Cardiac Cycle and Heart Sounds

diastole (dī-ĂS-tō-lē)	**9–82** The cardi/ac cycle refers to the events of one complete heartbeat. Each contraction, or systole, of the heart is followed by a period of relaxation, or diastole. The normal period of heart contraction is called systole; the normal period of heart relaxation is called _____ .
systole (SĬS-tō-lē)	**9–83** When the heart is in the phase of relaxation, it is in diastole. When the heart is in the contraction phase, it is in _____ .
diastole (dī-ĂS-tō-lē) systole (SĬS-tō-lē)	**9–84** When the atria are in systole, they are pumping blood into the ventricles. At this time the ventricles are relaxed (in diastole), as they fill with blood. Write the medical term relating to the cardi/ac cycle that is in a period of relaxation: _____ contraction: _____
diastole (dī-ĂS-tō-lē) systole (SĬS-tō-lē)	**9–85** When the ventricles are in systole, the atria are in _____ . When the ventricles are in diastole, the atria are in _____ .
-graphy -gram	**9–86** Recall the suffixes meaning the process of recording: _____ record: _____
heart	**9–87** Electr/o/cardi/o/graphy is the process of recording electric/al activity generated by the _____ .
record heart	**9–88** An electr/o/cardi/o/gram is a _____ of electric/al activity generated by the _____ (Fig. 9–5).
electr/o/cardi/o/gram (ē-lĕk-trō-KĂR-dē-ō-grăm)	**9–89** **ECG** and **EKG** are abbreviations for electr/o/cardi/o/gram. To evaluate an abnormal cardi/ac rhythm, such as tachy/cardia, an **EKG** may be helpful. The abbreviations **ECG** and **EKG** refer to _____ / _____ / _____ / _____ / _____ .

tachy- brady-	**9–90** Remember that the prefix that means rapid is _____ ; the prefix that means slow is _____ .

rapid slow	**9–91** Tachy/cardia is a heart rate that is _____ ; brady/cardia is a heart rate that is _____ .

INFORMATION FRAME: This frame offers a brief, general interpretation of an ECG. A more comprehensive explanation of ECG abnormalities is beyond the scope of this book. Refer to Figure 9–5 as you read the paragraphs that follow.

A normal **ECG** rhythm strip shows five waves, or deflections, that represent electrical currents as they spread through the heart. The deflections are known as the **P, Q, R, S**, and **T** waves.

The **P** wave, which represents the transmission of electrical impulses from the **SA** node, indicates atrial contraction. The **QRS** waves represent the electrical impulses through the bundle of His and the Purkinje fiber system (during systole). The **T** wave represents the electrical recovery and relaxation of the ventricles.

electr / o / cardi / o / gram (ē-lĕk-trō-KĂR-dē-ō-grăm)	**9–92** Although the heart itself generates the heartbeat, factors such as hormones, drugs, and nervous system stimulation can also influence the heart rate. To evaluate a patient's heart rate, a physician may order an **EKG**, which is an abbreviation for _____ / _____ / _____ / _____ / _____ .

micr / o / cardi / a (mī-krō-KĂR-dē-ă)	**9–93** Micr/o/cardi/a, an underdevelopment of the heart, is usually not compatible with life. The medical term for a person with a small heart is _____ / _____ / _____ / _____ .

enlargement heart	**9–94** Megal/o/cardia is an enlargement of the heart. Cardi/o/megaly also means _____ of the _____ .

cardi / o / megaly (kăr-dē-ō-MĔG-ă-lē) megal / o / cardia (mĕg-ă-lō-KĂR-dē-ă)	**9–95** In people with high blood pressure, the heart must work very hard. As a result, it enlarges, like any other muscle, in response to work or exercise. A person who develops an enlarged heart has _____ / _____ / _____ or _____ / _____ / _____ .

cardi/o/rrhaphy
(kăr-dē-ŎR-ă-fē)

9–96 When valve replacement is performed (Fig. 9–4), the heart must be opened. After the valve is inserted, cardi/o/rrhaphy repairs the incision.

The word meaning suture of the heart is

_____ / _____ / _____ .

9–97 Using your medical dictionary, define *angina pectoris, arteriosclerosis, atherosclerosis*, and *lumen*.

_____

_____

_____

_____

_____

_____

ather/o

arteri/o

scler/o

my/o

cardi

9–98 Ather/o/scler/osis (Fig. 9–6), a form of arteri/o/scler/osis, is characterized by an abnormal accumulation of lipid substances and fibrous tissue in the vessel wall that leads to changes in arterial structure and function and reduction of blood flow to the my/o/cardi/um.

Identify the elements in this frame that mean

fatty plaque: _____ / _____

artery: _____ / _____

hardening: _____ / _____

muscle: _____ / _____

heart: _____

arteri/o/scler/osis
(ăr-tē-rē-ō-sklĕ-RŌ-sĭs)

ather/o/scler/osis
(ăth-ĕr-ō-sklĕ-RŌ-sĭs)

9–99 Build medical words that mean
an abnormal condition of arterial hardening:

_____ / _____ / _____ / _____

an abnormal condition of fatty plaque hardening:

_____ / _____ / _____ / _____

excision or removal

9–100 The combining form **necr/o** means death. Necr/ectomy is an

_____ of dead tissue.

necr/o/phobia
(nĕk-rē-FŌ-bē-ă)

9–101 Use -phobia to form a word meaning fear of death.

_____ / _____ / _____

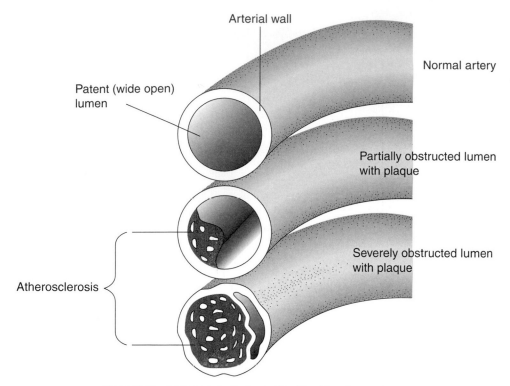

Figure 9–6. Atherosclerosis obstructing blood flow in an artery.

---

cardi/ac
(KĂR-dē-ăk)
necr/osis
(nĕ-KRŌ-sĭs)

9–102 Necr/osis of the my/o/cardi/um occurs when there is an insufficient blood supply to the heart. Eventually this may result in cardi/ac failure and death of the my/o/cardi/um.

Identify the words in this frame meaning

pertaining to the heart: _____ / _____

abnormal condition of death: _____ / _____

9–103 A my/o/cardi/al infarction (MI), or infarct, is caused by occlusion of one or more of the coronary arteries. **MI** is a medical emergency requiring immediate attention.

Using your medical dictionary, define *infarct*.

_____

_____

---

thromb/us
(THRŎM-bŭs)

9–104 Remember that the combining form **thromb/o** is used in words to refer to a clot, and **-us** to form a noun suffix.

Combine **thromb/o** and **-us** to form a word that means blood clot.

_____ / _____

---

thromb/us
(THRŎM-bŭs)

9–105 A blood clot that obstructs a blood vessel or a cavity of the heart is called a _____ / _____ .

thromb/ectomy
(thrŏm-BĔK-tō-mē)

9–106 The surgical excision of a blood clot is called

_____ / _____ .

---

anti-

9–107 Anti/coagulants are agents that prevent or delay blood coagulation; they are used in the prevention and treatment of a thrombus.

Write the element in this frame meaning against. _____

---

thromb/o/genesis
(thrŏm-bō-JĔN-ĕ-sĭs)

9–108 Use -genesis to form a word meaning producing or forming a blood clot:

_____ / _____ / _____

---

clot

9–109 If the anti/coagulant does not dissolve the clot, it may be surgically removed. A thromb/ectomy is an excision of a blood _____ .

---

anti/coagulant
(ăn-tī-kō-ĂG-ū-lănt)

9–110 To prevent blood coagulation, the physician uses an agent known as an

_____ / _____ .

---

thromb/o/lysis
(thrŏm-BŎL-ĭ-sĭs)

9–111 Use the surgical suffix -lysis to form a word meaning destruction or dissolving of a thrombus:

_____ / _____ / _____

---

thromb/o/lysis
(thrŏm-BŎL-ĭ-sĭs)

9–112 The surgical procedure to destroy or remove a clot is thromb/ectomy

or _____ / _____ / _____ .

---

aneurysm
(ĂN-ū-rĭzm)

9–113 An aneurysm (Fig. 9–7) is an abnormal dilation of the vessel wall caused by weakness that causes the vessel to balloon and eventually burst.

A ballooning out of the wall of the aorta is called an aort/ic

_____ .

---

aorta
(ā-OR-tă)

9–114 If a cerebr/al aneurysm ruptures, the hem/o/rrhage occurs in the cerebrum or brain. If an aort/ic aneurysm ruptures, the hem/o/rrhage occurs in

the _____ .

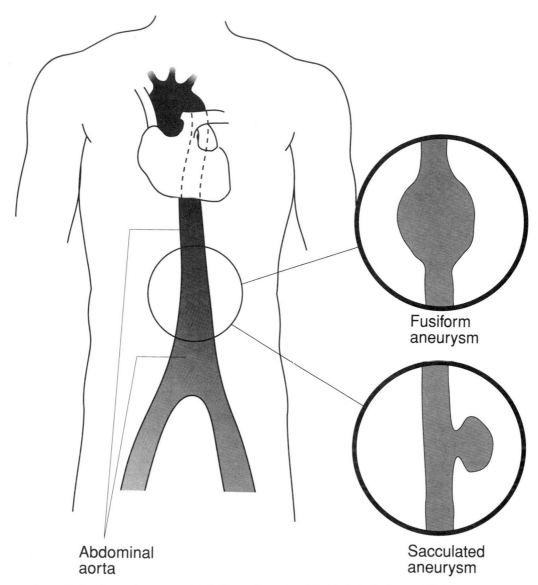

Figure 9–7. Types of aneurysm. (**A**) Fusiform: The walls of the blocked blood vessel dilate more or less equally, resulting in a tubular swelling. (**B**) Sacculated: The vessel yields at a weak spot (usually the result of a trauma) on one side. This results in a balloon-shaped swelling attached to the vessel by a narrow neck.

aort / ic
(ā-OR-tĭk)
hem / o / rrhage
(HĔM-ĕ-rĭj)
cerebr / al
(SĔR-ĕ-brăl)
aneurysm
(ĂN-ū-rĭzm)

9–115   Identify the words in Frame 9–114 meaning

pertaining to the aorta: _____ / _____

bursting forth (of) blood: _____ / ____ / _____

pertaining to the cerebrum: _____ / _____

dilation of a vessel caused by weakness: _____

Lymphatic System

The major parts of the lymphatic system include the lymph vessels, lymph nodes, and lymph fluid. Its functions in circulation are to drain excess fluid from the tissues, to return the tissue fluid back to the bloodstream, and to protect the body from impurities and foreign organisms.

The combining forms related to the lymphatic system are summarized here. Review this information before you begin to work the frames.

COMBINING FORMS

Combining Form	Meaning	Example	Pronunciation
aden/o	gland	aden/o/pathy disease	ă-dĕ-NŎP-ă-thē
lymph/o	lymph	lymph/o/poiesis formation, production	lĭm-fō-poy-Ē-sĭs
lymphaden/o	lymph node (gland)	lymphaden/itis inflammation	lĭm-făd-ĕn-Ī-tĭs
lymphangi/o	lymph vessel	lymphangi/oma tumor	lĭm-făn-jē-Ō-mă
splen/o	spleen	splen/o/megaly enlargement	splĕ-nō-MĔG-ă-lē

9–116 Like blood capillaries, **(1) lymph capillaries** are thin-walled tubes that carry lymph from the tissue spaces to larger **(2) lymph vessels**.
Label these structures in Figure 9–8.

---

lymph/o	**9–117** From lymph/oma construct the combining form that refers to lymph. _____ / _____
lymph (LĬMF)	**9–118** A lymph/o/cyte is a _____ cell.
vessels	**9–119** Recall that **angi/o** is used in words to denote either the blood or lymph _____ .
vessel	**9–120** Angi/ectasis is an expansion or dilation of a lymph or blood _____ .
lymphangi/o	**9–121** Combine **lymph/o** and **angi/o** to form a new element meaning lymph vessel: _____ / _____
lymphangi/oma (lĭm-făn-jē-Ō-mă)	**9–122** Use **lymphangi/o** to form a word meaning tumor composed of lymph vessels: _____ / _____

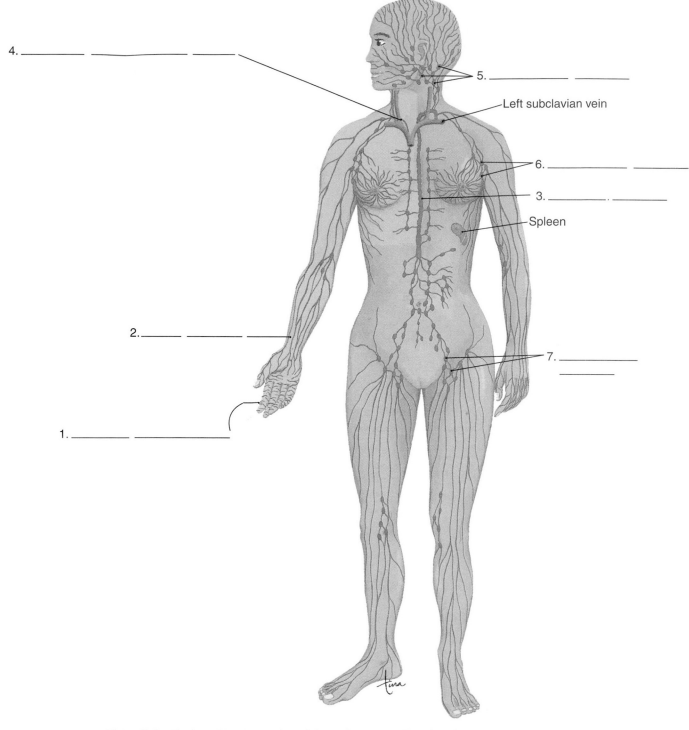

4. _____ _____ _____ _____

5. _____ _____

Left subclavian vein

6. _____ _____

3. _____. _____

Spleen

2. _____ _____ _____

7. _____

_____

1. _____ _____

Figure 9–8. System of lymph vessels and the major groups of lymph nodes. Lymph is returned to the blood in the right and left subclavian veins. (Adapted from Scanlon, VC, and Sanders, T: Understanding Human Structure and Function. FA Davis, Philadelphia, 1997, p 250, with permission.)

9–123 Use **angi/o** to develop medical words meaning

angi/o/rrhaphy
(ăn-jē-OR-ă-fē)

suture of a vessel: _____ / ___ / _____

angi/o/plasty
(ĂN-jē-ō-plăs-tē)

surgical repair of a vessel: _____ / ___ / _____

angi/o/rrhexis
(ăn-jē-or-ĔK-sĭs)

rupture of a vessel: _____ / ___ / _____

9–124 Like veins, lymph vessels contain valves that keep lymph flowing in one direction, toward the thorac/ic cavity.

chest

Thorac/ic means pertaining to the _____ .

9–125 The **(3) thoracic duct** and the **(4) right lymphatic duct** carry lymph into veins in the upper thoracic region.

Label these two ducts in Figure 9–8.

lymph/oid
(LĬM-foyd)

9–126 Use -oid to form a word meaning resembling lymph:

_____ / _____ .

lymph/o/pathy
(lĭm-FŎP-ă-thē)

9–127 The word meaning any disease of the lymphat/ic system is

_____ / _____ / _____ .

lymph/o/cytes
(LĬM-fō-sīts)

9–128 Small round structures called **lymph nodes** not only produce lymph/o/cytes, but also filter and purify lymph by removing harmful substances such as bacteria or cancerous cells.

Lymph cells are known as _____ / _____ / _____ .

9–129 The major lymph node sites are the **(5) cervical nodes**, the **(6) axillary nodes**, and the **(7) inguinal nodes**.

Label the three major lymph node sites in Figure 9–8.

cervical
(SĔR-vĭ-kăl)
axillary
(ĂK-sĭ-lăr-ē)

inguinal
(ĬNG-gwĭ-năl)

9–130 Write the name of the lymph node located in

the neck: _____

the armpit: _____

the groin area (depression between the thigh and trunk):

_____

VALIDATION FRAME: Check your labeling of Figure 9–8 in Appendix B, Answer Key.

Review

Select the element(s) that match(es) the meaning.

angi/o   my/o   -lysis
aort/o   necr/o   -megaly
cardi/o   thromb/o   -oma
cerebr/o   -al   -pathy
electr/o   -cyte   -plasty
hem/o   -ic   -rrhaphy
lymph/o   -gram   -rrhexis
                -graphy   -stenosis

a. _____ aorta

b. _____ blood

c. _____ blood clot

d. _____ cell

e. _____ cerebrum (brain)

f. _____ death

g. _____ disease

h. _____ electric

i. _____ enlargement

j. _____ heart

k. _____ lymph

l. _____ muscle

m. _____ process of recording

n. _____ record

o. _____ pertaining to

p. _____ rupture

q. _____ separation, destruction, loosening

r. _____ stricture, narrowing

s. _____ surgical repair

t. _____ suture

u. _____ tumor

v. _____ vessel (usually blood or lymph)

Check your answers with the Review Answer Key on the following page.

Review Answer Key

a. aort/o

b. hem/o

c. thromb/o

d. -cyte

e. cerebr/o

f. necr/o

g. -pathy

h. electr/o

i. -megaly

j. cardi/o

k. lymph/o

l. my/o

m. -graphy

n. -gram

o. -al, -ic

p. -rrhexis

q. -lysis

r. -stenosis

s. -plasty

t. -rrhaphy

u. -oma

v. angi/o

REINFORCEMENT FRAME: If you are not satisfied with your level comprehension, go back to Frame 9–73 and rework the frames.

Additional Pathological Conditions

CARDIOVASCULAR SYSTEM

arrhythmia (ă-RĬTH-mē-ă): irregularity or loss of rhythm of the heartbeat; dysrhythmia.

arteriosclerosis (ăr-tē-rē-ō-sklē-RŌ-sĭs): thickening, hardening, and loss of elasticity of arterial walls. This results in altered function of tissues and organs; also called hardening of the arteries.

atherosclerosis (ăth-ĕ-rō-sklē-RŌ-sĭs): the most common form of arteriosclerosis, caused by an accumulation of fatty substances within the walls of the arteries (see Fig. 9–6).

bruit (BRWĒ): soft blowing sound heard on auscultation caused by turbulent blood flow.

congestive heart failure (CHF) (kŏn-JĔS-tĭv HĂRT FĀL-yĕr): pathological condition of the heart in which there is a reduced outflow of blood from the left side of the heart. Results in lung congestion, dyspnea, and fatigue, and may cause edema.

deep vein thrombosis (DVT) (DĒP VĀN thrŏm-BŌ-sĭs): formation of a blood clot in a deep vein of the body, occurring most frequently in the iliac and femoral veins.

embolus (ĔM-bō-lŭs): a mass of undissolved matter present in a blood or lymphatic vessel brought there by the blood or lymph current. Emboli may be solid, liquid, or gaseous. Occlusion of vessels from emboli usually results in the development of infarcts.

fibrillation (fĭ-brĭl-Ā-shŭn): abnormal quivering or contraction of the heart fibers. Untreated ventricular fibrillation leads to cardiac arrest and then death. Defibrillation equipment to convert the heart to a normal beat is necessary.

hypertension (hī-pĕr-TĔN-shŭn): consistently elevated blood pressure that is higher than normal causing damage to the blood vessels and ultimately the heart.

ischemia (ĭs-KĒ-mē-ă): a local and temporary deficiency of blood supply to tissue caused by constriction or occlusion of a blood vessel.

mitral valve prolapse (MVP) (MĪ-trăl VĂLV PRŌ-lăps): condition in which the leaflets of the mitral valve prolapse into the left atrium during systole, resulting in incomplete closure and backflow of blood.

murmur (MĔR-mĕr): an abnormal sound heard on auscultation, caused by defects in the valves or chambers of the heart.

myocardial infarction (MI) (mī-ō-KĂR-dē-ăl ĭn-FĂRK-shŭn): caused by partial or complete occlusion of one or more of the coronary arteries; heart attack.

patent ductus arteriosus (PĂT-ĕnt DŬK-tŭs ăr-tē-rē-Ō-sĭs): failure of the ductus arteriosus to close after birth, resulting in an abnormal opening between the pulmonary artery and the aorta.

Raynaud's disease (rā-NŌZ dĭs-ZĒZ): vascular disorder in which the fingers and toes become cold, numb, and painful as a result of temporary blood vessel constriction in the skin.

rheumatic heart disease (rū-MĂT-ĭk HĂRT dĭ-ZĒZ): streptococcal infection that causes damage to the heart valves and heart muscle.

stroke (STRŌK): sudden loss of consciousness followed by paralysis caused by one of several different mechanisms including hemorrhage into brain; formation of an embolus or thrombus that occludes an artery; or rupture of an extracerebral artery causing subarachnoid hemorrhage; also known as cerebrovascular accident (CVA).

transient ischemic attack (TIA) (TRĂN-shĕnt ĭs-KĒ-mĭk ă-TĂK): temporary interference with blood supply to the brain, causing no permanent brain damage.

varicose veins (VĂR-ĭ-kōs VĀNS): swollen, distended veins caused by incompetent venous valves; most often seen in the lower legs.

LYMPHATIC SYSTEM

acquired immunodeficiency syndrome (AIDS) (ă-KWĪRD ĭm-ū-nō-dē-FĬSH-ĕn-sē SĬN-drōm): caused by human immunodeficiency virus (HIV) that results in immune cell ineffectiveness, increasing susceptibility to infections, malignancies, and neurological diseases; it is transmitted sexually or through contaminated blood exposure.

Hodgkin's disease (HŎJ-kĭns dĭ-ZĒZ): disease causing malignant solid tumors that may originate in lymphoid tissue. Other organs and areas will be invaded if the disease is left untreated.

lymphadenitis (lĭm-făd-ĕn-Ī-tĭs): inflammation and enlargement of the lymph nodes usually as a result of infection.

lymphosarcoma (lĭm-fō-săr-KŌ-mă): malignant neoplastic disorder of lymphatic tissue that is not related to Hodgkin's disease; non-Hodgkin's lymphoma.

mononucleosis (mŏn-ō-nū-klē-Ō-sĭs): acute infection caused by the Epstein-Barr virus (EBV) characterized by a sore throat, fever, fatigue, and enlarged lymph nodes.

Medical Record

The following medical reports are related to the medical specialty called cardiology and vascular surgery.

MEDICAL RECORD 9–1. Myocardial Infarction (MI)

Dictionary Exercise

Underline the following terms in the reading exercise. Use a medical dictionary and Appendix E, Abbreviations, to write a definition of each word in the list. This exercise helps you master the terminology in the medical record.

anxiety _____

apnea _____

atrial fibrillation _____

desiccated _____

dyspnea _____

EKG _____

malaise _____

mg _____

MI _____

myocardial infarction _____

postoperatively _____

radial pulse _____

sinus tachycardia _____

syncopal _____

syncope _____

tachycardia _____

thyroidectomy _____

thyroiditis _____

Word Elements Exercise

dyspnea	thyroidectomy
apnea	atrial
thyroiditis	myocardial

Reading Exercise

Read the case study out loud.

A 70-year-old white woman was admitted to the hospital for evaluation of a syncopal episode. She states that most recently she has experienced generalized malaise, increased shortness of breath while at rest, and dyspnea followed by periods of apnea and syncope.

Her past history includes recurrent episodes of thyroiditis, which led her to have a thyroidectomy 6 years ago while she was under the care of Dr. Knopp. At the time of surgery, the results of her EKG were interpreted as sinus tachycardia with nonspecific ST-T wave (see Fig. 9–5) changes. The tachycardia was attributed to preoperative anxiety and thyroiditis. Postoperatively, under the direction of Dr. Knopp, the patient was treated with a daily dose of 50 mg of desiccated thyroid and has been symptom free until this admission.

Upon clinical examination, the patient's radial pulse was found to be irregular, and the EKG demonstrated uncontrolled atrial fibrillation with evidence of a recent myocardial infarction (MI).

MEDICAL RECORD EVALUATION 9–1. Myocardial Infarction

1. What symptoms did the patient experience before admission to the hospital?

2. What was found during clinical examination?

3. What is the danger of atrial fibrillation?

4. Did the patient have prior history of heart problems? If so, describe them.

5. Was the patient's prior heart problem related to her current one?

MEDICAL RECORD 9–2. Carotid Angiogram

Dictionary Exercise

Underline the following terms in the reading exercise. Use a medical dictionary and Appendix E, Abbreviations, to write a definition of each word in the list. This exercise helps you master the terminology in the medical record.

angiographic _____

AP _____

asymptomatic _____

atherosclerotic _____

bifurcation _____

carotid _____

congenital _____

distal _____

femoral _____

fluoroscopic _____

hemodynamically _____

oblique _____

percutaneously _____

plaque _____

proximal _____

scan _____

stenosis _____

subclavian _____

artery _____

subjacent _____

vertebral _____

Reading Exercise

Read the case study out loud.

Clinical Indication: Asymptomatic right carotid bruit shows 90% stenosis on duplex scan.

Angiographic Technique: A polyethylene catheter was percutaneously inserted into the right femoral artery and guided under fluoroscopic control into each common carotid artery. Contrast injections were followed by imaging of the right common carotid bifurcation in both oblique and lateral projections and the right intracranial circulation in AP and lateral projection. The left carotid circulation was similarly studied, with only one oblique projection of the carotid bifurcation. The catheter was replaced with a multiple side-hole catheter, and an oblique aortic arch arteriogram was obtained.

Angiographic Findings: The left proximal internal carotid artery shows an irregular posterior plaque with a possible ulceration at the superior margin. This narrows the lumen of the vessel approximately 30%. The right distal common carotid artery shows a short segment area of narrowing of 80% to 90%. This is immediately subjacent to the carotid bifurcation. No definite ulceration is seen. The right vertebral is large. The left vertebral artery is absent. There are irregular atherosclerotic changes (see Fig. 9–6) in the left subclavian artery with stenosis approximately 50% or greater. The two anterior cerebral arteries fill from the left-sided injection. No posterior cerebral artery fills from the internal carotid arteries. There is no definite demonstration of the right A–1 segment.

Impression: There is 80% to 90% stenosis of the distal right common carotid artery just below the bifurcation. It is not possible to determine whether the filling of the right anterior cerebral artery from the left side is a congenital variant or is due to hemodynamically decreased flow in the right internal carotid artery. Approximately 30% stenosis of the proximal left internal carotid artery. Greater than 50% stenosis of the left subclavian artery. Large right vertebral artery and absent left vertebral artery.

MEDICAL RECORD EVALUATION 9–2. Carotid Angiogram

1. What is a catheter?

2. How did they insert the catheter into the femoral artery?

3. What type of x-ray examination did the physicians use to guide the catheter into the common carotid artery?

4. To what did the physician attribute the narrowing of the internal carotid lumen?

5. What part of the arterial branch showed the most narrowing?

6. Do the physicians suspect that the person was born with the stenosis?

Abbreviations

Abbreviation	Meaning	Abbreviation	Meaning
CARDIOVASCULAR			
AS	aortic stenosis	IAS	interatrial septum
ASD	atrial septal defect	IVC	inferior vena cava; intravenous cholangiography
ASHD	arteriosclerotic heart disease		
AV	atrioventricular, arteriovenous	IVS	interventricular septum
BBB	bundle-branch block	LA	left atrium
BP	blood pressure	LV	left ventricle
CAD	coronary artery disease	MI	myocardial infarction
CC	cardiac catheterization; chief complaint	MVP	mitral valve prolapse
		RA	right atrium, rheumatoid arthritis
CHF	congestive heart failure	RV	right ventricle
CPR	cardiopulmonary resuscitation	SA	sinoatrial (node)
CV	cardiovascular	SVC	superior vena cava
ECG, EKG	electrocardiogram	VSD	ventricular septal defect
LYMPHATIC			
AIDS	acquired immunodeficiency syndrome	KS	Kaposi's sarcoma
		PCP	*Pneumocystis carinii* pneumonia
HIV	human immunodeficiency virus		
HSV	herpes simplex virus		

Audiocassette Exercise

The audiocassette tape helps you master the pronunciation of medical words. Listen to the tape for instructions to complete this exercise. You may also use this list without the audiotape to practice correct pronunciation and spelling of the terms.

Frame	Word	Pronunciation	Spelling Exercise
9–113	[] aneurysm	(ĂN-ū-rĭzm)	_____
9–120	[] angiectasis	(ăn-jē-ĔK-tā-sĭs)	_____
9–97	[] angina pectoris	(ăn-JĪ-nă PĔK-tŏr-ĭs)	_____
9–58	[] angioma	(ăn-jē-Ō-mă)	_____
9–123	[] angioplasty	(ĂN-jē-ō-plăs-tē)	_____
9–123	[] angiorrhaphy	(ăn-jē-ŌR-ă-fē)	_____
9–123	[] angiorrhexis	(ăn-jē-ŏr-ĔK-sĭs)	_____
9–107	[] anticoagulant	(ăn-tī-kō-ĂG-ū-lănt)	_____
Reading Exercise	[] anxiety	(ăng-ZĪ-ĕ-tē)	_____
9–61	[] aorta	(ā-ŌR-tă)	_____
9–63	[] aortomalacia	(ā-ŏr-tō-mă-LA-shē-ă)	_____
9–62	[] aortopathy	(ā-ŏr-TŎP-ă-thē)	_____
Reading Exercise	[] apnea	(ăp-NĒ-ă)	_____
9–64	[] arteriole	(ăr-TĒ-rē-ōl)	_____
9–42	[] arteriolith	(ăr-TĒ-rē-ō-lĭth)	_____
9–45	[] arteriopathy	(ăr-tē-rē-ŎP-ă-thē)	_____
9–45	[] arteriorrhaphy	(ăr-tē-rē-ŌR-ă-fē)	_____
9–45	[] arteriorrhexis	(ăr-tē-rē-ō-RĔK-sĭs)	_____
9–42	[] arteriosclerosis	(ăr-tē-rē-ō-sklĕ-RŌ-sĭs)	_____
9–45	[] arteriospasm	(ăr-TĒ-rē-ō-spăzm)	_____
9–19	[] atria	(Ā-trē-ă)	_____
9–15	[] atrioventricular	(ā-trē-ō-vĕn-TRĬK-ū-lăr)	_____
9–9	[] atrium	(Ā-trē-ŭm)	_____
9–130	[] axillary	(ĂK-sĭ-lăr-ē)	_____
9–19	[] bacterium	(băk-TĒ-rē-ŭm)	_____
9–19	[] bacteria	(băk-TĒ-rē-ă)	_____
9–36	[] bicuspid	(bī-KŬS-pĭd)	_____
9–26	[] bradycardia	(brăd-ē-KĂR-dē-ä)	_____
9–27	[] bradyphagia	(brăd-ē-FĂ-jē-ă)	_____
9–27	[] bradypnea	(brăd-ĭp-NĒ-ă)	_____
9–67	[] capillaries	(KĂP-ĭ-lă-rēz)	_____
9–19	[] cardia	(KĂR-dē-ă)	_____
9–94	[] cardiomegaly	(kăr-dē-ō-MĔG-ă-lē)	_____
9–96	[] cardiorrhaphy	(kăr-dē-ŌR-ă-fē)	_____
9–114	[] cerebral	(SĔR-ĕ-brăl)	_____
9–130	[] cervical	(SĔR-vĭ-kăl)	_____
Reading Exercise	[] desiccated	(DĔS-ĭ-kā-tĕd)	_____
9–82	[] diastole	(dī-ĂS-tō-lē)	_____

Frame	Word	Pronunciation	Spelling Exercise
Reading Exercise	[] dyspnea	(dĭsp-NĒ-ă)	_____
9–88	[] electrocardiogram	(ē-lĕk-trō-KĂR-dē-ō-grăm)	_____
9–87	[] electrocardiography	(ē-lĕk-trō-kăr-dē-ŎG-ră-fē)	_____
9–3	[] endocardium	(ĕn-dō-KĂR-dē-ŭm)	_____
9–3	[] epicardium	(ĕp-ĭ-KĂR-dē-ŭm)	_____
Additional Pathological Conditions	[] fibrillation	(fĭ-brĭl-Ā-shŭn)	_____
9–60	[] hcmangicctasis	(hē-măn-jē-ĔK-tă-sĭs)	_____
9–59	[] hemangioma	(hē-măn-jē-Ō-mă)	_____
9–57	[] hematologist	(hē-mă-TŎL-ō-jĭst)	_____
9–57	[] hematology	(hē-mă-TŎL-ō-jē)	_____
9–114	[] hemorrhage	(HĔM-ĕ-rĭj)	_____
9–103	[] infarction	(ĭn-FĂRK-shŭn)	_____
9–130	[] inguinal	(ĬNG-gwĭ-năl)	_____
9–21	[] interatrial	(ĭn-tĕr-Ā-trē-ăl)	_____
9–20	[] interventricular	(ĭn-tĕr-vĕn-TRĬK-ū-lăr)	_____
9–122	[] lymphangioma	(lĭm-făn-jē-Ō-mă)	_____
9–118	[] lymphocyte	(LĬM-fō-sīt)	_____
9–126	[] lymphoid	(LĬM-foyd)	_____
9–117	[] lymphoma	(lĭm-FŌ-mă)	_____
9–127	[] lymphopathy	(lĭm-FŎP-ă-thē)	_____
Reading Exercise	[] malaise	(mă-LĀZ)	_____
9–94	[] megalocardia	(mĕg-ă-lō-KĂR-dē-ă)	_____
9–93	[] microcardia	(mī-krō-KĂR-dē-ă)	_____
9–54	[] mitral	(MĪ-trăl)	_____
9–3	[] myocardium	(mī-ō-KĂR-dē-ŭm)	_____
9–100	[] necrectomy	(nĕ-KRĔK-tō-mē)	_____
9–101	[] necrophobia	(nĕk-rō-FŌ-bē-ă)	_____
9–102	[] necrosis	(nĕ-KRŌ-sĭs)	_____
9–6	[] pericardiectomy	(pĕr-ĭ-kăr-dē-ĔK-tō-mē)	_____
9–7	[] pericardiorrhaphy	(pĕr-ĭ-kăr-dē-ŎR-ă-fē)	_____
9–5	[] pericarditis	(pĕr-ĭ-kăr-DĪ-tĭs)	_____
9–5	[] pericardium	(pĕr-ĭ-KĂR-dē-ŭm)	_____
9–52	[] phleborrhaphy	(flĕb-ŎR-ă-fē)	_____
9–52	[] phleborrhexis	(flĕb-ō-RĔK-sĭs)	_____
9–52	[] phlebostenosis	(flĕb-ō-stĕ-NŌ-sĭs)	_____
9–39	[] pulmonary	(PŬL-mō-nĕ-rē)	_____
9–80	[] Purkinje	(pŭr-KĬN-jē)	_____
9–19	[] septa	(SĔP-tă)	_____
9–19	[] septum	(SĔP-tŭm)	_____
9–73	[] sinoatrial	(sīn-ō-Ā-trē-āl)	_____
Reading Exercise	[] sinus	(SĪ-nŭs)	_____
Reading Exercise	[] syncopal	(SĬN-kō-păl)	_____

Frame	Word	Pronunciation	Spelling Exercise
Reading Exercise	[] syncope	(SĬN-kō-pē)	_____
9–83	[] systole	(SĬS-tō-lē)	_____
9–23	[] tachycardia	(tăk-ē-KĂR-dē-ă)	_____
9–28	[] tachyphagia	(tăk-ē-FĀ-jē-ă)	_____
9–24	[] tachypnea	(tăk-ĭp-NĒ-ă)	_____
9–124	[] thoracic	(thō-RĂS-ĭk)	_____
9–112	[] thrombectomy	(thrŏm-BĔK-tō-mē)	_____
9–108	[] thrombogenesis	(thrŏm-bō-JĔN-ĕ-sĭs)	_____
9–111	[] thrombolysis	(thrŏm-BŎL-ĭ-sĭs)	_____
9–104	[] thrombus	(THRŎM-bŭs)	_____
9–106	[] thyroidectomy	(thī-royd-ĔK-tō-mē)	_____
Reading Exercise	[] thyroiditis	(thī-royd-Ī-tĭs)	_____
9–34	[] tricuspid	(trī-KŬS-pĭd)	_____
9–30	[] vena cava	(VĒ-nă KĂ-vă)	_____
9–53	[] venosclerosis	(vē-nō-sklĕ-RŌ-sĭs)	_____
9–53	[] venospasm	(VĒ-nō-spăzm)	_____
9–53	[] venotomy	(vē-NŎT-ō-mē)	_____
9–13	[] ventricle	(VĔN-trĭk-l)	_____
9–16	[] ventricular	(věn-TRĬK-ū-lăr)	_____
9–14	[] ventriculotomy	(věn-trĭk-ū-LŎT-ō-mē)	_____
9–64	[] venule	(VĔN-ūl)	_____

Unit Exercises

DEFINITIONS

Review Unit Summary (pages 423–424) before completing this exercise. Write the meaning for each element.

SUFFIXES, PREFIXES, AND COMBINING FORMS

Element	Meaning
SUFFIXES	
1. -cyte	_____
2. -ectasis	_____
3. -gram	_____
4. -lith	_____
5. -lysis	_____
6. -malacia	_____
7. -megaly	_____
8. -oid	_____
9. -ole, -ule	_____
10. -osis	_____
11. -pathy	_____
12. -phagia	_____
13. -phobia	_____
14. -rrhexis	_____
15. -spasm	_____
16. -stenosis	_____
17. -um	_____
PREFIXES	
18. anti-	_____
19. bi-	_____
20. brady-	_____
21. endo-	_____
22. epi-	_____
23. micro-	_____
24. peri-	_____
25. tachy-	_____
26. tri-	_____

COMBINING FORMS RELATED TO CIRCULATORY SYSTEM

27. angi / o	_____
28. aort / o	_____
29. arteri / o	_____

Element	Meaning
30. ~~arti/o~~ atri/o	_____
31. cardi/o	_____
32. electr/o	_____
33. hemat/o, hem/o	_____
34. lymph/o	_____
35. phleb/o	_____

VALIDATION FRAME: Check your answers in Index of Medical Word Elements, Appendix A.

If you scored less than _____ %,* review Unit Summary (pages 423–424). To obtain a percentage score, multiply the number of correct answers times 2.86.

Number of Correct Answers: _____   **Percentage Score:** _____

*Enter the percentage required by your instructor to complete this course.

Vocabulary

Fill in the correct word(s) from the list that match(es) the definitions in the statements that follow.

aneurysm	capillaries	myocardial infarction (MI)
angiectasis	cardiomegaly	myocardium
angina pectoris	desiccated	pacemaker
anticoagulants	diastole	systole
arteriosclerosis	EKG	tachyphagia
anxiety	hemangioma	tachypnea
arterioles	malaise	

1. _____ Muscular layer of the heart.

2. _____ Rapid breathing.

3. _____ Disease characterized by an abnormal hardening of the arteries.

4. _____ A feeling of apprehension, worry, uneasiness, especially of the future.

5. _____ Contraction phase of the heart.

6. _____ Relaxation phase of the heart.

7. _____ Record of the electrical impulses of the heart.

8. _____ A vague feeling of bodily discomfort, which may be the first indication of an infection or disease.

9. _____ Dried thoroughly; rendered free from moisture.

10. _____ An enlarged heart.

11. _____ A weakness in the vessel wall that balloons and eventually bursts.

12. _____ Severe pain and constriction about the heart caused by an insufficient supply of oxygenated blood to the heart.

13. _____ Necrosis of an area of muscular heart tissue following cessation of blood supply.

14. _____ Agents or drugs that are used to prevent blood clotting.

15. _____ Rapid eating or swallowing.

16. _____ Dilation of a lymph or blood vessel.

17. _____ Smallest vessels of the circulatory system.

18. _____ Tumor composed of blood vessels.

19. _____ Small arteries.

20. _____ Maintains primary responsibility for initiating the heartbeat.

VALIDATION FRAME: Check your answers in Appendix B, Answer Key. If you scored less than _____ %, review the vocabulary and retake the exercise.

To obtain your percentage score, multiply the number of correct answers by 5.

Number of Correct Answers: _____   **Percentage Score:** _____

Additional Pathological Conditions

Match the medical term(s) that follow with the definitions in the numbered list.

AIDS
arrhythmia
atherosclerosis
bruit
congestive heart failure (CHF)
DVT
embolus
fibrillation

Hodgkin's disease
hypertension
ischemia
lymphadenitis
lymphosarcoma
mitral valve prolapse
mononucleosis

myocardial infarction (MI)
patent ductus arteriosus
Raynaud's disease
rheumatic heart disease
stroke
transient ischemic attack (TIA)
varicose veins

1. _____ Swollen, distended veins most often seen in the lower legs.

2. _____ Acute infection caused by the Epstein-Barr virus (EBV) characterized by a sore throat, fever, fatigue, and enlarged lymph nodes.

3. _____ A heart attack caused by partial or complete occlusion of one or more of the coronary arteries.

4. _____ Blood vessel obstruction caused by a traveling mass of undissolved matter.

5. _____ Inflammation and enlargement of the lymph nodes.

6. _____ Formation of a blood clot in a deep vein of the body.

7. _____ Blood pressure that is consistently higher than normal.

8. _____ Irregularity or loss of heartbeat rhythm.

9. _____ Temporary interference of blood supply to the brain without permanent damage.

10. _____ Soft blowing sound caused by turbulent blood flow.

11. _____ Heart condition also known as cerebrovascular accident (CVA).

12. _____ Streptococcal infection that causes damage to heart valves and muscle.

13. _____ Heart disease caused by an accumulation of fatty substances within the arterial walls.

14. _____ Non-Hodgkin's lymphoma.

15. _____ Vascular disorder in which the fingers and toes become cold, numb, and painful.

16. _____ Local, temporary deficiency of blood supply to tissue, caused by constriction or occlusion of a blood vessel.

17. _____ Malignant solid tumors of the lymphatic system.

18. _____ Transmissible infection caused by human immunodeficiency virus (HIV).

19. _____ Caused by a reduced outflow of blood from the left side of the heart. Results in lung congestion, dyspnea, and fatigue and may cause edema.

20. _____ Abnormal contraction of the heart fibers.

VALIDATION FRAME: Check your answers in Appendix B, Answer Key. If you scored less than _____ %, review the vocabulary and retake the exercise.

To obtain your percentage score, multiply the number of correct answers by 5.

Number of Correct Answers: _____   **Percentage Score:** _____

Unit Summary

COMBINING FORMS RELATED TO THE CARDIOVASCULAR AND LYMPHATIC SYSTEMS

Combining Form	Pronunciation	Meaning
angi/o	ăn-jē-ō	vessel (usually blood or lymph)
aort/o	ā-ōr-tō	aorta
arteri/o	ār-tē-rē-ō	artery
atri/o	ā-trē-ō	atrium
cardi/o	kār-dē-ō	heart
electr/o	ē-lěk-trō	electric
lymph/o	lĭm-fō	lymph
phleb/o ven/o	flěb-ō věn-o	vein
thromb/o	thrŏm-bō	clot
ventricul/o	věn-trĭk-ū-lō	ventricle (of brain or heart)

OTHER COMBINING FORMS IN UNIT 9

Combining Form	Pronunciation	Meaning
cerebr/o	sěr-ě-brō	cerebrum (brain)
my/o	mī-ō	muscle
necr/o	něk-rō	death
hem/o	hē-mō	blood
scler/o	sklě-rō	hardening, sclera (white of the eye)

SUFFIXES AND PREFIXES

Suffix (Prefix)	Pronunciation	Meaning
SURGICAL SUFFIXES		
-ectomy	ěk-tō-mē	excision, removal
-lysis	lĭ sĭs	separation, destruction, loosening
-plasty	plăs-tē	surgical repair
-rrhaphy	ră-fē	suture
-tomy	tō-mē	incision, cut into
OTHER SUFFIXES		
-al -ic	ăl ĭk	pertaining to
-cyte	sīt	cell
-ectasis	ěk-tă-sĭs	expansion, dilation

Suffix (Prefix)	Pronunciation	Meaning
-genesis	jĕn-ĕ-sĭs	producing, forming
-gram	grăm	record
-graphy	gră-fē	process of recording
-lith	lĭth	stone, calculus
-malacia	mă-lā-shē-ă	softening
-megaly	mĕg-ă-lē	enlargement
-oid	oyd	resemble
-ole -ule	ō-lē ūl	small
-oma	ō-mă	tumor
-osis	ō-sĭs	abnormal condition
-pathy	pă-thē	disease
-phagia	fă-jē-ă	swallow, eat
-phobia	fō-bē-ă	fear
-pnea	nē-ă	breathing
-rrhexis	rĕk-sĭs	rupture
-spasm	spăzm	involuntary contraction, twitching
-stenosis	stĕn-ō-sĭs	stricture, narrowing
-um	ŭm	noun ending
PREFIXES		
anti-	ăn-tĭ	against
bi-	bī	two, double
brady-	brăd-ĭ	slow
endo-	ĕn-dō	within
epi-	ĕp-ĭ	above, upon
micro-	mī-krō	small
peri-	pĕr-ĭ	around
tachy-	tăk-ē	rapid
tri-	trī	three

Special Senses: The Eyes and Ears

The eyes and their accessory structures are the receptor organs that enable us to see. As one of the most important sense organs of the body, the eyes provide us not only with most of the information about what we see but also of what we learn from printed material.

The ears and their accessory structures are the receptor organs that enable us to hear and to maintain our balance.

The Eye

The combining forms related to the eye are summarized here. Review this information before you begin to work the frames.

COMBINING FORMS

Combining Form	Meaning	Example	Pronunciation
blephar/o	eyelid	blephar/o/spasm twitching	BLĔF-ă-rō-spăzm
choroid/o	choroid	choroid/o/pathy disease	kō-roy-DŎP-ă-thē
corne/o	cornea	corne/itis inflammation	kōr-nē-Ī-tĭs
kerat/o		kerat/o/plasty surgical repair	KĔR-ă-tō-plăs-tē
dacry/o	tear, lacrimal sac	dacry/o/rrhea flow, discharge	dăk-rē-ō-RĒ-ă
dipl/o	double	dipl/opia vision	dĭp-LŌ-pē-ă
irid/o	iris	irid/o/plegia paralysis	ĭr-ĭd-ō-PLĒ-jē-ă
ocul/o	eye	intra/ocul/ar within pertaining to	ĭn-trā-ŎK-ū-lăr
ophthalm/o		ophthalm/o/scope instrument to view	ŏf-THĂL-mō-skōp
retin/o	retina	retin/o/pathy disease	rĕt-ĭn-ŎP-ă-thē
scler/o	hardening, sclera (white of the eye)	scler/itis inflammation	sklĕ-RĪ-tĭs

10–1 Use the Index of Medical Word Elements, Part A of Appendix A, to define the following word elements.

English Term	Medical Word Element
hardening, sclera	_____ / _____
eye	_____ / _____
eyelid	_____ / _____
choroid	_____ / _____
retina	_____ / _____
yellow	_____ / _____

---

pain, eye

10–2 **Ophthalm /o** is used to construct words that refer to the eye.

Ophthalm /algia is a _____ in the _____ .

---

of-THALM-o
(ŏf-THĂL-mō)

10–3 Words with **ophthalm /o** may be difficult to pronounce when you first encounter them. To avoid confusion, write the pronunciation of **ophthalm /o** as it is listed in the answer column, then practice saying it.

_____ .

---

instrument

10–4 An ophthalm /o /scope is an _____ for examining the interior of the eye.

---

ophthalm /o /scopy
(ŏf-thăl-MŎS-kō-pē)

10–5 The word meaning visual examination of the eye is

_____ / _____ / _____ .

---

ophthalm /algia
(ŏf-thăl-MĂL-jē-ă)

10–6 High blood pressure may cause ophthalm /o /dynia or

_____ / _____ .

---

eye(s)

10–7 An ophthalm /o /logist is a physician who specializes in disorders and treatment of the _____ .

---

ophthalm /ectomy
(ŏf-thăl-MĔK-tō-mē)
ophthalm /o /malacia
(ŏf-thăl-mō-mă-LĀ-shē-ă)
ophthalm /o /plegia
(ŏf-thăl-mō-PLĒ-jē-ă)

10–8 Use **ophthalm /o** to build words meaning

surgical excision of the eye: _____ / _____

softening of the eye: _____ / _____ / _____

paralysis of the eye: _____ / _____ / _____

ophthalm/o/plegia (ŏf-thăl-mō-PLĒ-jē-ă)	**10–9** A stroke can prevent eye movement and cause paralysis of the eye muscles. A person with paralysis of the eye (muscles) has a condition called _____ / ____ / _____ .
blephar/o	**10–10** The combining form **blephar/o** is used in words to refer to the eyelid. From blephar/o/spasm, identify the combining form for eyelid. _____ / ____ .
eyelid(s)	**10–11** Blephar/edema is a swelling and baggy appearance of the _____ .
blephar/o/plasty (BLĔF-ă-rō-plăs-tē)	**10–12** Blephar/o/plasty, also called an eye tuck, is a surgical procedure to remove wrinkles from the eyelids for cosmetic reasons. A surgical repair of the eyelid(s) is known as _____ / ____ / _____ .
blephar/o/plasty (BLĔF-ă-rō-plăs-tē)	**10–13** When a person has an eye tuck, small portions of the eyelids are removed to tighten the skin, thus removing wrinkles. The surgical procedure for an eye tuck is called _____ / ____ / _____ .
blephar/ectomy (blĕf-ă-RĔK-tō-mē) blephar/o/tomy (blĕf-ă-RŎT-ō-mē) blephar/o/spasm (BLĔF-ă-rō-spăzm) blephar/o/plegia (blĕf-ă-rō-PLĒ-jē-ă)	**10–14** Form medical words meaning excision of part or all of the eyelid: _____ / _____ surgical incision of the eyelid: _____ / ____ / _____ twitching or spasm of the eyelid: _____ / ____ / _____ paralysis of an eyelid: _____ / ____ / _____

10–15 In Figure 10–1, label each structure with its combining form as you read the following information.

1. **scler/o**   Means hardening and also refers to the sclera (white of the eye). The sclera serves as a protective shield for delicate inner layers of tissue.
2. **choroid/o**   Refers to the choroid, which provides the blood supply for the entire eye.
3. **retin/o**   Refers to the retina, which is composed of nerve endings that are responsible for the reception and transmission of light impulses.
4. **kerat/o**   Refers to the cornea, which is transparent and thus permits the entrance of light into the interior of the eye.
5. **irid/o**   Refers to the iris, which is the colored muscular layer that surrounds the pupil.

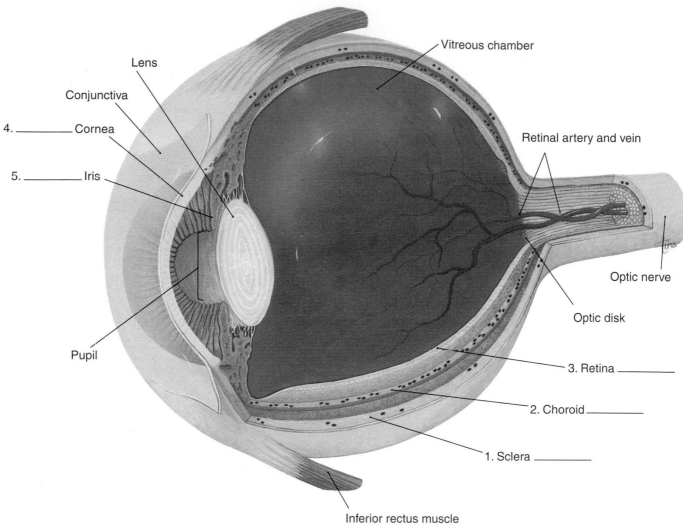

Figure 10–1. Internal anatomy of the eyeball. (Adapted from Scanlon, VC, and Sanders, T: Understanding Human Structure and Function. FA Davis, Philadelphia, 1997, p 164, with permission.)

scler /o	**10–16** The combining form that means either hardening or sclera is _____ / _____ .

scler /itis (sklĕ-RĪ-tĭs) choroid /itis (kō-royd-Ī-tĭs) retin /itis (rĕt-ĭ-NĪ-tĭs)	**10–17** The eyeball is a globe-shaped hollow structure with walls made up of three layers: the sclera, the choroid, and the retina. Use the information in Frame 10–15 to develop medical words meaning inflammation of the sclera: _____ / _____ inflammation of the choroid: _____ / _____ inflammation of the retina: _____ / _____

VALIDATION FRAME: Check your labeling of Figure 10–1 in Appendix B, Answer Key.

10-18 Kerat/itis, which is a vision-threatening infection, can occur if contact lenses are not cleaned and disinfected properly.

From kerat/itis, construct the combining form for cornea.

_____ / _____

kerat/o

10-19 Develop a word meaning rupture of the cornea:

_____ / _____ / _____

kerat/o/rrhexis
(kĕr-ă-tō-RĔK-sĭs)

10-20 Form medical words meaning

inflammation of the sclera: _____ / _____

softening of the sclera: _____ / _____ / _____

scler/itis
(sklĕ-RĪ-tĭs)
scler/o/malacia
(sklĕ-rō-mă-LĀ-shē-ă)

10-21 A kerat/o/tome is an instrument for incising the _____ .

cornea
(KŌR-nē-ă)

10-22 In some cases, laser kerat/o/tomy is being used to correct vision, thus eliminating the need for contact lenses or glasses.

The surgical procedure to incise the cornea is called

_____ / _____ / _____ .

kerat/o/tomy
(kĕr-ă-TŎT-ō-mē)

10-23 Use the information in Frame 10-15 to construct medical words meaning

disease of the choroid: _____ / _____ / _____

disease of the retina: _____ / _____ / _____

inflammation of the choroid: _____ / _____

choroid/o/pathy
(kō-roy-DŎP-ă-thē)
retin/o/pathy
(rĕt-ĭn-ŎP-ă-thē)
choroid/itis
(kō-royd-Ī-tĭs)

10-24 The suffix -opia is used in words to mean vision.
Erythr/opia is a condition in which objects that are not red appear to be

_____ .

Xanth/opia is a condition in which objects that are not yellow appear to be

_____ .

red

yellow

10-25 The combining form **dipl/o** means double. Dipl/opia occurs when both eyes are used but are not in focus.

A person with double vision has a condition called

_____ / _____ .

dipl/opia
(dĭp-LŌ-pē-ă)

dipl/opia
(dĭp-LŌ-pē-ă)

10–26 Dipl/opia can occur with brain tumors, strokes, head trauma, and even migraine headaches.

Write the word in this frame that means double vision.

_____ / _____

hyper-

-opia

10–27 Two common vision defects are my/opia, which is nearsightedness and hyper/opia, which is farsightedness (Fig. 10–2).
Write the element in this frame that means

excessive: _____

vision: _____

nearsightedness

10–28 Hyper/opia is a farsightedness; my/opia is _____ .

hyper/opia
(hī-pĕr-Ō-pē-ă)

10–29 The opposite of my/opia is _____ / _____ .

my/opia
(mī-Ō-pē-ă)

10–30 If the eyeball is too long, the image falls in front of the retina (Fig. 10–2). This condition is called nearsightedness, or _____ / _____ .

hyper/opia
(hī-pĕr-Ō-pē-ă)

10–31 If the eyeball is too short, the image falls behind the retina (Fig. 10–2). This condition is called farsightedness, or _____ / _____ .

blephar/o/plasty
(BLĔF-ă-rō-plăs-tē)
blephar/o/spasm
(BLĔF-ă-rō-spăzm)
blephar/o/ptosis
(blĕf-ă-rō-TŌ-sĭs)

10–32 Eyelids shade the eyes during sleep, protect them from excessive light and foreign objects, and spread lubricating secretions over the eyeballs.

Use **blephar/o** (eyelid) to construct medical words meaning

plastic surgery of the eyelid: _____ / _____ / _____

twitching of an eyelid: _____ / _____ / _____

prolapse of an eyelid: _____ / _____ / _____

blephar/o

-ptosis

10–33 Blephar/o/ptosis is often seen after a stroke because the muscles leading to the eyelids become paralyzed.

Denote the elements in this frame that mean

eyelid: _____ / _____

dropping, falling: _____

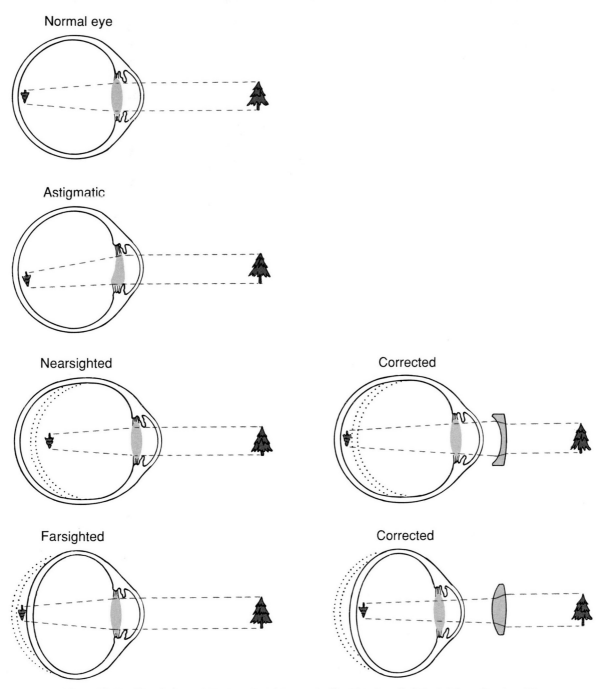

Normal eye

Astigmatic

Nearsighted

Corrected

Farsighted

Corrected

Figure 10–2. Myopia (nearsightedness) and hyperopia (farsightedness). (Adapted from Scanlon, VC, and Sanders, T: Understanding Human Structure and Function. FA Davis, Philadelphia, 1997, p 167, with permission.)

10–34 The **(1) lacrimal glands** (Fig. 10–3) are located above the outer corner of each eye. These glands produce tears, which keep the eyeballs moist. The **(2) lacrimal ducts** collect and drain tears into the **(3) lacrimal sacs**.

Label the lacrimal structures in Figure 10–3.

tears

10–35 The combining form **dacry/o** is used in words to mean tear.

Dacry/o/rrhea is an excessive flow of _____ .

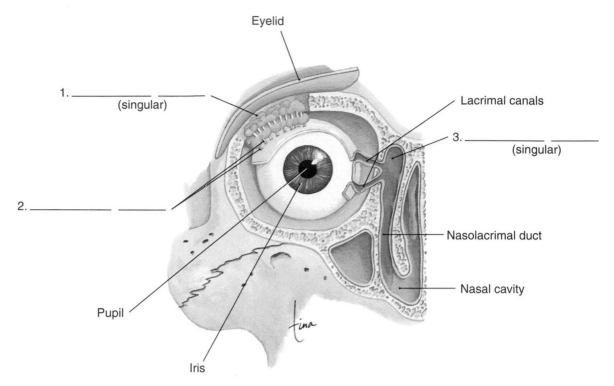

Eyelid

1. _____ _____
(singular)

2. _____ _____

Pupil

Iris

Lacrimal canals

3. _____ _____
(singular)

Nasolacrimal duct

Nasal cavity

Figure 10–3. The anterior view of the eye. (Adapted from Scanlon, VC, and Sanders, T: Understanding Human Structure and Function. FA Davis, Philadelphia, 1997, p 162, with permission.)

pain	**10–36** Dacry/aden/algia is a _____ in a tear gland.

tear gland	**10–37** Dacry/aden/itis is an inflammation of a _____ _____ .

VALIDATION FRAME: Check your labeling of Figure 10–3 Appendix B, Answer Key.

The Ear

The ear consists of three divisions: the external ear, the middle ear, and the inner ear. The external and middle ear conduct sound waves through the ear; the inner ear contains auditory structures that receive sound waves and transmit them to the brain. It also contains the receptor that maintains equilibrium.

The combining forms related to the ear are summarized here. Review this information before you begin to work the frames.

COMBINING FORMS

Combining Form	Meaning	Example	Pronunciation
acous/o	hearing	acous/tic pertaining to	ă-KOOS-tik
audi/o		audi/o/meter instrument to measure	aw-dē-ŎM-ĕ-tĕr
myring/o	tympanic membrane	myring/o/tomy incision, cut into	mĭr-ĭn-GŎT-ō-mē
tympan/o		tympan/o/plasty surgical repair	tĭm-păn-ō-PLĂS-tē
ot/o	ear	ot/o/rrhea flow, discharge	ō-tō-RĒ-ă
salping/o	eustachian (auditory) tube, fallopian (uterine) tube	salping/itis inflammation	săl-pĭn-JĪ-tĭs

---

ot/o

10–38 The combining form **ot/o** is used in words to refer to the ear. From ot/o/sclero/sis, determine the combining form for the ear. _____ / _____

---

ot/o

scler

-osis

10–39 Ot/o/scler/osis is a condition characterized by chronic progressive deafness, especially for low tones.

Write the element in this frame that means

    ear: _____ / _____

    hardening: _____

    abnormal condition: _____

---

pain, ear

10–40 The inner ear contains the receptors for two senses—hearing and equilibrium. Ot/o/dynia is a _____ in the _____ .

---

ot/algia
(ō-TĂL-jē-ă)

10–41 Ot/o/dynia is also known as an earache. Can you think of another term for pain in the ear? _____ / _____ .

---

ot/o/scope
(Ō-tō-skōp)

10–42 When the physician wants an instrument to examine the ear, he or she will ask for an _____ / _____ / _____ .

| ot/o/scopy
(ō-TŎS-kō-pē) | **10–43** Ear infections can be readily diagnosed with an ot/o/scope. A visual examination of the ear is known as _____ / _____ / _____ . |

| ot/o/plasty
(Ō-tō-plăs-tē) | **10–44** Plastic surgery of the ear (to correct defects and deformities) is called _____ / _____ / _____ . |

10–45 The ear can be divided into three anatomical sections: external, middle, and inner. The external ear includes the **(1) auricle**, which receives and directs sound waves from the **(2) ear canal** to the **(3) tympanic membrane** (eardrum).

Label Figure 10–4 as you learn about the ear.

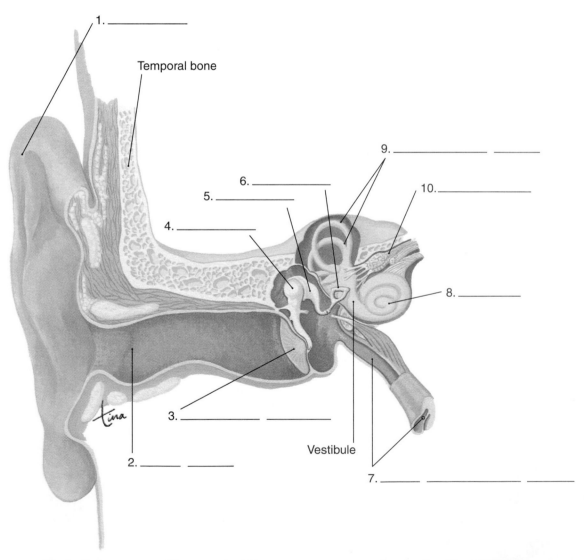

Figure 10–4. Anatomy of the external, middle, and inner ear. (Adapted from Scanlon, VC, and Sanders, T: Understanding Human Structure and Function. FA Davis, Philadelphia, 1997, p 169, with permission.)

ot / algia (ō-TĂL-jē-ă)	**10–46** Swimmer's ear (external and middle ear infections) can cause severe ot / o / dynia or _____ / _____ .

eardrum	**10–47** The combining forms **tympan / o** and **myring / o** both refer to the tympanic membrane or eardrum. Tympan / itis is an inflammation of the tympanic membrane or _____ .

tympan / o, myring / o	**10–48** The tympan / ic membrane is stretched across the end of the ear canal, and vibrates when sound waves strike it. The combining forms for the tympanic membrane or eardrum are _____ / _____ and _____ / _____ .

10–49 The vibrations of the tympanic membrane are transmitted to the three auditory bones in the middle ear: the **(4) malleus,** the **(5) incus**, and the **(6) stapes**. The **(7) eustachian (auditory) tube** leads from the middle ear to the nasopharynx, and permits air to enter or leave the middle ear cavity.

Label the structures of the middle ear in Figure 10–4.

salping / itis (săl-pĭn-JĪ-tĭs)	**10–50** The combining form **salping / o** is used in words to refer to the eustachian (auditory) tube or fallopian (uterine) tube. The medical word meaning inflammation of the eustachian tube is _____ / _____ .

salping / o / scope
(săl-PĬNG-gō-skōp)
 	
salping / o / scopy
(săl-pĭng-ŎS-kō-pē)
 	
salping / o / stenosis
(săl-pĭng-gō-stĕn-NŌ-sĭs)
	10–51 The eustachian tube equalizes the air pressure in the middle ear with that of the outside atmosphere. Air pressure must be equalized for the eardrum to vibrate properly.
	
	Build medical words meaning
	    an instrument to examine the eustachian tube:
	
	    _____ / _____ / _____
	
	    visual examination of the eustachian tube:
	
	    _____ / _____ / _____
	
	    a stricture or narrowing of the eustachian tube:
	
	    _____ / _____ / _____

10–52 Components of the inner ear include the **(8) cochlea** for hearing, the **(9) semicircular canals** for equilibrium, and the **(10) vestibule**, which is a chamber that joins the cochlea and semicircular canals.

Label the components of the inner ear in Figure 10–4.

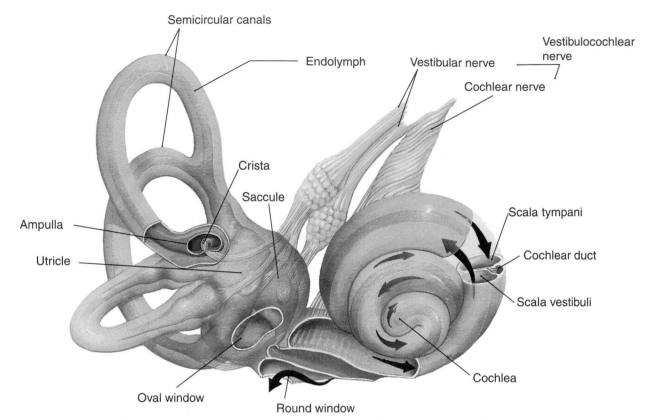

Figure 10–5. Inner ear structures. (From Scanlon, VC, and Sanders, T: Understanding Human Structure and Function. FA Davis, Philadelphia, 1997, p 170, with permission.)

10–53 The inner ear is sometimes referred to as the labyrinth (Fig. 10–5) because of its complicated mazelike structures.

Using your medical dictionary, define *labyrinth*.

_____

_____

VALIDATION FRAME: Check your labeling of Figure 10–4 in Appendix B, Answer Key.

Review

Select the element(s) that match(es) the meaning.

aden/o ✓
blephar/o ✓
choroid/o ✓
dacry/o ✓
dipl/o ✓
erythr/o ✓
irid/o ✓
kerat/o
myring/o ✓
ophthalm/o ✓
ot/o ✓
retin/o ✓
salping/o ✓
scler/o ✓✓
tympan/o
xanth/o ✓

-edema ✓
-logist ✓
-malacia ✓
-opia ✓
-ptosis ✓
-rrhexis ✓
-spasm ✓
-stenosis ✓

hyper- ✓

a. _____hyper-_____ excessive
b. _____choroid/o_____ choroid
c. _____kerat/o_____ cornea
d. _____dipl/o_____ double
e. _____ot/o_____ ear
f. _____salping/o_____ eustachian tube (auditory tube)
g. _____ophthalm/o_____ eye
h. _____blephar/o_____ eyelid
i. _____aden/o_____ gland
j. _____scler/o_____ hardening, sclera (white of the eye)
k. _____-spasm_____ involuntary contraction, twitching
l. _____irid/o_____ iris
m. _____-ptosis_____ prolapse, falling, dropping
n. _____erythr/o_____ red
o. _____retin/o_____ retina
p. _____-rrhexis_____ rupture
q. _____-malacia_____ softening
r. _____-logist_____ specialist in the study of
s. _____-stenosis_____ stricture, narrowing
t. _____-edema_____ swelling
u. _____dacry/o_____ tear
v. _____myring/o_____ tympanic membrane
w. _____scler/o_____ hardening
x. _____-opia_____ vision
y. _____xanth/o_____ yellow

Check your answers with the Review Answer Key on the following page.

Review Answer Key

a. hyper-

b. choroid/o

c. kerat/o

d. dipl/o

e. ot/o

f. salping/o

g. ophthalm/o

h. blephar/o

i. aden/o

j. scler/o

k. -spasm

l. irid/o

m. -ptosis

n. erythr/o

o. retin/o

p. -rrhexis

q. -malacia

r. -logist

s. -stenosis

t. -edema

u. dacry/o

v. tympan/o, myring/o

w. scler/o

x. -opia

y. xanth/o

REINFORCEMENT FRAME: If you are not satisfied with your level of comprehension, go back to Frame 10–1 and rework the frames.

Additional Pathological Conditions

THE EYE

achromatopsia (ă-krō-mă-TŎP-sē-ă): condition of color blindness that is more common in men.

astigmatism (ă-STĬG-mă-tĭzm): abnormal curvature of the cornea, which causes light rays to focus unevenly over the retina rather than being focused on a single point, resulting in a distorted image.

cataract (KĂT-ă-răkt): opacity (cloudiness) of the lens as a result of protein deposits on its surface that slowly build up until vision is lost. The common form is a result of the aging process. Treatment usually consists of surgical removal of the lens.

conjunctivitis (kŏn-jŭnk-tĭ-VĪ-tĭs): inflammation of the conjunctiva that can be caused by bacteria, allergy, irritation, or a foreign body; pinkeye.

diabetic retinopathy (dī-ă-BĔT-ĭk rĕt-ĭn-ŎP-ă-thē): retinal blood vessel disorder that occurs in people with diabetes, manifested by small hemorrhages, edema, and formation of new vessels leading to scarring and eventual loss of vision.

esotropia (ĕs-ō-TRŌ-pē-ă): strabismus in which there is deviation of the visual axis of one eye toward that of the other eye, resulting in diplopia; also called cross-eye and convergent strabismus (Fig. 10–6).

exotropia (ĕks-ō-TRŌ-pē-ă): strabismus in which there is deviation of the visual axis of one eye away from that of the other, resulting in diplopia; also called wall-eye and divergent strabismus (see Fig. 10–6).

glaucoma (glaw-KŌ-mă): increased intraocular pressure caused by the failure of the aqueous humor to drain, which results in atrophy of the optic nerve and may eventually lead to blindness.

hordeolum (hōr-DĒ-ō-lŭm): a small purulent inflammatory infection of a sebaceous gland of the eyelid; sty.

macular degeneration (MĂK-ū-lăr dē-jĕn-ĕr-Ā-shŭn): breakdown of the tissues in the macula resulting in loss of central vision. This condition is the most common cause of visual impairment in persons over age 50.

photophobia (fō-tō-FŌ-bē-ă): unusual intolerance and sensitivity to light. Occurs in diseases such as meningitis, inflammation of the eyes, measles, and rubella.

retinal detachment (RĔT-ĭ-năl dē-TĂCH-mĕnt): separation of the retina from the choroid, which disrupts vision and results in blindness if not repaired. May follow trauma, choroidal hemorrhages, or tumors and may be associated with diabetes mellitus.

strabismus (stră-BĬZ-mŭs): a muscular eye disorder in which the eyes turn from the normal position so that they deviate in different directions. In children, strabismus is associated with the lazy eye syndrome. Various forms of strabismus are spoken of as tropias, their direction being indicated by the appropriate prefix, as esotropia and exotropia (see Fig. 10–6).

THE EAR

acoustic neuroma (a-KOOS-tĭk nū-RŌ-mă): a benign tumor of the 8th cranial nerve sheath that can cause symptoms from pressure exerted on surrounding tissue.

anacusis (ăn-ă-KŪ-sĭs): total deafness; complete hearing loss.

conductive hearing loss: hearing loss due to an impairment in the transmission of sound because of an obstruction of the ear canal or damage to the eardrum or ossicles.

Ménière's disease (mān-ē-ĀRZ dĭ-ZĕZ): a rare disorder of unknown etiology within the labyrinth of the inner ear that can lead to a progressive loss of hearing. Symptoms include vertigo, hearing loss, tinnitus, and the sensation of pressure in the ear.

otitis media (ō-TĪ-tĭs MĒ-dē-ă): middle ear infection, usually a result of bacterial infection; most frequently seen in children.

otosclerosis (ō-tō-sklĕ-RŌ-sĭs): progressive deafness due to ossification in the bony labyrinth of the inner ear. A stapedectomy is often successful in permanently restoring hearing.

presbycusis (prĕz-bĭ-KŪ-sĭs): impairment of hearing resulting from old age.

tinnitus (tĭn-Ī-tĭs): a ringing in the ears.

vertigo (VĔR-tĭ-gō): sensation of moving around in space; a feeling of spinning or dizziness; usually results from inner ear structure damage associated with balance and equilibrium.

Esotropia

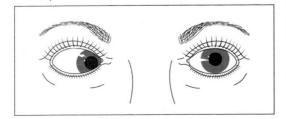

Exotropia

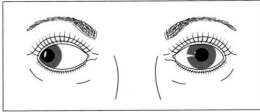

Figure 10–6. Strabismus: (left) esotropia; (right) exotropia.

Medical Record

The following medical reports are related to the medical specialty called ophthalmology, otolaryngology, and ENT (ear, nose, throat). Ophthalmologists, otolaryngologists, and ENT physicians specialize in medical and surgical treatment of diseases and disorders of the ear, nose, and throat.

MEDICAL RECORD 10–1. Otitis Media

Dictionary Exercise

Underline the following terms in the reading exercise. Use a medical dictionary and Appendix E, Abbreviations, to write a definition of each word in the list. This exercise helps you master the terminology in the medical record.

adhesive _____

cholesteatoma _____

chronic _____

diagnosis _____

ENT _____

general anesthetic _____

mucoserous _____

otitis media _____

postoperatively _____

Word Element Exercise

Break down the following words into their basic elements.

mastoid
otitis
tympanoplasty

VALIDATION FRAME: Check your answers in Appendix B, Answer Key.

Reading Exercise

Read the case study out loud.

A 25-year-old white woman with a diagnosis of mucoserous otitis media on the right ear was seen by the ENT specialist. The patient was admitted to City Hospital and developed cholesteatoma. A tube was inserted for the chronic adhesive otitis media with secondary cholesteatoma. The patient progressed favorably postoperatively, but the cholesteatoma continued to enlarge in size. Currently she has been admitted to the hospital for a right tympanoplasty performed under general anesthesia.

MEDICAL RECORD EVALUATION 10–1. Otitis Media

1. Where was the patient's infection located?

2. What complication developed while the patient was hospitalized?

3. What is the purpose of the tube placement?

4. What surgery is being performed to resolve the cholesteatoma?

5. Will the patient be asleep during the surgery?

MEDICAL RECORD 10–2. Retinal Detachment

Dictionary Exercise

Underline the following terms in the reading exercise. Use a medical dictionary and Appendix E, Abbreviations, to write a definition of each word in the list. This exercise helps you master the terminology in the medical record.

akinesia _____

cannula _____

conjuctival _____

detachment _____

disk _____

EKG _____

infusion _____

IV _____

loculated _____

perfusion _____

retinal _____

retinitis _____

retrobulbar _____

sclera _____

sclerotomy _____

vitrectomy _____

vitreous _____

Word Element Exercise

Break down the following words into their basic elements.

retinal   sclerotomy
retinitis   vitrectomy
conjunctival

VALIDATION FRAME: Check your answers in Appendix B, Answer Key.

Reading Exercise

Read the case study out loud.

Diagnosis: Total retinal detachment (Fig. 10–7), left eye, secondary to complications of retinitis.

The patient was taken to the operating room, placed on the operating table, IV line begun, EKG lead monitor attached, and retrobulbar anesthetic given, achieving good anesthesia and akinesia. The patient was scrubbed, prepped, and draped in a standard sterile fashion for retinal surgery. A 360-degree conjunctival opening was made and 2–0 silks were placed around each rectus muscle. Four millimeters from the limbus a mark in the sclera was made and preplaced 5–0 Mersiline suture was passed, MVR stab incision made, and 4 mm infusion cannula was slipped into position and visualized inside the eye. Similar sclerotomy sites were made superior nasally and superior temporally. Trans pars plana vitrectomy was undertaken. Dense vitreous hemorrhage and debris were found, which were removed. There was incomplete posterior vitreous attachment. The retina was almost totally detached, and a small amount of nasal retina was still attached. A linear retinal break was seen just above the disk along a vessel. Gradually all the peripheral vitreous was removed.

The air-fluid exchange was performed with some difficulty because some sort of vitreous was found anteriorly, which loculated the bubble. It gave me a peculiar view, but slowly the retina became totally flat and we treated the retinal break with the diode laser. A 240 band was wrapped around the eye and fixed with the Watke's sleeve superior temporally. The sclerotomies were all sewn closed. Before the last sclerotomy was closed, the air was exchanged for silicone. The eye was left rather soft because the patient had poor perfusion.

MEDICAL RECORD EVALUATION 10–2. Retinal Detachment

1. Where is the retina located?

2. Was the anesthetic administered behind or in front of the eyeball?

3. How much movement remained in the eye following anesthesia?

4. Where was the hemorrhage located?

5. What type of vitrectomy was undertaken?

6. Why was the eye left soft?

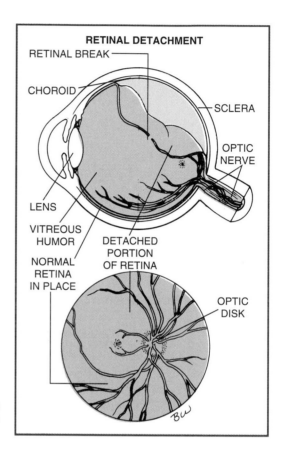

Figure 10–7. Retinal detachment. (Adapted from Taber's Cyclopedic Medical Dictionary, ed 18. FA Davis, Philadelphia, 1997, p 1672, with permission.)

Abbreviations

EYE

Abbreviation	Meaning	Abbreviation	Meaning
ARMD	age-related macular degeneration	OD	right eye (Latin, oculus dexter)
Astigm	astigmatism	OS	left eye (Latin, oculus sinister)
D	diopter (lens strength)	OU	each eye (Latin, oculus uterque)
EOM	extraocular movement	REM	rapid eye movement
IOL	intraocular lens	ST	esotropia
IOP	intraocular pressure	VA	visual acuity
mix astig	mixed astigmatism	VF	visual field
Myop.	myopia	XT	exotropia

EAR

Abbreviation	Meaning	Abbreviation	Meaning
AD	right ear (Latin, auris dextra)	ENT	ear, nose, and throat
AS	left ear (Latin, auris sinistra)		

Audiocassette Exercise

The audiocassette tape helps you master the pronunciation of medical words. Listen to the tape for instructions to complete this exercise. You may also use this list without the audiotape to practice correct pronunciation and spelling of the terms.

Frame	Word	Pronunciation	Spelling Exercise
Reading Exercise	[] akinesia	(ă-kĭn-Ē-zē-ă)	_____
Reading Exercise	[] anesthetic	(ăn-ĕs-THĔT-ĭk)	_____
10–45	[] auricle	(AW-rĭ-kl)	_____
10–14	[] blepharectomy	(blĕf-ă-RĔK-tō-mē)	_____
10–11	[] blepharedema	(blĕf-ăr-ĕ-DĒ-mă)	_____
10–12	[] blepharoplasty	(BLĔF-ă-rō-plăs-tē)	_____
10–14	[] blepharoplegia	(blĕf-ă-rō-PLĒ-jē-ă)	_____
10–32	[] blepharoptosis	(blĕf-ă-rō-TŌ-sĭs)	_____
10–10	[] blepharospasm	(BLĔF-ă-rō-spăzm)	_____
10–14	[] blepharotomy	(blĕf-ă-RŎT-ō-mē)	_____
Reading Exercise	[] cannula	(KĂN-ū-lă)	_____
Reading Exercise	[] cholesteatoma	(kō-lē-stē-ă-TŌ-mă)	_____
10–17	[] choroiditis	(kō-royd-Ī-tĭs)	_____
10–23	[] choroidopathy	(kō-roy-DŎP-ă-thē)	_____
Reading Exercise	[] conjunctival	(kŏn-jŭnk-TĪ-văl)	_____
10–36	[] dacryadenalgia	(dăk-rē-ăd-ĕn-ĂL-jē-ă)	_____
10–37	[] dacryadenitis	(dăk-rē-ăd-ĕ-NĪ-tĭs)	_____
10–35	[] dacryorrhea	(dăk-rē-ō-RĒ-ă)	_____
Reading Exercise	[] diagnosis	(dī-ăg-NŌ-sĭs)	_____
10–25	[] diplopia	(dĭp-LŌ-pē-ă)	_____
10–24	[] erythropia	(ĕr-ĭ-THRŌ-pē-ă)	_____
10–27	[] hyperopia	(hī-pĕr-Ō-pē-ă)	_____
Reading Exercise	[] infusion	(ĭn-FŪ-zhŭn)	_____
10–18	[] keratitis	(kĕr-ă-TĪ-tĭs)	_____
10–21	[] keratotome	(kĕr-ĂT-ō-tōm)	_____
10–19	[] keratorrhexis	(kĕr-ă-tō-RĔKS-ĭs)	_____
10–22	[] keratotomy	(kĕr-ă-TŎT-ō-mē)	_____
10–53	[] labyrinth	(LĂB-ĭ-rĭnth)	_____
Reading Exercise	[] loculated	(LŎK-ū-lāt-ĕd)	_____
Reading Exercise	[] mucoserous	(mū-kō-SĒR-ŭs)	_____
10–27	[] myopia	(mī-Ō-pē-ă)	_____
10–2	[] ophthalmalgia	(ŏf-thăl-MĂL-jē-ă)	_____
10–8	[] ophthalmectomy	(ŏf-thăl-MĔK-tō-mē)	_____
10–6	[] ophthalmodynia	(ŏf-thăl-mō-DĬN-ē-ă)	_____
10–8	[] ophthalmomalacia	(ŏf-thăl-mō-mă-LĀ-shē-ă)	_____
10–8	[] ophthalmoplegia	(ŏf-thăl-mō-PLĒ-jē-ă)	_____
10–4	[] ophthalmoscope	(ŏf-THĂL-mō-skōp)	_____
10–5	[] ophthalmoscopy	(ŏf-thăl-MŎS-kō-pē)	_____

Frame	Word	Pronunciation	Spelling Exercise
10–41	[] otalgia	(ō-TĂL-jē-ă)	_____
10–40	[] otodynia	(ō-tō-DĬN-ē-ă)	_____
10–44	[] otoplasty	(Ō-tō-plăs-tē)	_____
10–42	[] otoscope	(Ō-tō-skōp)	_____
10–43	[] otoscopy	(ō-TŎS-kō-pē)	_____
Case Study	[] perfusion	(pĕr-FŪ-zhŭn)	_____
Reading Exercise	[] postoperatively	(pōst-ŎP-ĕr-ă-tĭv-lē)	_____
Reading Exercise	[] retinal	(RĔT-ĭ-năl)	_____
Reading Exercise	[] retrobulbar	(rĕt-rō-BŪL-băr)	_____
Reading Exercise	[] retinitis	(rĕt-ĭn-Ī-tĭs)	_____
10–23	[] retinopathy	(rĕt-ĭn-ŎP-ă-thē)	_____
10–50	[] salpingitis	(săl-pĭng-JĪ-tĭs)	_____
10–51	[] salpingostenosis	(săl-pĭng-gō-stĕn-Ō-sĭs)	_____
10–51	[] salpingoscope	(săl-PĬNG-gō-skōp)	_____
10–51	[] salpingoscopy	(săl-pĭng-GŎS-kō-pē)	_____
10–16	[] sclera	(SKLĔR-ă)	_____
10–17	[] scleritis	(sklĕ-RĪ-tĭs)	_____
10–20	[] scleromalacia	(sklĕ-rō-mă-LĀ-shē-ă)	_____
Reading Exercise	[] sclerotomy	(sklĕr-ŎT-ō-mē)	_____
10–45	[] tympanic	(tĭm-PĂN-ĭk)	_____
10–47	[] tympanitis	(tĭm-păn-Ī-tĭs)	_____
Reading Exercise	[] vitrectomy	(vĭ-TRĔK-tō-mē)	_____
Reading Exercise	[] vitreous	(VĬT-rē-ŭs)	_____
10–24	[] xanthopia	(zăn-THŌ-pē-ă)	_____

Unit Exercises

DEFINITIONS

Review Unit Summary (pages 453–454) before completing this exercise. Write the meaning for each word part.

SUFFIXES AND PREFIXES

Element	Meaning
1. -dynia	_____
2. -ectomy	_____
3. -edema	_____
4. -logist	_____
5. -malacia	_____
6. -opia	_____
7. -pathy	_____
8. -ptosis	_____
9. -rrhexis	_____
10. -scope	_____
11. -spasm	_____
12. -stenosis	_____
13. -tomy	_____

COMBINING FORMS

Element	Meaning
14. aden/o	_____
15. blephar/o	_____
16. choroid/o	_____
17. dacry/o	_____
18. dipl/o	_____
19. irid/o	_____
20. kerat/o	_____
21. myring/o	_____
22. ophthalm/o	_____
23. ot/o	_____
24. retin/o	_____
25. salping/o	_____
26. tympan/o	_____
27. scler/o	_____

OTHER COMBINING FORMS

28. erythr/o   _____

29. my/o   _____

30. xanth/o   _____

VALIDATION FRAME: Check your answers in Index of Medical Word Elements, Appendix A. If you scored less than

_____ %,* review Unit Summary (pages 453–454).

To obtain a percentage score, multiply the number of correct answers times 3.33.

Number of Correct Answers: _____   **Percentage Score:** _____

*Enter the percentage required by your instructor to complete this course.

Vocabulary

Match the medical word(s) below with the definitions in the numbered list.

blepharoptosis	general anesthetic	ophthalmologist
cholesteatoma	hyperopia	otitis media
chronic	keratitis	postoperatively
dacryorrhea	labyrinth	salpingostenosis
diagnosis	mastoid surgery	sclera
diplopia	mucoserous	tympanic membrane
eustachian tube	myopia	

1. _____ Double vision.

2. _____ White of the eye.

3. _____ Eardrum; it vibrates when sound waves strike it.

4. _____ An excessive flow of tears.

5. _____ A structure that equalizes the air pressure in the middle ear with that of the outside atmosphere.

6. _____ Inflammation of the cornea due to a vision-threatening infection; sometimes occurs when contact lenses are not cleaned and disinfected properly.

7. _____ Process of determining the cause and nature of a pathological condition; to recognize a disease.

8. _____ Composed of mucus and serum.

9. _____ Inflammation of the middle ear.

10. _____ A tumor-like sac filled with keratin debris most commonly found in the middle ear.

11. _____ Operation on the mastoid process of the temporal bone.

12. _____ Anesthesia that affects the entire body with loss of consciousness.

13. _____ A physician who specializes in the treatment of eye disorders.

14. _____ Of long duration; designating a disease showing little change or of slow progression.

15. _____ Farsightedness.

16. _____ Occurring after or following a surgical operation.

17. _____ A system of intercommunicating canals, especially of the inner ear.

18. _____ Prolapse of an eyelid.

19. _____ A narrowing or stricture of the eustachian tube.

20. _____ Nearsightedness.

VALIDATION FRAME: Check your answers in Appendix B, Answer Key. If you scored less than _____ %, review the vocabulary and retake the exercise.

To obtain a percentage score, multiply the number of correct answers times 5.

Additional Pathological Conditions

Match the medical term(s) below with the definitions in the numbered list.

anacusis
achromatopsia
acoustic neuroma
astigmatism
cataract
conductive hearing loss
conjunctivitis

diabetic retinopathy
glaucoma
hordeolum
macular degeneration
Ménière's disease
otitis media
otosclerosis

photophobia
presbycusis
retinal detachment
strabismus
tinnitus
vertigo

1. _____ Ringing in the ears.

2. _____ Progressive deafness due to ossification in the bony labyrinth of the inner ear.

3. _____ Color blindness.

4. _____ Rare disorder characterized by progressive deafness, vertigo, and tinnitus, possibly due to swelling of membranous structures within the labyrinth.

5. _____ Disorder in which both eyes cannot focus on the same point resulting in the looking in different directions at the same time; also called *lazy eye* or *cross eyes*.

6. _____ Total deafness.

7. _____ Middle ear infection that is most commonly seen in young children.

8. _____ Pinkeye.

9. _____ Intolerance or unusual sensitivity to light.

10. _____ Hearing loss due to old age.

11. _____ Increased intraocular pressure caused by the failure of the aqueous humor to drain, which results in atrophy of the optic nerve and may eventually lead to blindness.

12. _____ Feeling of spinning or dizziness.

13. _____ Separation of the retina from the choroid.

14. _____ Sty.

15. _____ Abnormal curvature of the cornea, which causes light rays to focus unevenly over the retina rather than focus on a single point, resulting in a distorted image.

16. _____ Benign tumor of the 8th cranial nerve that may or may not produce symptomatic changes.

17. _____ Hearing loss caused by an impairment in sound transmission because of damage to the eardrum or ossicles or obstruction of the ear canal.

18. _____ Opacity (cloudiness) of the lens as a result of protein deposits on its surface.

19. _____ Eye disorder characterized by edema, small hemorrhages, and formation of vessels in the retina.

20. _____ Macular tissue breakdown causing loss of central vision. This condition is the most common cause of visual impairment in persons over age 50.

VALIDATION FRAME: Check your answers in Appendix B, Answer Key. If you scored less than _____ %, review the vocabulary and retake the exercise.
    To obtain a percentage score, multiply the number of correct answers times 5.

Unit Summary

COMBINING FORMS RELATED TO THE SPECIAL SENSES

Combining Form	Meaning
acous/o audi/o	hearing
aden/o	gland
blephar/o	eyelid
choroid/o	choroid
corne/o kerat/o	cornea
dacry/o	tear, lacrimal
dipl/o	double
irid/o	iris
myring/o tympan/o	tympanic membrane
ocul/o ophthalm/o	eye
ot/o	ear
retin/o	retina
salping/o	eustachian (auditory) tube; fallopian (uterine) tube
scler/o	hardening, sclera (white of the eye)

OTHER COMBINING FORMS

Combining Form	Meaning
erythr/o	red
my/o	muscle
xanth/o	yellow

SUFFIXES AND PREFIXES

Suffix (Prefix)	Meaning
Suffixes	
-algia -dynia	pain
-ectomy	excision, removal
-edema	swelling
-itis	inflammation
-logist	specialist in the study of
-malacia	softening

Suffix (Prefix)	Meaning
-opia	vision
-pathy	disease
-ptosis	prolapse, falling, dropping
-rrhexis	rupture
-scope	instrument to view
-spasm	involuntary contraction, twitching
-stenosis	stricture, narrowing
-tomy	incision, cut into
Prefix	
hyper-	excessive

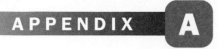

Index of Medical Word Elements

PART A: Medical Terms—Meaning

Medical Word Element	Pronunciation	Meaning	Frame
a-, an-	ă	without, not	3–114
acr / o	ăk-rō	extremities	7–28
aden / o	ăd-ē-nō	gland	3–72
adip / o	ăd-ĭ-pō	fat	4–27
adren / o	ăd-rē-nō	adrenal glands	7–58
adrenal / o	ă-drĕn-ăl-ō	adrenal glands	7–58
aer / o	ĕr-ō	air	2–100
-al	ăl	pertaining to	1–74
-algia	ăl-jē-ă	pain	2–10
angi / o	ăn-jē-ō	vessel (usually blood or lymph)	9–58
anter / o	ăn-tĕr-ō	front, anterior	7–9
anti-	ăn-tē	against	9–107
aort / o	ā-or-tō	aorta	9–62
append / o	ăp-ĕnd-ō	appendix	1–53
-ar	ăr	pertaining to	6–74
arteri / o	ăr-tē-rē-ō	artery	9–40
arthr / o	ăr thrō	joint	8–41
-ary	ĕr-ē	pertaining to	2–24
atri / o	ā-trē-ō	atrium	9–10
auto-	aw-tō	self	4–98
bi-	bī	two, double	9–36
blephar / o	blĕf-ă-rō	eyelid	10–10
brady-	brăd-ē	slow	6–99
bronchi / o	brŏng-kē-ō	bronchus (plural, bronchi)	6–49
bronch / o	brŏng-kō	bronchus (plural, bronchi)	6–49
calcane / o	kăl-kā-nē-ō	calcaneum (heel bone)	8–48
calc / o	kăl-kō	calcium	7–46
carcin / o	kăr-sĭ-nō	cancer	2–85
cardi / o	kăr-dē-ō	heart	9–3
carp / o	kār-pō	carpus (wrist bones)	8–48
-cele	sēl	hernia, swelling	3–97
-centesis	sĕn-tē-sĭs	surgical puncture	6–68
cephal / o	sĕf-ăl-ō	head	8–49
cerebr / o	sĕr-ē-brō	cerebrum (brain)	7–99

Medical Word Element	Pronunciation	Meaning	Frame
cervic / o	sĕr-vĭ-kō	neck, cervix uteri (neck of uterus)	5–52
chol / e	kō-lē	bile, gall	2–171
cholecyst / o	kō-lē-sĭs-tō	gallbladder	2–163
choledoch / o	kō-lē-dō-kō	bile duct	2–181
chondr / o	kŏn-drō	cartilage	6–37
choroid / o	kō-roy-dō	choroid	10–15
col / o	kō-lō	colon	2–131
colon / o	kō-lŏn-ō	colon	2–156
colp / o	kŏl-pō	vagina	5–30
cost / o	kŏs-tō	ribs	8–48
crani / o	krā-nē-ō	cranium (skull)	8–48
cutane / o	kū-tā-nē-ō	skin	4–8
cyan / o	sī-ă-nō	blue	4–67
cyst / o	sĭs-tō	bladder	2–168
-cyte	sīt	cell	4–71
cyt / o	sī-tō	cell	4–71
dacry / o	dăk-rē-ō	tear, lacrimal	10–35
dent / o	dĕnt-ō	teeth	1–27
-derma	dĕr-mă	skin	4–13
dermat / o	dĕr-mă-tō	skin	4–8
derm / o	dĕr-mō	skin	4–5
dia-	dī-ă	through	2–17
dipl / o	dĭp-lō	double	10–25
-dipsia	dĭp-sē-ă	thirst	7–82
dist / o	dĭs-tō	far, farthest	8–32
duoden / o	doo-ŏd-ĕ-nō	duodenum	2–71
-dynia	dĭ-nē-ă	pain	2–10
dys-	dĭs	bad, painful, difficult	2–96
-ectasis	ĕk-tă-sĭs	dilation, expansion	3–40
-ectomy	ĕk-tŏ-mē	excision, removal	2–75
-edema	ĕd-ĕ-mă	swelling	3–16
electr / o	ē-lĕk-trō	electric	9–75
-emesis	ĕm-ĕ-sĭs	vomiting	2–91
-emia	ēm-ē-ă	blood	4–77
en-	ĕn	in	8–52
encephal / o	ĕn-sĕf-ă-lō	brain	7–91
enter / o	ĕn-tĕr-ō	intestine (usually small)	1–37
epi-	ĕp-ē	above, upon	2–90
-er	ĕr	one who	1–44
erythr / o	ē-rĭth-rō	red	3–102
esophag / o	ē-sŏf-ă-gō	esophagus	2–63
eu-	ū	good, normal	6–95
femor / o	fĕm-ō-rō	femur (thigh bone)	8–48
fibul / o	fĭb-ū-lō	fibula	8–48
gastr / o	găs-trō	stomach	1–37
-gen	jĕn	producing, forming	7–72
-genesis	jĕn-ĕ-sĭs	producing, forming	5–101
gingiv / o	jĭn-jĭ-vō	gum	2–54
-glia	glē-ă	glue or gluelike; neuroglial tissue (binding, supportive tissue of nervous system)	7–113
glomerul / o	glō-mĕr-ū-lō	glomerulus	3–84
gluc / o	gloo-kō	sugar, glucose	7–72
glyc / o	glī-kō	sugar, glucose	7–72

Medical Word Element	Pronunciation	Meaning	Frame
-gram	grăm	record	2–214
-graphy	gră-fē	process of recording	2–214
-gravida	grăv-ĭ-dă	pregnant woman	5–82
gynec / o	gĭ-nē-kō or jĭ-nē-kō	woman, female	5–57
hemangi / o	hē-măn-jē-ō	blood vessel	9–59
hemat / o	hē-mă-tō	blood	2–91
hemi-	hĕm-ē	half, partly	8–102
hem / o	hē-mō	blood	5–26
hepat / o	hĕp-ă-tō	liver	2–163
hidr / o	hī-drō	sweat	4–21
humer / o	hū-mĕr-ō	humerus (upper arm bone)	8–48
hydr / o	hī-drō	water	4–23
hyper-	hī-pĕr	excessive	2–92
hypo-	hī-pō	under, below	4–11
hyster / o	hĭs-tĕr-ō	uterus	5–14
-ia	ē-ă	condition	2–225
-iasis	ī-ă-sĭs	abnormal condition (produced by something specified)	2–194
-ic	ĭk	pertaining to	1–65
ile / o	ĭl-ē-ō	ileum	2–104
in-	ĭn	not	3–126
inter-	ĭn-tĕr	between	8–56
intra-	ĭn-tră	within	3–88
irid / o	ĭr-ĭ-dō	iris	10–15
-is	ĭs	noun ending	4–14
-ism	ĭzm	condition	5–105
-ist	ĭst	specialist	2–37
-itis	ī-tĭs	inflammation	2–6
jejun / o	jĕ-joo-nō	jejunum	2–104
kerat / o	kĕr-ă-tō	cornea, hard tissue	10–15, 4–43
laryng / o	lă-rĭng-gō	larynx (voice box)	6–25
leuk / o	loo-kō	white	3–102
lingu / o	lĭng-gwō	tongue	2–22
lip / o	lĭ-pō	fat	4–27
-lith	lĭth	stone, calculus	2–176
lith / o	lĭ-thō	stone, calculus	2–193
lob / o	lō-bō	lobe	6–74
log / o	lō-gō	study of	2–40
-logist	lŏ-jĭst	specialist in the study of	2–40
-logy	lŏ-jē	study of	2–40
lumb / o	lŭm-bō	lower back, loin	8–77
lymphangi / o	lĭm-făn-jē-ō	lymph vessel	9–122
lymph / o	lĭm-fō	lymph	9–117
-lysis	lī-sĭs	separation, destruction, loosening	7–68
macro-	măk-rō	large	6–57
-malacia	mă-lā-shē-ă	softening	4–61
mamm / o	măm-ō	breast	5–72
mast / o	măs-tō	breast	5–70
maxill / o	măk-sĭ-lō	jaw	2–23
megal / o	mĕg-ă-lō	enlargement	2–219
-megaly	mĕg-ă-lē	enlargement	2–220
melan / o	mĕl-ă-nō	black	4–67
mening / o	mĕ-nĭng-gō	meninges	7–106

Medical Word Element	Pronunciation	Meaning	Frame
meningi / o	mĕ-nĭn-jē-ō	meninges	7–106
men / o	mĕn-ō	menses, menstruation	5–62
-meter	mĕ-tĕr	measure, instrument for measuring	8–49
metacarp / o	mĕt-ă-kăr-pō	metacarpus (bones of the hand)	8–48
metr / o	mĕt-rō	uterus	5–17
micro-	mī-krō	small	6–57
muc / o	mū-kō	mucus	5–42
myc / o	mī-kō	fungus	2–34
myel / o	mī-ĕl-ō	spinal cord, bone marrow	7–93
my / o	mī-ō	muscle	6–40
myring / o	mĭ-rĭng-gō	tympanic membrane (eardrum)	10–47
nas / o	nā-zō	nose	6–3
nat / o	nā-tō	birth	5–79
necr / o	nĕk-rō	death	4–93
neo-	nē-ō	new	5–80
nephr / o	nĕf-rō	kidney	3–4
neur / o	noo-rō	nerve	7–17
noct / o	nŏk-tō	night	3–123
odont / o	ō-dŏn-tō	teeth	2–47
-oid	oyd	resembling	5–43
-ole	ōl	small	6–113
olig / o	ŏl-ĭ-gō	scanty, little	2–117
-oma	ō-mă	tumor	2–88
onych / o	ŏn-ĭ-kō	nail	4–59
oophor / o	ō-ŏf-ō-rō	ovary	5–4
ophthalm / o	ŏf-thăl-mō	eye	10–2
-opia	ō-pē-ă	vision	10–24
orchid / o	ŏr-kĭ-dō	testis	5–111
orchi / o	ŏr-kē-ō	testis	5–111
or / o	or-ō	mouth	2–4
orth / o	or-thō	straight	2–49
-osis	ō-sĭs	abnormal condition	2–32
oste / o	ŏs-tē-ō	bone	8–2
ot / o	ō-tō	ear	10–38
-ous	ŭs	pertaining to	2–86
pancreat / o	păn-krē-ă-tō	pancreas	2–163
para-	păr-ă	near, beside, around	7–49
patell / o	pă-tĕl-ō	knee cap	8–48
-pathy	pă-thē	disease	3–21
-pause	pawz	cessation	5–66
pelv / i	pĕl-vē	pelvis	8–48
pelv / o	pĕl-vō	pelvis	8–48
-penia	pē-nē-ă	decrease	4–74
-pepsia	pĕp-sē-ă	digestion	2–96
peri-	pĕr-ē	around	2–52
-pexy	pĕk-sē	fixation	3–34
-phagia	fā-jē-ă	swallow, eat	2–99
phalang / o	fā-lăng-gō	phalanges (finger and toe)	8–48
pharyng / o	fă-rĭng-gō	pharynx (throat)	6–17
-phasia	fā-zē-ă	speech	7–105
phleb / o	flĕb-ō	vein	9–51
-phobia	fō-bē-ă	fear	3–121
-plasia	plā-zē-ă	formation, growth	5–132
-plasm	plăzm	formation, growth	5–124

Medical Word Element	Pronunciation	Meaning	Frame
-plasty	plăs-tē	surgical repair	2–73
-plegia	plē-jē-ă	paralysis	6–19
pleur / o	ploo-rō	pleura	6–78
-pnea	nē-ă	breathing	6–89
pneum / o	noo-mō	lung, air	6–63, 6–10
pneumon / o	noo-mŏn-ō	lung, air	6–63, 6–10
poly-	pŏl-ē	many, much	3–120
polyp / o	pŏl-ĭp-ō	polyp	p. 261
post-	pōst	after, behind	1–72
poster / o	pŏs-tĕr-ō	back (of body), behind, posterior	7–9
pre-	prē	before	1–73
proct / o	prŏk-tō	anus, rectum	2–146
prostat / o	prŏs-tă-tō	prostate gland	5–114
proxim / o	prŏk-sĭ-mō	near, nearest	8–33
-ptosis	tō-sĭs	prolapse, falling, dropping	3–31
pyel / o	pī-ĕ-lō	renal pelvis	3–81
py / o	pī-ō	pus	3–109
quadri-	kwŏd-rī	four	8–100
radi / o	rā-dē-ō	x-rays, radiation	7–13
rect / o	rĕk-tō	rectum	2–139
ren / o	rē-nō	kidney	3–4
retin / o	rĕt-ĭ-nō	retina	10–15
rhin / o	rī-nō	nose	6–3
roentgen / o	rĕnt-gĕn-ō	x-rays	8–21
-rrhage	răj	bursting forth (of)	5–24
-rrhagia	ră-jē-ă	bursting forth (of)	5–24
-rrhaphy	ră-fē	suture	2–117
-rrhea	rē-ă	flow, discharge	2–15
-rrhexis	rĕk-sĭs	rupture	8–87
sacr / o	săk-rō	sacrum	8–81
salping / o	săl-pĭn-gō or săl-pĭn-jō	fallopian (uterine) tube eustachian (auditory) tube	5–7 10–50
scler / o	sklē-rō	hardening, sclera (white of the eye)	3–24
-scope	skōp	instrument to view	2–150
-scopy	skŏ-pē	visual examination	2–150
sial / o	sī-ă-lō	saliva, salivary glands	2–13
sigmoid / o	sĭg-moyd-ō	sigmoid colon	2–136
-spasm	spăzm	involuntary contraction, twitching	2–149
spermat / o	spĕr-mă-tō	sperm	5–99
spin / o	spī-no	spine	7–112
spondyl / o	spŏn-dĭ-lō	vertebra (backbone)	8–62
-stenosis	stĕn-ō-sĭs	stricture, narrowing	2–144
stern / o	stĕr-nō	sternum (breastbone)	8–48
stomat / o	stō-mă-tō	mouth	2–4
-stomy	stō-mē	forming a new opening or mouth	2–109
sub-	sŭb	under, below	4–11
supra-	soo-pră	above	3–23
tachy-	tăk-ē	rapid	6–97
tend / o	tĕn-dō	tendon	8–98
test / o	tĕs-tō	testis	5–96
-therapy	thĕr-ă-pē	treatment	6–12
therm / o	thĕr-mō	heat	2–207

Medical Word Element	Pronunciation	Meaning	Frame
thorac / o	thō-răk-ō	chest	6–86
thromb / o	thrŏm-bō	blood clot	7–95
thym / o	thī-mō	thymus gland	7–85
thyr / o	thī-rō	thyroid gland	7–36
thyroid / o	thī-royd-ō	thyroid gland	7–36
tibi / o	tĭb-ē-ō	tibia	8–48
-tome	tōm	instrument to cut	2–75
-tomy	tō-mē	incision, cut into	2–75
toxic / o	tŏks-ĭ-kō	poison	2–212
tox / o	tŏks-ō	poison	2–211
trache / o	trā-kē-ō	trachea (windpipe)	6–33
tri-	trī	three	9–34
trich / o	trĭk-ō	hair	4–55
-tripsy	trĭp-sē	crushing	3–45
tympan / o	tĭm-pă-nō	tympanic membrane (eardrum)	10–47
-ule	ūl	small	9–64
-um	ŭm	noun ending	8–39
ureter / o	ū-rē-tĕr-ō	ureter	3–39
urethr / o	ū-rē-thrō	urethra	3–64
-uria	ū-rē-ă	urine, urination	3–102
ur / o	ū-rō	urine	3–104
uter / o	ū-tĕr-ō	uterus	5–17
vagin / o	vă-jĭ-nō	vagina	5–30
vascul / o	văs-kū-lō	blood vessel	7–99
vas / o	vă-sō	vas deferens, vessel	5–137
ven / o	vē-nō	vein	3–90
ventricul / o	vĕn-trĭk-ū-lō	ventricle (of brain or heart)	9–14
vesic / o	vĕs-ĭ-kō	bladder	3–47
vertebr / o	vĕr-tē-brō	vertebra (backbone)	8–48
vulvo	vŭl-vō	vulva	5–47
xanth / o	zăn-thō	yellow	4–67
xer / o	zē-rō	dry	4–63
-y	ē	noun ending	2–208

PART B: English Term—Medical Word Element

English Term	Medical Word Element	Pronunciation	Frame
abnormal condition	-osis	ō-sĭs	2–32
abnormal condition (produced by something specified)	-iasis	ī-ă-sĭs	2–194
above, upon	epi-	ĕp-ē	2–90
above	supra-	soo-pră	2–23
adrenal glands	adren / o	ăd-rē-nō	7–58
adrenal glands	adrenal / o	ă-drĕn-ăl-ō	7–58
after, behind	post-	pōst	1–72
against	anti-	ăn-tē	9–107
air	aer / o	ĕr-ō	2–100
air, lung	pneum / o	noo-mō	6–3 6–10
air, lung	pneumon / o	noo-mŏn-ō	6–10 6–63
anterior, front	anter / o	ăn-tĕr-ō	7–9
anus, rectum	proct / o	prŏk-tō	2–146
aorta	aort / o	āor-tō	9–62
appendix	append / o	ăp-ĕnd-ō	1–53
around, near, beside	para-	păr-ă	7–49
around	peri-	pĕr-ē	2–52
artery	arteri / o	ăr-tē-rē-ō	9–40
atrium	atri / o	ā-trē-ō	9–10
back (of body), behind, posterior	poster / o	pŏs-tĕr-ō	7–9
bad, painful, difficult	dys-	dĭs	2–96
before	pre-	prē-	1–73
behind	poster / o	pŏs-tĕr-o	7–9
behind, after	post-	pōst	1–72
behind, posterior, back of (body)	poster / o	pŏs-tĕr-ō	7–9
below, under	sub-	sŭb	4–11
below, under	hypo-	hī-pō	4–11
beside, around, near	para-	păr-ă	7–49
between	inter-	ĭn-tĕr	8–56
bile, gall	chol / e	kō-lē	2–171
bile duct	choledoch / o	kō-lē-dō-kō	2–181
birth	nat / o	nā-tō	5–79
black	melan / o	mĕl-ă-nō	4–67
bladder	vesic / o	vĕs-ĭ-kō	3–47
bladder	cyst / o	sĭs-tō	2–168
blood vessel	hemangi / o	hē-măn-jē-ō	9–59
blood vessel	vascul / o	văs-kū-lō	7–99
blood	-emia	ēm-ē-ă	4–77
blood	hemat / o	hē-mă-tō	2–91
blood	hem / o	hē-mō	5–26
blood clot	thromb / o	thrŏm-bō	7–95
blue	cyan / o	sī-ă-nō	4–67
bone	oste / o	ŏs-tē-ō	8–2
bone marrow, spinal cord	myel / o	mī-ĕl-ō	7–93
brain	encephal / o	ĕn-sĕf-ă-lō	7–91
breast	mamm / o	măm-ō	5–72

English Term	Medical Word Element	Pronunciation	Frame
breast	mast / o	măs-tō	5–70
breastbone (sternum)	stern / o	stĕr-nō	8–48
breathing	-pnea	nē-ă	6–89
bronchus	bronchi / o (plural, bronchi)	brŏng-kē-ō	6–49
bronchus	bronch / o (plural, bronchi)	brŏng-kō	6–49
bursting forth (of)	-rrhage, -rrhagia	răj, ră-jē-ă	5–24
calcaneum (heel bone)	calcane / o	kăl-kā-nē-ō	8–48
calcium	calc / o	kăl-kō	7–46
calculus, stone	-lith, lith / o	lĭth, lĭthō	2–176, 2–193
cancer	carcin / o	kăr-sĭ-nō	2–85
carpus (wrist bones)	carp / o	kăr-pō	8–48
cartilage	chondr / o	kŏn-drō	6–37
cell	-cyte	sīt	4–71
cell	cyt / o	sī-tō	4–71
cerebrum (brain)	cerebr / o	sĕr-ē-brō	7–99
cervix uteri (neck of uterus), neck	cervic / o	sĕr-vĭ-kō	5–52
cessation	-pause	pawz	5–66
chest	thorac / o	thō-răk-ō	6–86
choroid	choroid / o	kō-roy-dō	10–15
colon	col / o	kō-lō	2–131
colon	colon / o	kō-lŏn-ō	2–156
condition	-ia	ē-ă	2–225
condition	-ism	ĭzm	5–105
cornea	kerat / o	kĕr-ă-tō	10–15
cranium (skull)	crani / o	krā-nē-ō	8–48
crushing	-tripsy	trĭp-sē	3–45
cut into, incision	-tomy	tō-mē	2–75
death	necr / o	nĕk-rō	4–93
decrease	-penia	pē-nē-ă	4–74
destruction, loosening, separation	-lysis	lī-sĭs	7–68
difficult, bad, painful	dys-	dĭs	2–96
digestion	-pepsia	pĕp-sē-ă	2–96
dilation, expansion	-ectasis	ĕk-tă-sĭs	3–40
discharge, flow	-rrhea	rē-ă	2–15
disease	-pathy	pă-thē	3–21
double, two	dipl / o	dĭp-lō	9–36
dropping, falling, prolapse	-ptosis	tō-sĭs	3–31
dry	xer / o	zē-rō	4–63
duodenum	duoden / o	doo-ōd-ĕ-nō	2–71
ear	ot / o	ō-tō	10–38
eardrum (tympanic membrane)	myring / o	mĭ-rĭng-gō	10–47
eat, swallow	-phagia	fā-jē-ă	2–98
electric	electr / o	ē-lĕk-trō	9–75
enlargement	-megaly	mĕg-ă-lē	2–220
enlargement	megal / o	mĕg-ă-lō	2–219
esophagus	esophag / o	ē-sŏf-ă-gō	2–63
eustachian (auditory) tube	salping / o	săl-pĭn-gō or săl-pĭn-jō	10–50
excessive	hyper-	hī-pĕr	2–92

English Term	Medical Word Element	Pronunciation	Frame
excision, removal	-ectomy	ĕk-tō-mē	2–75
expansion	-ectasis	ĕk-tă-sĭs	3–40
extremities	acr / o	ăk-rō	7–28
eye	ophthalm / o	ŏf-thŏl-mō	10–2
eyelid	blephar / o	blĕf-ă-rō	10–10
falling, prolapse, dropping	-ptosis	tō-sĭs	3–31
fallopian (uterine) tube	salping / o	săl-pĭn-gō or săl-pĭn-jō	5–7
far, farthest	dist / o	dĭs-tō	8–32
fat	adip / o, lip / o	ăd-ĭ-pō, lĭp-ō	4–27
fear	-phobia	fō-bē-ă	3–121
female, woman	gynec / o	gĭ-nē-kō or jĭ-nē-kō	5–57
femur (thigh bone)	femor / o	fĕm-ō-rō	8–48
fibula	fibul / o	fĭb-ū-lō	8–48
finger or toe (phalanges)	phalang / o	fā-lăng-gō	8–48
fixation	-pexy	pĕk-sē	3–34
flow, discharge	-rrhea	rē-ă	2–15
formation, growth	-plasm	plăzm	5–124
formation, growth	-plasia	plā-zē-ă	5–132
forming, producing	-gen	jĕn	7–72
forming, producing	-genesis	jĕn-ĕ-sis	5–101
forming a new opening or mouth	-stomy	stō-mē	2–109
four	quadri-	kwăd-rī	8–100
front, anterior	anter / o	ăn-tĕr-ō	7–9
fungus	myc / o	mī-kō	2–34
gall, bile	chol / e	kō-lē	2–171
gallbladder	cholecyst / o	kō-lē-sĭs-tō	2–163
gland	aden / o	ăd-ē-nō	3–72
glomerulus	glomerul / o	glō-mĕr-ū-lō	3–84
glucose, sugar	gluc / o	gloo-kō	7–72
glucose, sugar	glyc / o	glī-kō	7–72
glue, gluelike; neuroglial tissue (binding, supportive tissue of nervous system)	-glia	glē-ă	7–113
good, normal	eu-	ū	6–95
process of recording	-graphy	gră-fē	2–214
growth, formation	-plasia	plā-zē-ă	5–132
growth, formation	-plasm	plăzm	5–124
gum	gingiv / o	jĭn-jĭ-vō	2–54
hair	trich / o	trĭk-ō	4–55
half, partly	hemi-	hĕm-ē	8–102
hardening, sclera	scler / o	sklē-rō	3–24
head	cephal / o	sĕf-ăl-ō	8–49
heart	cardi / o	kăr-dē-ō	9–3
heat	therm / o	thĕr-mō	2–207
heel bone (calcaneum)	calcane / o	kăl-kā-nē-ō	8–48
hernia, swelling	-cele	sēl	3–97
humerus (upper arm bone)	humer / o	hū-mĕr-ō	8–48
ileum	ile / o	ĭl-ē-ō	2–104
in	en-	ĕn	8–52
incision, cut into	-tomy	tō-mē	2–75
inflammation	-itis	ī-tĭs	2–6
instrument to cut	-tome	tōm	2–75
instrument for measuring	-meter	mĕ-tĕr	8–51
instrument to view	-scope	skōp	2–150
intestine (usually small)	enter / o	ĕn-tĕr-ō	1–37

English Term	Medical Word Element	Pronunciation	Frame
involuntary contraction, twitching	-spasm	spăzm	1–149
iris	irid / o	ĭr-ĭ-dō	10–15
jaw	maxill / o	măk-sĭ-lō	2–23
jejunum	jejun / o	jĕ-joo-nō	2–104
joint	arthr / o	ăr-thrō	8–41
kidney	nephr / o	nĕf-rō	3–4
kidney	ren / o	rē-nō	3–4
knee cap	patell / o	pă-tĕl-ō	8–48
lacrimal, tear	dacry / o	dăk-rē-o	10–35
large	macro-	măk-rō	6–57
larynx (voice box)	laryng / o	lă-rĭng-gō	6–25
little, scanty	olig / o	ŏl-ĭ-gō	3–117
liver	hepat / o	hĕp-ă-tō	2–163
lobe	lob / o	lō-bō	6–73
loin, lower back	lumb / o	lŭm-bō	8–77
loosening, destruction, separation	-lysis	lī-sĭs	7–68
lower back, loin	lumb / o	lŭm-bō	8–77
lung, air	pneum / o	noo-mō	6–10
lung, air	pneumon / o	noo-mŏn-ō	6–10
lymph	lymph / o	lĭm-fō	9–117
lymph vessel	lymphangi / o	lĭm-făn-jē-ō	9–122
many, much	poly-	pŏl-ē	3–120
measure, instrument for measuring	-meter	mĕ-tĕr	8–51
meninges	meningi / o	mĕ-nĭn-jē-ō	7–106
meninges	mening / o	mĕ-nĭng-gō	7–106
menses	men / o	mĕn-ō	5–62
menstruation	men / o	mĕn-ō	5–62
metacarpus (bones of the hand)	metacarp / o	mĕt-ă-kăr-pō	8–48
mouth, forming a new opening	-stomy, stomat / o	stŏ-mē, stō-mă-tō	2–120 2–4
mouth	or / o	or / ō	2–4
mucus	muc / o	mū-kō	5–42
muscle	my / o	mī-ō	6–40
nail	onych / o	ŏn-ĭ-kō	4–59
narrowing, stricture	-stenosis	stĕn-ō-sĭs	2–144
near, nearest	proxim / o	prŏk-sĭ-mō	8–33
near, beside, around	para-	păr-ă	7–49
neck, cervix uteri (neck of the uterus)	cervic / o	sĕr-vĭ-kō	5–52
nerve	neur / o	noo-rō	7–17
new	neo-	nē-ō	5–80
night	noct / o	nŏk-tō	3–123
normal, good	eu-	ū	6–95
nose	rhin / o	rī-nō	6–3
nose	nas / o	nā-zō	6–3
not	an-	ăn	3–114
noun ending	-um	ŭm	8–39
noun ending	-y	ē	2–208
one who	-er	ĕr	1–44
ovary	oophor / o	ō-ŏf-ō-rō	5–4
pain	-algia	ăl-jē-ă	2–10

English Term	Medical Word Element	Pronunciation	Frame
pain	-dynia	dĭ-nē-ă	2–10
painful, bad, difficult	dys-	dĭs	2–96
pancreas	pancreat / o	păn-krē-ă-tō	2–163
paralysis	-plegia	plē-jē-ă	6–19
partly, half	hemi-	hĕm-ē	8–102
pelvis	pelv / o	pĕl-vō	8–48
pelvis	pelv / i	pĕl-vē	8–48
pertaining to	-al	ăl	1–74
pertaining to	-ic	ĭk	2–25
pertaining to	-ous	ŭs	2–86
pertaining to	-ary	ĕr-ē	2–25
pertaining to	-ar	ăr	6–74
phalanges (fingers or toes)	phalang / o	fā-lăng-gō	8–48
pharynx (throat)	pharyng / o	fă-rĭng-gō	6–17
pleura	pleur / o	ploo-rō	6–78
poison	toxic / o, tox / o	tŏk-ĭ-kō, tŏks-ō	2–212 2–211
polyp	polyp / o	pŏl-ĭ-pō	p. 261
posterior, behind, back (of body)	poster / o	pŏs-tĕr-ō	7–9
pregnant woman	-gravida	grăv-ĭ-dă	5–82
process of recording	-graphy	grăf-ē	2–214
producing, forming	-gen	jĕn	7–72
producing, forming	-genesis	jĕn-ĕ-sĭs	5–101
prolapse, falling, dropping	-ptosis	tō-sĭs	3–24
prostate gland	prostat / o	prŏs-tă-tō	5–114
pus	py / o	pī-ō	3–110
radiation, x-rays	radi / o	rā-dē-ō	7–13
rapid	tachy-	tăk-ē	6–97
record	-gram	grăm	2–214
rectum	rect / o	rĕk-tō	2–139
rectum, anus	proct / o	prŏk-tō	2–146
red	erythr / o	ē-rĭth-rō	3–102
removal, excision	-ectomy	ĕk-tō-mē	2–75
renal pelvis	pyel / o	pī-ĕ-lō	3–81
resembling	-oid	oyd	5–43
retina	retin / o	rĕt-ĭ-nō	10–15
ribs	cost / o	kŏs-tō	8–48
rupture	-rrhexis	rĕk-sĭs	8–87
sacrum	sacr / o	săk-rō	8–81
saliva, salivary glands	sial / o	sī-ă-lō	2–13
salivary glands, saliva	sial / o	sī-ă-lō	2–13
scanty, little	olig / o	ŏl-ĭ-gō	3–117
sclera (white of the eye), hardening	scler / o	sklē-rō	3–24
self	auto-	aw-tō	4–98
separation, loosening, destruction	-lysis	lĭ-sĭs	7–68
sigmoid colon	sigmoid / o	sĭg-moyd-ō	2–136
skin	cutane / o	kū-tā-nē-ō	4–8
skin	-derma	dĕr-mă	4–13
skin	dermat / o	dĕr-mă-tō	4–8
skin	derm / o	dĕr-mō	4–5
skull	crani / o	krā-nē-ō	8–48

English Term	Medical Word Element	Pronunciation	Frame
slow	brady-	brăd-ē	6–99
small	-ole	ōl	6–113
small	-ule	ūl	9–64
small	micro-	mī-krō	6–37
softening	-malacia	mă-lā-shē-ă	4–61
specialist in the study of	-logist	lŏ-jĭst	2–40
specialist	-ist	ĭst	2–37
speech	-phasia	fā-zē-ă	7–105
sperm	spermat / o	spĕr-mă-tō	5–99
spinal cord, bone marrow	myel / o	mī-ĕl-ō	7–93
spine	spin / o	spī-nō	7–112
sternum (breastbone)	stern / o	stĕr-nō	8–48
stomach	gastr / o	găs-trō	1–37
stone, calculus	-lith, lith / o	lĭth, lĭ-thō	2–176 2–193
straight	orth / o	or-thō	2–47
stricture, narrowing	-stenosis	stĕn-ō-sĭs	2–144
study of	-logy	lŏ-jē	2–40
sugar, glucose	gluc / o	gloo-kō	7–72
sugar, glucose	glyc / o	glī-kō	7–72
surgical puncture	-centesis	sĕn-tē-sĭs	6–68
surgical repair	-plasty	plăs-tē	2–73
suture	-rrhaphy	ră-fē	2–117
swallow, eat	-phagia	fā-jē-ă	2–98
sweat	hidr / o	hī-drō	4–21
swelling	-edema	ĕd-ē-mă	3–16
swelling, hernia	-cele	sēl	3–97
tear, lacrimal	dacry / o	dăk-rē-ō	10–35
teeth	dent / o	dĕnt-ō	1–27
teeth	odont / o	ō-dŏnt-tō	2–47
tendon	tend / o	tĕn-dō	8–98
testis	test / o	tĕs-tō	5–96
testis	orchi / o	ŏr-kē-ō	5–111
testis	orchid / o	ŏr-kĭ-dō	5–111
thirst	-dipsia	dĭp-sē-ă	7–82
three	tri-	trī	9–34
through	dia-	dī-ă	2–17
thymus gland	thym / o	thī-mō	7–85
thyroid gland	thyro, thyroid / o	thī-rō, thī-royd-ō	7–36
tibia	tibi / o	tĭb-ē-ō	8–48
tongue	lingu / o	lĭng-gwō	2–22
trachea (windpipe)	trache / o	trā-kē-ō	6–33
treatment	-therapy	thĕr-ă-pē	6–12
tumor	-oma	ō-mă	2–88
twitching, involuntary contraction	-spasm	spăzm	2–149
two, double	bi-	bī	9–36
tympanic membrane (eardrum)	tympan / o	tĭm-pă-nō	10–47
tympanic membrane (eardrum)	myring / o	mĭ-rĭng-gō	10–47
under, below	sub-	sŭb	4–11
under, below	hypo-	hī-pō	4–11
upon, above	epi-	ĕp-ē	2–90

English Term	Medical Word Element	Pronunciation	Frame
ureter	ureter / o	ū-rē-tĕr-ō	3–39
urethra	urethr / o	ū-rē-thrō	3–64
urine, urination	-uria	ū-rē-ă	3–102
urine	ur / o	ū-rō	3–104
uterus	hyster / o	hĭs-tĕr-ō	5–14
uterus	metr / o	mĕt-rō	5–17
uterus	uter / o	ū-tĕr-ō	5–17
vagina	colp / o	kŏl-pō	5–30
vagina	vagin / o	vă-jĭ-nō	5–30
vas deferens, vessel	vas / o	vă-sō	5–137
vein	phleb / o	flĕb-ō	9–51
vein	ven / o	vē-nō	3–90
ventricle (of brain or heart)	ventricul / o	vĕn-trĭk-ū-lō	9–14
vertebra (backbone)	spondyl / o	spŏn-dĭ-lō	8–62
vertebra (backbone)	vertebr / o	vĕr-tĕ-brō	8–48
vessel	angi / o	ăn-jē-ō	9–58
vessel, vas deferens	vas / o	vă-sō	5–137
vision	-opia	ō-pē-ă	10–24
visual examination	-scopy	skŏ-pē	2–150
vomiting	-emesis	ĕm-ĕ-sĭs	2–91
vulva	vulv/o	vŭl-vō	5–47
water	hydr / o	hī-drō	4–23
white	leuk / o	loo-kō	3–102
within	intra-	ĭn-tră	3–88
without, not	an-, a-	ăn, ă	3–114
woman, female	gynec / o	gĭ-nē-kō or jĭ-nē-kō	5–57
x-rays	roentgen / o	rĕnt-gĕn-ō	8–21
x-rays, radiation	radi / o	rā-dē-ō	7–13
yellow	xanth / o	zăn-thō	4–67

Answer Key

UNIT 1: Introduction to Programmed Learning

Answers to Frame 1–53

Word	Combining Form (root + vowel)	Root	Suffix
dermat/itis		dermat	-itis
append/ix		append	-ix
vagin/itis		vagin	-itis
oste/o/arthr/itis	oste/o	arthr	-itis
gastr/o/enter/itis	gastr/o	enter	-itis
orth/o/ped/ic	orth/o	ped	-ic

REVIEW A ANSWER KEY

Basic Elements of a Medical Word

Prefix	Combining Form(s) (root + vowel)	Word Root(s)	Suffix
peri-		dent	-al
ab-		norm	-al
		hepat	-itis
supra-		ren	-al
trans-		vagin	-al
	gastr / o	intestin	-al
macro-		cephal	-ic
	ren / o		-pathy
	therm / o		-meter
	hepat / o		-megaly
sub-		stern	-al
hypo-		insulin	-ism
	gastr / o, enter / o		-pathy
	arteri / o	scler	-osis
hypo-		derm	-ic

REVIEW B ANSWER KEY

peridental, abnormal, hepatitis, suprarenal, transvaginal, gastrointestinal, macrocephalic, renopathy, thermometer, hepatomegaly, substernal, hypoinsulinism, gastroenteropathy, arteriosclerosis, hypodermic

REVIEW C ANSWER KEY

Singular	Plural	Rule
1. sarcoma	sarcomata	Retain the *ma* and add *ta*
2. thrombus	thrombi	Drop *us* and add *i*
3. appendix	appendices	Drop *ix* and add *ices*
4. diverticulum	diverticula	Drop *um* and add *a*
5. ovary	ovaries	Drop *y* and add *ies*
6. diagnosis	diagnoses	Drop *is* and add *es*
7. lumen	lumina	Drop *en* and add *ina*
8. vertebra	vertebrae	Retain the *a* and add *e*
9. thorax	thoraces	Drop the *x* and add *ces*
10. spermatozoon	spermatozoa	Drop *on* and add *a*

UNIT 2: Digestive System

Figure 2–2.

1. oral cavity
2. sublingual
3. submaxillary
4. parotid
5. esophagus
6. stomach
7. duodenum
8. jejunum
9. ileum
10. ascending colon
11. transverse colon
12. descending colon
13. sigmoid colon
14. rectum
15. anus
16. liver
17. gallbladder
18. pancreas

Figure 2–5.

1. hepatic duct
2. cystic duct
3. pancreatic duct
4. common bile duct
5. duodenum

Word Element Exercise 2–1: Rectal Bleeding

dys/phagia
dia/rrhea
hemat/emesis
enter/itis
col/o/nic
ile/o/stomy
append/ectomy
sigmoid/o/scopy
an/o/rect/al
rect/al
carcin/oma

**Medical Record Evaluation 2–1:
Rectal Bleeding**

1. What is the patient's symptom that made him seek medical help?
   Weight loss of 40 pounds since his last examination.
2. What surgical procedures were performed on the patient for his regional enteritis?
   Ileostomy and appendectomy.
3. What abnormality was found with the sigmoidoscopy?
   Dark blood and rectal bleeding.
4. What is causing the rectal bleeding?
   It could be due to a polyp, bleeding, diverticulum, or rectal carcinoma.
5. Write the plural form of diverticulum.
   diverticula

Word Element Exercise 2–2: Carcinosarcoma of the Esophagus

carcin/o/sarc/oma
dys/phagia

esophag/o/scopy
path/o/logy
polyp/oid
esophag/eal

**Medical Record Evaluation 2–2.
Carcinosarcoma of the Esophagus**

1. What surgery was performed on this patient?
   Resection of the esophagus with anastomosis of the stomach; lymph node excision.
2. What diagnostic testing confirmed malignancy?
   Pathology tests on the biopsy.
3. Where was the carcinosarcoma located?
   Middle third of the esophagus.
4. Why was the adjacent lymph node excised?
   Metastasis was suspected.

Vocabulary (page 79)

1. gastroscopy
2. dyspepsia
3. hematemesis
4. cholecystogram
5. salivary glands
6. alimentary canal
7. stomatalgia
8. duodenotomy
9. hepatomegaly
10. dysphagia
11. cholecystectomy
12. linguogingival
13. sigmoidotomy
14. rectoplasty
15. stomach
16. ileostomy
17. cholelithiasis
18. friable
19. choledoch
20. sigmoid colon

Pathological Conditions (page 81)

1. volvulus
2. hernia
3. anorexia
4. cirrhosis
5. hematochezia
6. ascites
7. bulimia
8. borborygmus
9. ulcer
10. jaundice
11. irritable bowel syndrome
12. dysentery
13. hemorrhoids
14. inflammatory bowel disease (IBD)
15. Crohn's disease

UNIT 3: Urinary System

Figure 3–2. Urinary System

1. kidney
2. ureter
3. bladder
4. urethra
5. nephron
6. calyx (plural: calyces)
7. renal pelvis

Figure 3–5. Urinary System

1. glomerulus
2. collecting tubule
3. Bowman's capsule

Word Element Exercise 3–1: Cystitis

pelv/ic
cyst/o/scopy

cyst/itis
noct/uria
epi/gastr/ic
poly/uria
hemat/uria
chol/e/lith/iasis
chol/e/doch/o/lith/iasis **or**
   choledoch/o/lith/iasis
chol/e/cyst/ectomy **or** cholecyst/ectomy
chol/e/doch/o/lith/o/tomy **or**
   choledoch/o/lith/o/tomy
append/ectomy

Medical Record Evaluation 3–1: Cystitis

1. What was found when the patient had a cystoscopy?
   Cystitis.

2. What are the symptoms of cystitis?
Nocturia, urinary frequency, pelvic pain, and hematuria, in this case.
3. What is the patients' past surgical history?
Cholecystectomy, choledocholithotomy, and incidental appendectomy.
4. What is the treatment for cystitis?
Antibiotics and taking in a lot of fluids.
5. What are the dangers of untreated cystitis?
The spreading of infection to the kidneys or to the bloodstream (sepsis).
6. What instrument is used to perform a cystoscopy?
A cystoscope.

Word Element Exercise 3–2: Benign Prostatic Hypertrophy

pneum/o/thorax
col/ectomy
trans/urethr/al
retin/al
carcin/oma
hydr/o/cele
hyper/trophy

Medical Record Evaluation 3–2: Benign Prostatic Hypertrophy

1. What was wrong with the patient's prostate?
It was enlarged.

2. Did it cause him any urinary difficulty?
No significant difficulty.
3. Why did the surgeon call in Dr. Moriarty?
The doctor was unable to pass a catheter.
4. Did the patient have any previous surgery on his prostate?
No.
5. Where was the patient's hernia?
In the groin and scrotum (hydrocele).
6. Was the patient's past medical history contributory for his present urological problem?
No.

Vocabulary (page 133)

1. malignant
2. nephrons
3. Bright's disease
4. renal pelvis
5. IVP
6. diuretics
7. edema
8. benign
9. nephrolithotomy
10. acute renal failure
11. nephroptosis
12. ureteropyeloplasty
13. spasm
14. nocturia
15. urinary incontinence
16. hematuria
17. polyuria
18. oliguria
19. anuria
20. cystocele

Pathological Conditions (page 135)

1. phimosis
2. Wilms' tumor
3. azoturea
4. dysuria
5. diuresis
6. end-stage renal disease
7. hypospadias
8. interstitial nephritis
9. uremia
10. enuresis

UNIT 4: Integumentary System

Figure 4–2. Integumentary System

1. epidermis
2. dermis
3. hair follicle
4. sebaceous glands (oil glands)
5. sudoriferous glands (sweat glands)
6. subcutaneous tissue

Word Element Exercise 4–1: Compound Nevus

chron/ic
sinus/itis
abdomin/al
histi/o/cyt/omas
col/itis
enter/itis

Medical Record Evaluation 4–1: Compound Nevus

1. What is a nevus?
A mole; a type of skin tumor.
2. Locate the vermilion border on your lip and tell where it is located?
It is the edge of the red portion of the upper or lower lip.

3. Was the lesion limited to a certain area?
Yes, the right side of the lower lip.
4. In the impression, the pathologist has ruled out melanoma. What does this mean?
The nevus is not cancerous even though it appears to be.
5. What is unusual about a melanoma?
It is made up of pigmented cells and is malignant.
6. Is a melanoma a dangerous condition? If so, explain why.
Yes, it metastasizes rapidly.

Medical Record Evaluation 4–2: Psoriasis

1. What causes psoriasis?
The etiology is unknown, but heredity is a significant determining factor.
2. On what parts of the body does psoriasis typically occur?
Scalp; elbows; knees; sacrum; around the nails, arms, and legs.
3. How is psoriasis treated?
Mild to moderate psoriasis is treated with corticosteroids and phototherapy.
4. What is a histiocytoma?
A tumor containing histiocytes, a macrophage present in all loose connective tissue.

Vocabulary (page 175)

1. subcutaneous
2. hidrorrhea; diaphoresis
3. trichopathy
4. autograft
5. Kaposi's sarcoma
6. suction lipectomy
7. macules
8. decubitus ulcer
9. leukemia
10. ecchymosis
11. psoriasis
12. hirsutism
13. pustule
14. papules
15. diabetes mellitus
16. xeroderma
17. melanoma
18. lipocele
19. vulgaris
20. onychomalacia

Additional Pathological Conditions (page 177)

1. wart
2. vitiligo
3. tinea
4. pustule
5. fissure
6. eczema
7. impetigo
8. urticaria
9. wheal
10. vesicle
11. scales
12. scabies
13. nodule
14. alopecia
15. comedo
16. laceration
17. cyst
18. contusion
19. papule
20. petechia

UNIT 5: Reproductive System

Figures 5–2 and 5–3.

1. ovary (singular)
2. fallopian tube (singular)
3. uterus
4. vagina
5. labia majora
6. labia minora
7. clitoris
8. Bartholin's glands
9. cervix

Figure 5–5.

1. testis (singular)
2. scrotum
3. epididymis
4. vas deferens or ductus deferens
5. seminal vesicles
6. prostate gland
7. Cowper's glands or bulbourethral glands
8. penis
9. glans penis
10. foreskin or prepuce

Word Element Exercise 5–1: Postmenopausal Bleeding

dia/gnos/tic
post/men/o/paus/al
vagin/al
neo/plast/ic
mast/ectomy

Medical Record Evaluation 5–1. Postmenopausal Bleeding

1. How many times has the patient been pregnant? How many children has the patient given birth to?
   Four; four.
2. Why is the patient being admitted to the hospital?
   To have a gynecological laparoscopy and diagnostic D&C, to rule out the neoplastic process.
3. What is a D&C?
   Dilation and curettage; a surgical procedure that expands the cervical canal of the uterus so that the surface lining of the uterine wall can be scraped.
4. What is the patient's past surgical history?
   Simple mastectomy last year.
5. At what sites did the patient have malignant growth?
   Left breast with metastases to the axilla, liver, and bone.

Medical Record Evaluation 5–2: Bilateral Vasectomy

1. What is the end result of a bilateral vasectomy?
   Sterilization.

2. What structure does vas refer to?
   The vas deferens or ductus deferens.
3. Was the patient awake during the surgery? What type of anesthesia was used?
   Yes, 1% Xylocaine.
4. What was used to prevent bleeding?
   Hemostat.
5. Did the patient have any complications during surgery?
   No.
6. What type of suture material was used to close the incision?
   2-0 chromic.
7. What was the patient given for pain relief at home?
   Darvocet-N100.
8. Why is it important for the patient to go for a follow-up visit?
   To analyze his semen and confirm sterilization.

Vocabulary (page 227)

1. prostatomegaly
2. testopathy
3. testosterone
4. amenorrhea
5. estrogen, progesterone
6. oophoritis
7. aspermatism
8. gravida 4
9. uterus
10. prostatic cancer
11. epididymis
12. hydrocele
13. vas deferens
14. para 4
15. cervix uteri
16. dysmenorrhea
17. postmenopausal
18. aplasia
19. vasectomy
20. pelvic inflammatory disease (PID)

Additional Pathological Conditions (page 229)

1. cryptorchidism
2. pyosalpinx
3. sterility
4. anorchism
5. candidiasis
6. chlamydia
7. balanitis
8. benign prostatic hypertrophy
9. leukorrhea
10. endometriosis
11. fibroids
12. gonorrhea
13. syphilis
14. toxic shock syndrome
15. trichomoniasis
16. urethritis
17. phimosis
18. impotence
19. oligospermia
20. retroversion

UNIT 6: Respiratory System

Figure 6–2.

1. nasal cavity
2. pharynx (throat)
3. larynx (voice box)
4. epiglottis
5. trachea (windpipe)
6. bronchus
7. bronchioles
8. alveoli
9. pulmonary capillaries
10. lung
11. pleura
12. diaphragm

Word Element Exercise 6–1: Papillary Carcinoma

carcin/oma
polyp/oid
polyp/ectomy
hem/o/rrhage
nas/al
pneumon/ia

Medical Record Evaluation 6–1: Papillary Carcinoma

1. What type of patients are at risk for nasal polyps?
Those with chronic inflammation of the nasal and sinus mucosa that is usually due to allergies.
2. When is a polypectomy indicated?
When the patient fails to respond to medical treatment or if there is severe nasal obstruction.
3. Were the nasal polyps cancerous?
No, polyps are benign.
4. What contributed to the patient's expiration?
Papillary carcinoma that metastasized to the lymph node.
5. Why was a biopsy of the liver performed?
To check for metastasis.

Medical Record Evaluation 6–2: Lobar Pneumonia

1. What physical examination techniques are useful in this case?
Inspection, palpation, percussion, and auscultation.
2. What explains the unilateral chest expansion?
The affected lung doesn't expand with inspiration.
3. What explains the decrease in resonance and increase in tactile fremitus?
The tissue underlying the chest wall in the affected region is dense.
4. What is the significance of bronchial breath sounds in this case?
They are consistent with lung consolidation.
5. What laboratory data are useful to confirm the diagnosis?
Chest x-ray, arterial blood gas analysis, sputum Gram stain with culture and sensitivity and complete blood count.

Vocabulary (page 271)

1. necropsy
2. meatus
3. asthma
4. croup
5. polyp
6. diagnosis
7. apnea
8. aerophagia
9. aspiration
10. chondroma
11. hepatocarcinoma
12. neopathy
13. pharyngoplegia
14. pleurisy
15. *Pneumocystis carinii*
16. snare
17. rhinoplasty
18. tuberculosis (TB)
19. chronic obstructive lung disease (COLD)
20. anesthesia

Additional Pathological Conditions (page 273)

1. stridor
2. epistaxis
3. influenza
4. acidosis
5. coryza
6. cystic fibrosis (CF)
7. lung cancer
8. pleural effusion
9. pneumothorax
10. rales
11. empyema
12. adult respiratory distress syndrome (ARDS)
13. croup
14. atelectasis
15. epiglottitis
16. pertussis
17. wheezes
18. sudden infant death syndrome (SIDS)
19. hypoxia
20. rhonchi

UNIT 7: Endocrine and Nervous Systems

Figure 7–5.

1. pituitary gland (hypophysis)
2. thyroid gland
3. parathyroid glands
4. adrenal (suprarenal) glands
5. pancreas
6. pineal gland
7. thymus gland
8. ovaries
9. testes

Word Elements Exercise 7–1: Cerebrovascular Accident

aden/o/carcin/oma
cardi/o/vascul/ar
chole/cyst/o/jejun/o/stomy
jejun/o/jejun/o/stomy

Medical Record Evaluation 7–1: Cerebrovascular Accident

1. What is a CVA?
Cerebrovascular accident is a stroke and refers to any occurrence that deprives the brain of oxygen.
2. Did the patient have a history of cardiovascular problems?
No.
3. What symptoms did the patient experience just prior to her CVA?
Paralysis of the right arm and left leg, aphasia, and diplopia.
4. What is the primary site of this patient's cancer?
Head of the pancreas.

5. What is cerebrovascular disease?
   A disorder resulting from a change within the blood vessel(s) of the brain.
6. What is the probable cause of the patient's CVA?
   Metastatic lesion of the brain or cerebrovascular disease.

Medical Record Evaluation 7–2: Diabetes Mellitus

1. What symptoms of DM did the patient experience before his office visit?
   Increased appetite, polydipsia, and polyuria.
2. What confirmed the patient's new diagnosis of DM?
   Elevated blood sugar and glycosuria.
3. What conditions had to be met before the patient could be discharged from the hospital?
   He had to be able to draw up and give his own insulin and perform fingersticks.
4. How many times a day does the patient have to take insulin?
   Two times, once in the morning and once in the afternoon.
5. Why does the patient have to perform fingersticks four times a day?
   To monitor his blood sugar levels closely and make sure they are within the normal range.
6. What is an ADA 2000-calorie diet? Why is it important?
   A 2000-calorie diet designed by the American Diabetic Association. Maintaining the same number of calories each day will help to control blood sugar levels.

Vocabulary (page 323)

1. acromegaly	14. thyrotoxicosis
2. pancreatolysis	15. adrenalectomy
3. adenohypophysis	16. adrenaline
4. cerebral palsy	17. glycogenesis
5. hypercalcemia	18. meningorrhagia
6. insulin	19. neuromalacia
7. neurohypophysis	20. pruritus
8. pancreatopathy	21. deglutition
9. polyphagia	22. vertigo
10. diabetes mellitus	23. jaundice
11. hyperglycemia	24. metastasis
12. pancreatolith	25. hormone
13. polydipsia	

Additional Pathological Conditions (page 325)

1. Bell's palsy	11. sciatica
2. cerebrovascular accident (CVA)	12. spina bifida
	13. hydrocephalus
3. epilepsy	14. neuroblastoma
4. exophthalmos	15. Alzheimer's disease
5. Graves' disease	16. shingles
6. insulinoma	17. pituitarism
7. myxedema	18. panhypopituitarism
8. pheochromocytoma	19. Huntington's chorea
9. Parkinson's disease	20. Cushing's syndrome
10. poliomyelitis	

UNIT 8: Musculoskeletal System

Figure 8–1.

1. crani/o	8. phalang/o
2. stern/o	9. pelv/i, pelv/o
3. cost/o	10. femor/o
4. vertebr/o	11. patell/o
5. humer/o	12. tibi/o
6. carp/o	13. fibul/o
7. metacarp/o	14. calcane/o

Figure 8–3.

1. diaphysis
2. bone marrow
3. medullary cavity (singular)
4. distal epiphysis
5. proximal epiphysis
6. articular cartilage
7. periosteum

Figure 8–5.

1. simple *or* closed fracture
2. open *or* compound fracture
3. greenstick fracture
4. impacted fracture

Figure 8–6.

1. intervertebral disks	5. thoracic vertebrae
2. cervical vertebrae	6. lumbar vertebrae
3. atlas	7. sacrum
4. axis	8. coccyx

Word Element Exercise 8–1: Degenerative, Intervertebral Disk Disease

bi/later/al
hyper/troph/ic
inter/vertebr/al
later/al
lumb/o/sacr/al
sacr/o/ili/ac
vertebr/al

Medical Record Evaluation 8–1: Degenerative, Intervertebral Disk Disease

1. Why does the x-ray show a decreased density at L5–S1?
   Appears that a bilateral laminectomy had been done.
2. What is the most common cause of degenerative intervertebral disk disease?

Aging; this is a common finding in individuals 50 years of age and older.

3. What happens to the gelatinous material of the disk as aging occurs?
The gelatinous material is replaced by harder fibrocartilage.

4. What is the probable cause of the narrowing of the L3-4 and L4-5 spaces?
Narrowing often occurs as a result of degenerative intervertebral disk disease.

Word Element Exercise 8–2: Rotator cuff tear, right shoulder

arthr/itis
arthr/o/scopy
oste/o/arthr/itis
sub/acromi/al
tendin/itis

Medical Record Evaluation 8–2: Rotator cuff tear, right shoulder

1. Locate the area and structures that make up the rotator cuff. Use the following references: Figure 8–7A (textbook), anatomy and physiology textbook, or a medical dictionary.
Supraspinatus, infraspinatus, teres minor and subcapularis muscles.

2. What type of arthritis did the patient have?
Degenerative.

3. Did the patient have calcium deposits in the right shoulder?
No.

4. Refer to Figure 8–1 (textbook), and observe the location of the clavicle. Now feel the outer end of your clavicle. What does it feel like?
Bony ridge.

5. What type of instrument did the doctor use to visualize the glenoid labrums?
Arthroscope.

6. What are labra?
Liplike structures; in this case edges or rims of bones.

7. Did the patient have any outgrowths of bone? If so, where?
Yes, spurs were found at the inferior and anterior acromioclavicular calcifications.

8. Did they find any deposits of calcium salts within the shoulder joint?
They were unable to visualize an intra-articular calcification.

Vocabulary (page 371)

1. radiology
2. diaphysis
3. AP
4. simple or closed fracture
5. bilateral
6. proximal
7. articulation
8. compound or open fracture
9. atlas
10. arthrocentesis
11. bone marrow
12. cephalometer
13. myelogram
14. myorrhexis
15. spondylomalacia
16. distal
17. roentgenologist
18. cervical vertebrae
19. intervertebral
20. quadriplegia

Additional Pathological Conditions (page 373)

1. osteoporosis
2. tendinitis
3. sprain
4. strain
5. kyphosis
6. Ewing's sarcoma
7. torticollis
8. gout
9. rheumatoid arthritis
10. Paget's disease
11. sequestrum
12. talipes
13. crepitation
14. myasthenia gravis
15. lordosis
16. muscular dystrophy
17. contracture
18. ankylosis
19. herniated disk
20. carpal tunnel syndrome

UNIT 9: Cardiovascular and Lymphatic Systems

Figure 9–2: Cardiovascular System

1. endocardium
2. myocardium
3. epicardium
4. pericardium

Figure 9–3: Cardiovascular System

1. right atrium (RA)
2. left atrium(LA)
3. right ventricle (RV)
4. left ventricle (LV)
5. interventricular septum (IVS)
6. superior vena cava (SVC)
7. inferior vena cava (IVC)
8. tricuspid valve
9. pulmonary valve
10. right pulmonary artery; left pulmonary arteries
11. right pulmonary veins; left pulmonary veins
12. mitral valve
13. aortic valve
14. aorta
15. branches of the aorta
16. descending aorta

Figure 9–5: Cardiovascular System

1. sinoatrial (SA) node
2. right atrium (RA)
3. atrioventricular (AV) node
4. Bundle of His
5. bundle branches
6. Purkinje fibers

Figure 9–8: Lymphatic System

1. lymph capillaries
2. lymph vessels
3. thoracic duct
4. right lymphatic duct
5. cervical nodes
6. axillary nodes
7. inguinal nodes

Word Element—Exercise 9–1: Myocardial Infarction

dys/pnea
a/pnea
thyroid/itis

thyroid/ectomy
atri/al
my/o/cardi/al

Medical Record Evaluation 9–1: Myocardial Infarction

1. What symptoms did the patient experience before admission to the hospital?
   Generalized malaise, increased shortness of breath (SOB) while at rest, and dyspnea followed by periods of apnea and syncope.
2. What was found during clinical examination?
   Irregular radial pulse, uncontrolled atrial fibrillation with evidence of a recent myocardial infarction (MI).
3. What is the danger of atrial fibrillation?
   A decrease in cardiac output and promotion of thrombus formation in the upper chambers.
4. Did the patient have prior history of heart problems? If so, describe them.
   Yes, sinus tachycardia attributed to preoperative anxiety and thyroiditis.
5. Was the patient's prior heart problem related to her current one?
   No.

Medical Record Evaluation 9–2: Carotid Angiogram

1. What is a catheter?
   A tube used to withdraw fluids from the body.
2. How did they insert the catheter into the femoral artery?
   Through the skin into the right femoral artery.
3. What type of x-ray did they use to guide the catheter into the common carotid artery?
   Fluoroscopic control.

4. To what did the doctor attribute the narrowing of the internal carotid lumen?
   Plaque with possible ulceration.
5. What part of the arterial branch showed the most narrowing?
   Right distal common carotid artery.
6. Do the physicians suspect that the person was born with the stenosis?
   It is a possibility.

Vocabulary (page 419)

1. myocardium
2. tachypnea
3. arteriosclerosis
4. anxiety
5. systole
6. diastole
7. EKG
8. malaise
9. desiccated
10. cardiomegaly
11. aneurysm
12. angina pectoris
13. myocardial infarction (MI)
14. anticoagulants
15. tachyphagia
16. angiectasis
17. capillaries
18. hemangioma
19. arterioles
20. pacemaker

Additional Pathological Conditions (page 421)

1. varicose veins
2. mononucleosis
3. myocardial infarction (MI)
4. embolus
5. lymphadenitis
6. DVT
7. hypertension
8. arrhythmia
9. transient ischemic attack (TIA)
10. bruit
11. stroke
12. rheumatic heart disease
13. atherosclerosis
14. lymphosarcoma
15. Raynaud's disease
16. ischemia
17. Hodgkin's disease
18. AIDS
19. congestive heart failure (CHF)
20. fibrillation

UNIT 10: Special Senses: The Eyes and Ears

Figure 10–1.

1. scler/o
2. choroid/o
3. retin/o
4. kerat/o
5. irid/o

Figure 10–3.

1. lacrimal gland
2. lacrimal ducts
3. lacrimal sac

Figure 10–4.

1. auricle
2. ear canal
3. tympanic membrane
4. malleus
5. incus
6. stapes
7. eustachian (auditory) tube
8. cochlea
9. semicircular canals
10. vestibule

Word Elements: Exercise 10–1: Otitis Media

mast/oid
ot/itis
tympan/o/plasty

Medical Record Evaluation 10–1: Otitis Media

1. Where was the patient's infection located?
   Right ear.
2. What complication developed while the patient was hospitalized?
   Cholesteatoma.
3. What is the purpose of the tube placement?
   It reduces the accumulation of fluid within the middle ear.
4. What surgery is being performed to resolve the cholesteatoma?
   Tympanoplasty, right ear.
5. Will the patient be asleep during the surgery?
   Yes, under general anesthesia.

Word Element: Exercise 10–2: Retinal Detachment

retin/al
retin/itis
conjuctiv/al
scler/o/tomy
vitr/ectomy

Medical Record Evaluation 10–2: Retinal Detachment

1. Where is the retina located?
   The retina is the innermost layer of the eye.
2. Was the anesthetic administered behind or in front of the eyeball?
   Behind the eyeball (retrobulbar).
3. How much movement remained in the eye following anesthesia?
   None; kinesia.
4. Where was the hemorrhage located?
   In the orbit of the eye behind the lens, where the vitreous humor is located.
5. What type of vitrectomy was undertaken?
   Trans pars plana vitrectomy
6. Why was the eye left soft?
   Because it had poor perfusion.

Vocabulary (page 449)

1. diplopia
2. sclera
3. tympanic membrane
4. dacryorrhea
5. eustachian tube
6. keratitis
7. diagnosis
8. mucoserous
9. otitis media
10. cholesteatoma
11. mastoid surgery
12. general anesthetic
13. ophthalmologist
14. chronic
15. hyperopia
16. postoperatively
17. labyrinth
18. blepharoptosis
19. salpingostenosis
20. myopia

Additional Pathological Conditions (page 451)

1. tinnitus
2. otosclerosis
3. achromatopsia
4. Menière's disease
5. strabismus
6. anacusis
7. otitis media
8. conjunctivitis
9. photophobia
10. presbycusis
11. glaucoma
12. vertigo
13. retinal detachment
14. hordeolum
15. astigmatism
16. acoustic neuroma
17. conductive hearing loss
18. cataract
19. diabetic retinopathy
20. macular degeneration

Diagnostic Procedures

CLINICAL, RADIOGRAPHICAL, AND LABORATORY

Diagnostic procedures are key components in determining and treating a person's illness. Clinical, radiographical, and laboratory procedures are performed to establish the nature of an illness, establish a diagnosis, and determine a type of treatment.

Clinical Procedures

The following are some of the clinical procedures used to assist the physician in an accurate diagnosis.

arthroscopy: Direct joint visualization by means of an arthroscope. Surgical instruments can be passed through the arthroscope to remove tissue and repair the joint.

aspiration: The act of withdrawing a fluid, such as mucus or serum, from the body by a suction device.

audiometry: Measurement of hearing acuity for the various frequencies of sound waves, using an audiometer.

biopsy: Excision of a small piece of tissue for microscopic examination. Usually performed to establish a diagnosis.

bronchoscopy: Visual examination of the bronchi, using a flexible bronchoscope that is inserted through the mouth and trachea into the bronchial tubes. In addition to visualization, the procedure can be used for suctioning, obtaining a biopsy, examining fluid or sputum, removing foreign bodies, and diagnostic purposes.

colonoscopy: Visual examination of the colon with a colonoscope. Biopsy and surgical excision can also be accomplished by using the colonoscope.

colposcopy: Visual examination of vaginal and cervical tissues with a colposcope.

culdoscopy: Visual examination of the female viscera. This procedure requires an incision in the posterior vaginal wall to admit a culdoscope. Culdoscopy is used in suspected ectopic pregnancy, in unexplained pelvic pain, and in the presence of undetermined pelvic masses.

cystoscopy: Visual examination of the urinary bladder by inserting a cystoscope into the urethra. In addition to visualization, cystoscopy is used to obtain biopsies of tumors or other growths and to remove polyps.

electrocardiograph: The instrument used in electrocardiography.

electrocardiography, electrocardiogram (ECG, EKG): A graphic record of electrical currents emanating from the heart muscle. Electrodes are placed on the patient to obtain a reading.

electroencephalography, electroencephalogram (EEG): A graphic record of electrical currents developed in the brain that are detected by placing electrodes on the skull.

endoscopy: Visual examination of any cavity of the body using an endoscope. Arthroscope, cystoscope, gastroscope, and colonoscope are examples of endoscopes.

esophagogastroduodenoscopy (EGD): Visual examination of the esophagus, stomach, and duodenum using an endoscope.

esophagoscopy: Visual examination of the esophagus using an esophagoscope. Usually done as a diagnostic procedure to locate and inspect disorders of the esophagus. After the esophagoscope has been inserted through the mouth, it is possible to obtain tissue samples for microscopic study. In some instances, the esophagoscope can be used to remove a foreign object that has become lodged in the esophagus.

gastroscopy: Visual examination of the interior of the stomach and upper part of the small intestine with a gastroscope, inserted through the mouth and esophagus.

Holter monitor: A small portable device to be worn by a patient during normal activity, to obtain a record of cardiac arrhythmia that would not be discovered by means of an ECG record of only a few minutes' duration. It consists of an electrocardiograph and a recording system capable of storing up to 24 hours of recording of the individual's electrocardiogram (ECG) record.

laparoscopy, peritoneoscopy: Visual examination of the abdominal cavity. This procedure requires a small incision in the abdominal wall to admit a laparoscope. Laparascopy is used to examine the ovaries or fallopian tubes and to perform gynecological sterilization techniques.

laryngoscopy: Direct or indirect visual examination of the larynx (voice box). Direct visual examination is performed with a speculum or laryngoscope. Indirect visual examination is performed with a laryngoscope that transmits an image of the larynx via a laryngeal mirror. In addition to providing a means for biopsies and sputum samples, this procedure is used to identify tumors and account for abnormal changes in the voice.

ophthalmoscopy: Visual examination of the interior of the eye using an ophthalmoscope. It is useful in detecting eye disorders as well as disorders of other organs that are reflected in the condition of the eyes.

otoscopy: Visual examination of the external auditory canal and the tympanic membrane (eardrum), using an otoscope.

palpation: Process in which the examiner feels the texture, size, consistency, and location of certain parts of the body with the hands.

proctosigmoidoscopy, sigmoidoscopy: Visual examination of the rectum and sigmoid colon using a sigmoidoscope or proctoscope. This instrument is used for excisional biopsies of small lesions, such as polyps, and for segmental biopsies of large lesions for diagnosis. This procedure is also used to determine such abnormalities as tumors, cancer, and diverticulitis.

pulmonary function tests (PFTs): A series of tests used to determine the capacity of the lungs to exchange oxygen and carbon dioxide efficiently, by using an instrument called a spirometer.

retinoscopy: Visual examination to evaluate refractive errors of the eye. The examiner projects light into the eyes and judges errors of refraction by movement of reflected light rays. The emerging path of the beam determines whether the eye is nearsighted or farsighted.

tonometry: Measurement of tension and pressure, usually of the eye for detection of glaucoma.

treadmill stress test: Used for noninvasive cardiac evaluation to aid in patient diagnosis and prognosis, usually includes an electrocardiogram (ECG) taken during controlled exercise stress conditions. During this test of increased stress and work, abnormal electrocardiographic tracings (that do not appear during an ECG taken when the patient is resting) may appear. The test is done in the presence of a physician, and the patient is constantly monitored.

urethroscopy: Visual examination of the urethra using a urethroscope.

visual acuity test: Part of an eye examination that evaluates the patient's ability to distinguish the form and detail of an object.

Radiographic Procedures

The following selected x-ray procedures use radioactive substances and various techniques of visualization to prevent, diagnose, and treat disease.

angiography, angiogram: Radiographic image of blood vessels following an injection of a radiopaque substance. Used to detect vascular abnormalities including tumors, occlusions, and aneurysms. Examples of this radiographic procedure include cardiac angiography, cerebral angiography, peripheral angiography, and pulmonary angiography.

arthrography: A series of radiographs taken after injection of a radiopaque substance or air into a joint cavity, usually the knee or shoulder, in order to outline the contour of the joint.

barium enema, lower GI: Radiographic examination of the colon (large bowel or large intestine). An enema using a liquid contrast medium called barium is administered and retained in the lower gastrointestinal (GI) tract during roentgenographical studies. Used for diagnosing obstructions, tumors, or other abnormalities.

barium swallow, upper GI: Radiographic examination of the upper gastrointestinal (GI) tract in order to visualize the esophagus, stomach, and duodenum after a liquid contrast medium called barium is swallowed.

bone scan: Radiographic image is taken as a camera scans the entire body. Used to evaluate skeletal involvement related to connective tissue disease, fracture, or bone infection.

bronchography, bronchogram: Radiographic image of the bronchi after installation of an opaque medium through a catheter into the trachea. Bronchoscopy is more frequently used to evaluate the bronchi.

cardiac catheterization: Passage of a tiny plastic tube (catheter) into the heart through a vein or artery. Samples of blood are withdrawn for testing; blood pressure and cardiac output are measured. Used to diagnose heart disorders and anomalies and to evaluate narrowing of the coronary arteries caused by atherosclerosis.

chest radiographs: Series of radiographs designed to evaluate the chest, heart, lungs, and rib cage.

cholangiography, cholangiogram: Radiographic image of the bile ducts after intravenous injection of a radiopaque dye as a contrast medium. Used to identify obstructions caused by a tumor or stone(s). If no obstruction is present, the biliary structures fill and rapidly empty into the intestinal tract.

cholecystography, cholecystogram, gallbladder series: Radiographic image of the gallbladder after administration of a radiopaque dye as a contrast medium. The dye is administered to patients in tablet form the evening before the x-ray films are made.

computerized axial tomography (CT) scan: Noninvasive x-ray technique that is more sensitive than a conventional x-ray examination, and shows the body in slices or cross-sections. A scanner and detector circle the patient's body, sending images to a monitor that allows a specialist to view any area of the body. This is most frequently used to visualize the brain, abdomen, and chest. Also called computerized tomography (CT) scan.

cystography, cystogram: X-ray image of the urinary bladder after administration of a radiopaque dye. This type of examination frequently is part of any excretory urographical procedure, as in retrograde pyelography. It is useful in diagnosing tumors or other defects in the bladder wall, vesicoureteral reflux, or stones, or other pathological conditions of the bladder.

Doppler ultrasonography: A noninvasive diagnostic test that evaluates blood flow in the major veins and arteries of arms, legs, and extracranial cerebrovascular system. A hand-held transducer directs high-frequency sound waves to the area being tested. See ultrasonography.

echocardiography, echocardiogram: A noninvasive diagnostic test using ultrasound to visualize internal cardiac structures and record images of the heart. Ultrasonic waves directed through the heart are reflected backward, or echoed, when they pass from one type of tissue to another, as from cardiac muscle to blood. The sound waves are transmitted from, and received by, a transducer and recorded on a strip chart. This test is useful in demonstrating, without danger to the patient, valvular and other structural deformities of the heart that formerly required cardiac catheterization or some other elaborate procedure for accurate diagnoses.

echoencephalography, echoencephalogram: The use of ultrasound to study and record the intracranial structures of the brain. Used to diagnose conditions that cause a shift in the midline structures of the brain. Less commonly used than a computerized tomography (CT) scan.

electromyography, electromyogram: Graphic record of electrical currents generated in an active muscle. Useful in diagnosing disorders of the nerves supplying the muscles and in disorders affecting the muscle tissue.

fluoroscopy: Immediate projection of internal organs by using x-rays. Useful in seeing organs in motion and guiding catheter insertions.

hysterosalpingography, hysterosalpingogram: X-ray image of the uterus and oviducts after a contrast medium is injected into those organs. Used to determine pathology in the uterine cavity, evaluate tubal patency, and determine the cause of fertility problems.

intravenous pyelography (IVP): Contrast medium is injected intravenously at designated intervals and x-ray examinations are taken as the medium is cleared from the blood by glomerular filtration. The renal calyces, renal pelvis, ureters, and urinary bladder are all visible on film.

magnetic resonance imaging (MRI): A nonionizing (no x-ray)–imaging technique using magnetic fields and radiofrequency waves to produce a cross-sectional multiplanar image of the entire body or specific body part. Useful in detecting various conditions affecting blood flow, tumors, infection, and any other type of tissue pathology because of its ability to produce images, through bone tissue and fluid-filled soft tissues. Also called nuclear magnetic resonance (NMR).

mammography, mammogram: An x-ray image of the breast to detect abnormalities of breast tissue.

myelography, myelogram: X-ray image of the spinal cord after injection of a contrast medium. Used to identify and study spinal distortions caused by tumors, cysts, herniated intervertebral disks, or other lesions.

nuclear scan studies: Procedures that use radiopharmaceuticals (radionuclides), radiation detectors with imaging devices, and computers to visualize organs and study the dynamic processes that differentiate normal from pathological tissues. Administration of a radionuclide, intravenously or orally, is followed by the measurement of the radiation emitted by a camera that converts the readings into a two-dimensional image.

percutaneous transhepatic cholangiography: A procedure for outlining the major bile transhepatic ducts. A radiopaque contrast material is injected via a needle through the skin into the liver.

phlebography, venography: Radiography of a vein filled with an injected contrast medium. Incomplete filling of a vein indicates obstruction.

phonocardiography: A procedure that provides a graphic display of the heart sounds during the cardiac cycle. It is used to identify, time, and differentiate heart sounds and murmurs. A specialized microphone is placed over the heart to detect sound, which is electronically amplified and graphically recorded on a monitor. An electrocardiogram (ECG) is simultaneously recorded on the monitor to provide a reference point for each of the sounds and their duration. In this procedure, abnormal acoustic events can be permanently recorded in order to evaluate treatment.

pyelography, pyelogram, urogram, urography: X-ray examination of the kidneys, ureters, and bladder after injection of a contrast medium, introduced by the intravenous (IVP) or retrograde method.

radiography, roentgenography: The making of x-ray images of any part of the body for diagnostic purposes. The most common diagnostic study used to assess musculoskeletal problems and to follow the progress and effectiveness of treatment.

radiotherapy, radiation therapy: Treatment of cancer and other diseases by the use of x-rays, radiation from radioactive substances, and other similar forms of radiant energy.

retrograde pyelography, retrograde pyelogram (RP): Contrast medium is introduced using a urinary catheter that is passed from the urethra, through the urinary bladder, into the ureters and calyces of the kidney pelves while being observed via x-ray images. This technique provides detailed visualization of the urinary collecting system and is useful in locating an obstruction in the urinary tract.

spleen scan: Radioactive material is injected intravenously. This medium is absorbed by the spleen cells to visualize the spleen. Abnormalities such as cysts, abscesses, tumors, splenomegaly, and ruptures can be diagnosed.

thyroid scan: After an intravenous injection of a radioactive iodine that collects in the thyroid gland, a scanning device produces an image of the gland. The ability of the thyroid gland to trap and retain iodine provides a measure of thyroid activity.

tomography, tomogram: Noninvasive special techniques of roentgenography designed to show detailed images of structures in a selected plane of tissue by blurring images of structures in all other planes. In computerized tomography (CT) and positron emission tomography (PET), the image is produced by a computer program.

ultrasonography, ultrasonogram: Use of ultrasound to produce an image or photograph of an organ or tissue. Ultrasonic echoes are recorded as they strike tissues of different densities. An example is the evaluation of the female reproductive system as well as the fetus in the obstetric patient. Another use of ultrasound is echography and the echogram.

xeromammography, xeromammogram: Xeroradiography of the breast.

xeroradiography, xerography: An x-ray technique in which an image is produced electrically rather than chemically, permitting lower exposure times and radiation of lower energy than that of ordinary x-ray examinations. It is especially beneficial in the diagnosis of breast tumors.

Laboratory Procedures

The following diagnostic laboratory procedures are only a sample of the many laboratory tests performed on a patient's urine, blood, tissue, and fluid.

alpha-fetoprotein (AFP): A blood sample is used to determine the presence of alpha-globulin protein. AFP measurements are used for early diagnosis of fetal neural defects, such as spina bifida and anencephaly. AFP is also used to monitor the effectiveness of cancer therapy because high levels of AFP are found in patients with certain malignancies.

arterial biopsy: Used to examine a specimen of an arterial vessel wall. Most frequently the temporal artery is selected, but other arteries may be biopsied as indicated. Arterial biopsy most often confirms inflammation of the vessel wall, or arteritis, a type of vasculitis.

arterial blood gas (ABG): A percutaneous arterial puncture is made to assess the gas exchange of oxygen and carbon dioxide in the lungs by measuring the partial pressure of oxygen and carbon dioxide.

aspiration biopsy cytology (ABC): Microscopic study of cells obtained from superficial or internal lesions by suction through a fine needle. It is used primarily as a diagnostic procedure, usually as a technique for detecting nuclear and cytoplasmic changes in cancerous tissue.

bleeding time: Time required for blood to stop flowing from a small wound or pin prick. This test is helpful in determining the functional capacity of platelets and of vasoconstriction. A prolonged bleeding time is found in patients with vascular abnormalities, with deficiencies in the platelet count, and with conditions in which there is a deficiency of fibrinogen.

blood urea nitrogen (BUN): Provides an estimate of kidney function by determining the nitrogen level in the blood. An increase in the BUN level usually indicates decreased renal function.

calcium test: Measures calcium in a blood sample to detect bone and parathyroid disorders. Hypercalcemia can indicate loss of calcium in the bones, parathyroid disorders, or cancer. Hypocalcemia may be associated with hypoparathyroidism and central nervous system (CNS) disorders. Symptoms of hypocalcemia include tetany and muscle spasms.

carcinoembryonic antigen (CEA): Blood samples are used to monitor the effectiveness of cancer therapy. CEA levels will fall within a month if treatment is successful. High levels of this antigen may be a sign of cancer.

cardiac enzyme studies: Serum studies that determine enzyme levels in the blood, along with a clinical evaluation and an ECG, help in establishing a diagnosis and extent of a myocardial infarction (MI).

complete blood count (CBC): Test performed on a blood sample, including hemoglobin, hematocrit, red and white blood counts, platelet count, and a differential white blood cell count.

CSF analysis, spinal puncture, spinal tap: Puncture of the spinal cavity with a needle to extract the spinal fluid for diagnostic purposes, to introduce anesthetic agents into the spinal canal, or to inject radiopaque substances for radiographical procedures.

differential white blood cell count: Performed to examine and enumerate the distribution of leukocytes (white blood cells) in a stained blood smear. The different kinds of white cells are counted and reported as a percentage of the total examined. The differential values change considerably in pathology, and this test is often used as a first step to diagnose a disease.

endometrial biopsy, endometrial smear: Used in screening high-risk patients for endometrial cancer. This procedure is done during the gynecological examination. Following the administration of a small amount of anesthetic, a thin, hollow curette is used to remove endometrial tissue for laboratory analysis.

erythrocyte sedimentation rate (ESR): Performed on a blood sample to measure the time it takes for erythrocytes (red blood cells) to settle at the bottom of a narrow tube. The rate of settlement increases in inflammatory diseases, cancer, and pregnancy and decreases in liver disease.

exfoliative cytology: Microscopic examination of desquamated cells for diagnostic purposes. The cells are obtained from lesions, sputum, secretions, urine, and other material by aspiration, scraping, a smear, or washings of the tissue.

fasting blood sugar (FBS): Measures circulating glucose level after a 12-hour fast.

glucose tolerance test (GTT): Performed by giving a certain amount of glucose (sugar) to a patient orally or intravenously. Blood samples are drawn at specified intervals and the blood glucose is determined in each sample. The GTT is most often used to assist in the diagnosis of diabetes or other disorders that affect carbohydrate metabolism.

hematocrit (Hct): Performed on a blood sample to measure the percentage of packed red blood cells in a whole blood sample. A low hematocrit often indicates anemia.

hemoglobin (Hgb, Hb): Performed on a blood sample to measure the amount of hemoglobin found in whole blood. A low hemoglobin level indicates anemia.

insulin tolerance test: Performed to determine the body's ability to use insulin, in which insulin is given and blood glucose is measured at regular intervals. In hypoglycemia, the glucose levels may drop lower and are slower to return to normal.

monospot: Performed on a blood sample to detect the presence of a nonspecific antibody called the heterophile antibody that is present in the serum of patients with infectious mononucleosis.

occult blood: Determines bleeding in gastrointestinal disorders; used primarily to detect colon cancer.

Papanicolaou test, Pap test: A simple smear method of examining exfoliative cells. Used most frequently to detect cancer of the cervix. The smear is usually obtained during a routine pelvic examination.

patch test: The simplest type of skin test. A small piece of gauze or filter paper is impregnated with a minute quantity of the substance to be tested (food, pollen, animal fur, and so on), and is applied to the skin, usually on the forearm. After a certain length of time the patch is removed and the reaction observed. If there is no reaction, the test result is said to be negative; if the skin is reddened or swollen, the result is positive. The patch test is used in testing for skin allergies, especially contact dermatitis.

phenylketonuria (PKU): A heelstick on an infant is done to collect 3 drops of blood for screening. This test is used to determine the presence of a congenital disease caused by a defect in the metabolism of the amino acid phenylalanine that, left untreated, results in mental retardation.

PPD (purified protein derivative) tuberculin test: Involves an intradermal injection of tuberculin antigen, which causes a delayed reaction in patients with active or dormant tuberculosis.

pregnancy test: Urinary or blood test to detect the presence of human chorionic gonadotropin (HGC), a hormone secreted by the placenta. Used to determine pregnancy.

prothrombin time: Performed on a blood sample to determine clotting time. Used to evaluate the effect of administration of anticoagulant drugs. When blood clotting is prolonged, the patient is at risk for hemorrhage.

red blood cell (count) (RBC): Performed on a blood sample to determine the number of red blood cells (RBCs). An abnormally low red blood cell count often indicates anemia; an increase may indicate polycythemia.

scratch test: A form of skin test used in testing for allergies. It is performed by placing a small quantity of a solution containing a suspected allergen on a lightly scratched area of the skin. If redness or swelling occurs at the scratch sites within 15 to 20 minutes, allergy to the substance is indicated and the test result is considered positive. If no reaction has occurred after 30 minutes, the substance is removed and the result is considered negative.

Schick test: One of the best-known intradermal tests. This skin test, in which diphtheria toxin is injected interdermally, is used to determine immunity to diphtheria. A positive reaction, indicating susceptibility, is marked by redness and swelling at the site of injection; a negative reaction, indicating immunity, is marked by absence of redness or swelling.

semen analysis: A sperm sample is analyzed for volume, sperm count, motility, and morphology. This test is also used to document adequate sterilization after a vasectomy. If sperm are seen 6 weeks after vasectomy, the adequacy of the surgery must be questioned.

serum bilirubin: May indicate excessive hemolysis, hepatic disorders, or obstructive conditions of the bile ducts. Serum bilirubin is formed from the breakdown of hemoglobin. In the liver, bilirubin is secreted into the bile and then excreted into the intestinal tract through the bile ducts.

skin tests: Used to determine the body's reaction to a substance by observing the results after the substance is applied to the skin or injected intradermally. Skin tests are used to detect allergens, to determine immunity, and to diagnose disease. Kinds of skin tests include the patch test, scratch test, Schick test, and tuberculin test.

sputum specimen, sputum culture: Microscopic examination of mucous secretions coughed up from the lungs and bronchi. The mucus is examined and cultured to identify the presence of microorganisms.

throat culture: Bacteriological test used to identify throat pathogens, especially group A strepococci. Strep infections must be treated with appropriate antibiotics because they may cause serious secondary disorders.

thyroid function tests: Used to evaluate evidence of thyroid dysfunction. Some tests include determination of thyroid hormones.

urinalysis (UA): Analysis of the urine, including microscopic examination for blood cells, bacteria, and casts, which are formed from protein precipitates in the renal tubules.

white blood cell (count) (WBC): Performed on a blood sample to determine the number of white blood cells (WBCs). An increase is often noted when infection is present. In leukemia the number of WBCs (leukocytes) is greatly increased. Chemotherapy and x-ray therapy often cause a decrease.

APPENDIX D

Drug Classifications

The following classifications of medication include prescription and over-the-counter drugs that are used for various medical purposes.

alkylate: Drugs used to treat certain types of malignancies.

analgesic, painkiller: Drugs that relieve pain. Aspirin, codeine, and morphine are examples of analgesics.

antacid: Agent that neutralizes excess acid in the stomach and helps relieve gastritis and ulcer pain. Antacids are also used to relieve indigestion and reflux esophagitis (heartburn).

antianginals: Agents used to relieve angina pectoris by expanding the blood vessels of the heart. The most common drug in this category is nitroglycerin.

antibiotic: Any of a variety of natural or synthetic substances that inhibit growth of or destroy microorganisms. Used extensively in treatment of infectious diseases in plants, animals, and humans.

anticoagulants: Agents that inhibit or delay the clotting process; used to prevent clots from forming in blood vessels.

anticonvulsant: Substance that prevents or reduces the severity of epileptic or other convulsive seizures.

antidepressant: Medicine or other mode of therapy that acts to prevent, cure, or alleviate mental depression.

antidiarrheals: Agent used to relieve diarrhea either by absorbing the excess fluids that cause diarrhea or by lessening intestinal motility (slowing the movement of fecal material through the intestine), which allows more time for absorption of water.

antiemetics, antinauseants: Agents that suppress nausea and vomiting, mainly by acting on the brain control to stop the nerve impulses. There are many uses for these drugs, including the treatment of motion sickness and of dizziness associated with inner ear infections. Some antihistamines and tranquilizers have antiemetic properties.

antihistamine: A drug that counteracts the effects of a histamine. Antihistamines are used to relieve the symptoms of allergic reactions, especially hay fever and other allergic disorders of the nasal passages.

antihyperlipidemics: Agents that lower cholesterol levels in the bloodstream, thereby helping to prevent atherosclerosis (fatty build-up in the blood vessels).

antihypertensives: Agents that lower blood pressure.

anti-infective, antibacterial, antifungal agents: Substances that eliminate or inhibit bacterial or fungal infections. They can be administered either topically or systemically.

anti-inflammatory, antipyretic: A nonnarcotic analgesic used for relief of pain and fever. Many of these drugs have anti-inflammatory effects as well and are used to treat arthritis and gout. These drugs are also called non-steroidal anti-inflammatory drugs (NSAIDs) when used for arthritis and gout.

anti-inflammatory, topical corticosteroids: These topically applied drugs relieve three common symptoms of skin disorders: pruritus or itching, vasodilation, and inflammation.

antimetabolites: Agents that interfere with the utilization of enzymes required for cell division.

antipruritics: Agents that prevent or relieve itching.

antiseptics: Topically applied agents that destroy bacteria, thus preventing or treating the development of infections in cuts, scratches, and surgical incisions.

antispasmodics: Agents that act on the autonomic nervous system to slow peristalsis, thereby relieving intestinal cramping.

astringents: Agents used to shrink the blood vessels locally, dry up secretions from seepy lesions, and lessen skin sensitivity.

antitussive: An agent that prevents or relieves coughing.

beta-adrenergic blocking agents: Drugs used to treat cardiac arrhythmias, angina pectoris, postmyocardial hypertension, and migraine headaches.

beta-adrenergics: Drugs used in the treatment of glaucoma that lower intraocular pressure by reducing the production of aqueous humor.

bronchodilator: An agent that caused dilation of the bronchi.

calcium channel blockers: Drugs that selectively block the flow of calcium ions in the heart and are used to treat angina pectoris and some arrhythmias. Also used to treat hypertension.

contraceptives: Any process, device, or method that prevents conception.

corticosteroids: Replacement hormones for adrenal insufficiency (Addison's disease). Corticosteroids are widely used for suppressing inflammation, controlling allergic reactions, reducing the rejection process in transplantation, and treating some cancers.

cycloplegics: Agents that paralyze the ciliary muscles and result in pupil dilation; used to facilitate certain eye examinations.

cytotoxics: Chemical agents that destroy cells or prevent their multiplication; used in cancer chemotherapy.

decongestant: Agent that reduces congestion or swelling, especially in the nasal passages.

diuretics: Agents that promote the excretion of urine.

emetics: Substances used to induce vomiting, especially in cases of poisoning.

estrogen hormones: Pharmaceutical preparation of the estrogen hormone. Used in oral contraceptives to provide a satisfactory replacement hormone to treat menopause and to palliate postmenopausal breast cancer and prostatic cancer. In the woman, its long-term, continued use may increase the risk of endometrial carcinoma.

expectorant: An agent that promotes the expulsion of mucus or exudate from the lungs, bronchi, and trachea.

fibrinolytics: Agents that trigger the body to produce plasmin, an enzyme that dissolves clots. Used to treat acute pulmonary embolism and, occasionally, deep vein thromboses.

gold therapy, chrysotherapy: The use of gold compounds as a medicine; employed in treating rheumatoid arthritis.

gonadotropin: Agent used to raise sperm count in infertility cases.

hemostatics: Any drug, medicine, or blood component that serves to stop bleeding.

hypnotic: Substance or procedure that induces sleep or hypnosis.

inotropics, cardiotonics: Drugs that affect the force of contraction of the heart. Used to treat cardiac arrhythmias and cardiac failure.

insulin: Major drug for diabetes that is administered by injection to lower glucose (sugar) level in the blood.

keratolytics: Agents used to destroy and soften the outer layer of skin so that it is sloughed off or shed. The strong keratolytics are effective for removing warts and corns. Milder preparations are used to promote the shedding of scales and crusts in eczema, psoriasis, and seborrheic dermatitis. Very weak keratolytics irritate inflamed skin, acting as tonics that speed up the healing process.

laxatives (cathartics, purgatives): Agents that promote bowel movements and/or defecation. When used in smaller doses, they relieve constipation. When used in larger doses, they evacuate the entire GI tract, for example, prior to surgery or intestinal radiologic examinations.

miotic: Any substance that causes constriction of the pupil of the eye. Such agents are used in the treatment of glaucoma.

mydriatic: Any drug that dilates the pupil. In certain eye diseases it is essential that the pupil be dilated during treatment to prevent adhesions of the pupils.

mucolytic: An agent that destroys or dissolves mucus so that it can be more readily coughed up.

nitrates: Drugs used to treat acute attacks of angina pectoris.

opiate: A narcotic drug that contains opium or its derivatives.

oral contraceptives: Pharmaceutically prepared chemicals that are quite similar to natural hormones and act by preventing ovulation. When taken according to instructions, these pills are almost 100% effective. Also called "the pill."

oxytocin: Pharmaceutically prepared chemicals that are similar to the pituitary hormone oxytocin. This hormone stimulates the uterus to contract, thus inducing labor, or to rid the uterus of an unexpelled placenta or a fetus that has died.

parasiticides: Agents that, in their oral forms, kill systemic parasites, pinworm, tapeworm.

protectives: Agents that function by covering, cooling, drying, or soothing inflamed skin. Protectives do not penetrate or soften the skin but form a long-lasting film that protects the skin from air, water, and clothing during the natural healing process.

psychotropic drugs: Drugs that affect and can alter psychic function, behavior, or experience. They are often employed in the management of psychotic disorders.

relaxants: Drugs that reduce tension and produce relaxation. For example, muscle relaxants provide therapeutic treatment that specifically relieves muscular tension.

sedative: An agent that exerts a soothing or tranquilizing effect.

spermicidals: Substances that destroy sperm and are used within the woman's vagina for contraceptive purposes. Spermicidals consist of jellies, creams, and foams and do not require a prescription.

topical anesthetics: Agents that are prescribed for pain on skin surfaces or mucous membranes that is caused by wounds, hemorrhoids, or sunburns. They relieve pain and itching by numbing the skin layers and mucous membranes. Applied directly by means of sprays, creams, gargles, suppositories, and other preparations. Also used to numb the skin to make the injection of medication more comfortable.

tranquilizers: Drugs used to calm anxious or agitated people, ideally without decreasing their consciousness.

uricosurics: Drugs that increase the urinary excretion of uric acid, thereby reducing the concentration of uric acid in the blood. Used in the treatment of gout.

vasoconstrictors: Drugs that cause a narrowing of blood vessels; used to decrease blood flow.

vasodilators: Drugs that expand blood vessels; used in the treatment of angina pectoris and hypertension.

Abbreviations

The use of medical and scientific abbreviations is time-saving and often a standard practice in the healthcare industry. A number of the abbreviations may appear with or without periods and with either capital or small letters.

Abbreviation	Meaning
AAMA	American Association of Medical Assistants
AB, ab	abortion
ABC	aspiration biopsy cytology
ABG	arterial blood gas
ac	before meals (ante cibum)
AC	air conduction
Acc	accommodation
ACG	angiocardiography
ACS	American Cancer Society
ACTH	adrenocorticotropic hormone
AD	right ear (auris dextra)
ad lib	as desired
adeno-CA	adenocarcinoma
ADH	antidiuretic hormone
AE	above the elbow
AFB	acid-fast bacillus
AFP	alpha-fetoprotein
AIDS	acquired immunodeficiency syndrome
AK	above the knee
AKA	above-knee amputation
ALL	acute lymphocytic leukemia
AMA	American Medical Association
AMI	acute myocardial infarction
ANS	autonomic nervous system
AP	anteroposterior
A&P	auscultation and percussion
ARDS	adult respiratory distress syndrome
ARMD	age-related macular degeneration
AS	aortic stenosis; left ear (auris sinistra)
ASD	atrial septal defect
ASHD	arteriosclerotic heart disease
Astigm	astigmatism
ATN	acute tubular necrosis
AV	atrioventricular; arteriovenous
AVR	aortic valve replacement
BaE	barium enema
baso	basophil

Abbreviation	Meaning
BBB	bundle-branch block
BE	below the elbow
bid	twice a day
BIN, bin	twice a night
BK	below the knee
BKA	below-knee amputation
BM	bowel movement
BMR	basal metabolic rate
BNO	bladder neck obstruction
BP	blood pressure
BPH	benign prostatic hyperplasia; benign prostatic hypertrophy
BT	bleeding time
BUN	blood urea nitrogen
bx	biopsy
$\bar{c}$	with (cum)
C1, C2 to C8	first cervical vertebra, second cervical vertebra through eighth cervical vertebra
CA, Ca	cancer, calcium
CAD	coronary artery disease
CAT, CT	computerized axial tomography
CBC	complete blood count
CC	cardiac catheterization; chief complaint
cc	cubic centimeter
CCU	coronary care unit
CDC	Centers for Disease Control
CDH	congenital dislocation of the hip
CEA	carcinoembryonic antigen
CHD	coronary heart disease
CHF	congestive heart failure
Cl	chlorine
cm	centimeter
CMA	certified medical assistant
CMML	chronic myelomonocytic leukemia
CNS	central nervous system
CO_2	carbon dioxide
COLD	chronic obstructive lung disease
COPD	chronic obstructive pulmonary disease
CP	cerebral palsy
CPD	cephalopelvic disproportion
CPR	cardiopulmonary resuscitation
CS, C-section	cesarean section

Abbreviation	Meaning
CSF	cerebrospinal fluid
CT	computed tomography
CT scan	computerized tomography scan
CTS	carpal tunnel syndrome
CV	cardiovascular
CVA	cerebrovascular accident
CVD	cardiovascular disease
CWP	childbirth without pain
CXR	chest x-ray
cysto	cystoscopy
D	diopter (lens strength)
dc	discontinue
/d	per day
D&C	dilation and curettage
DDS	Doctor of Dental Surgery
D&E	dilation and evacuation
Derm	dermatology
DI	diabetes insipidus; diagnostic imaging
diff	differential count (white blood cells)
DM	diabetes mellitus
DO	doctor of osteopathy
DOA	dead on arrival
DOB	date of birth
DPT	diphtheria, pertussis, tetanus
DRGs	diagnostic related groups
DUB	dysfunctional uterine bleeding
DVT	deep vein thrombosis
dx	diagnosis
EBV	Epstein-Barr virus
ECG, EKG	electrocardiogram
ECF	extracellular fluid; extended care facility
EDC	estimated or expected date of confinement
EEG	electroencephalogram
EENT	eye, ear, nose, and throat
Em	emmetropia
EMG	electromyogram
ENT	ear, nose, and throat
EOM	extraocular movement
eosin	eosinophil
ESR	erythrocyte sedimentation rate
EST	electric shock therapy
ET	esotropia
F	fahrenheit
FACP	Fellow, American College of Physicians
FACS	Fellow, American College of Surgeons
FBS	fasting blood sugar
FDA	Food and Drug Administration
FEF	forced expiratory flow
FEKG	fetal electrocardiogram
FEV	forced expiratory volume
FH	family history
FHR	fetal heart rate
FHT	fetal heart tone

Abbreviation	Meaning
FS	frozen section
FSH	follicle-stimulating hormone
FTND	full-term normal delivery
FUO	fever of undetermined origin
FVC	forced vital capacity
Fx	fracture
GB	gallbladder
GC	gonorrhea
GH	growth hormone
GI	gastrointestinal
gm	gram
gr	grain
GTT	glucose tolerance test
gtt	drops (guttae)
GU	genitourinary
Gyn	gynecology
H	hypodermic; hydrogen
h	hour
HCG	human chorionic gonadotropin
HCl	hydrochloric acid
HCO	bicarbonate
HCT, hct	hematocrit
HD	hip disarticulation; hemodialysis; hearing distance; Hodgkin's disease
HDL	high-density lipoprotein
HEENT	head, eyes, ears, nose, and throat
Hg	mercury
Hgb, Hb	hemoglobin
HIV	human immunodeficiency virus
HMD	hyaline membrane disease
HNP	herniated nucleus pulposus (herniated disk)
HP	hemipelvectomy
hs	at bedtime
HSG	hysterosalpingography
HSV	herpes simplex virus
hypo	hypodermically
IAS	interatrial septum
IBD	inflammatory bowel disease
ICF	intracellular fluid
ICSH	interstitial cell-stimulating hormone
ICU	intensive care unit
I&D	incision and drainage
ID	intradermal
IDDM	insulin-dependent diabetes mellitus
Ig	immunoglobulin
IH	infectious hepatitis
IM	intramuscular
inj	injection
IOL	intraocular lens
IOP	intraocular pressure
IPPB	intermittent positive-pressure breathing
IQ	intelligence quotient
IRDS	infant repiratory distress syndrome
IS	intercostal space

Abbreviation	Meaning	Abbreviation	Meaning
IUD	intrauterine device	OA	osteoarthritis
IV	intravenous	OB	obstetrics
IVC	inferior vena cava, intravenous cholangiography	OB-GYN	obstetrics and gynecology
		OCPs	oral contraceptive pills
IVF	in vitro fertilization	OD	right eye (oculus dexter); overdose
IVP	intravenous pyelogram	od	once a day
IVS	interventricular septum	OHS	open heart surgery
K	potassium	OR	operating room
KD	knee disarticulation	Ortho, ORTH	orthopedics
kg	kilogram	OS	left eye (oculus sinister)
KS	Kaposi's sarcoma	os	mouth; opening; bone
KUB	kidney ureter bladder	Oto	otology
l	liter	OU	both eyes (oculi unitas)
L1, L2 to L5	first lumbar vertebra, second lumbar vertebra through fifth lumbar vertebra	OV	office visit
		oz	ounce
LA	left atrium	P	pulse
L&A	light and accommodation	PA	posteroanterior
LAT, lat	lateral	Pap smear	Papanicolaou's smear
LB	large bowel	paren	parenterally
LDL	low-density lipoprotein	PAT	paroxysmal atrial tachycardia
LE	lupus erythematosus, lower extremity	Path	pathology
LH	luteinizing hormone	PBI	protein-bound iodine
LLQ	left lower quadrant	pc	after meals
LMP	last menstrual period	PCP	*Pneumocystis carinii* pneumonia
LP	lumbar puncture	PCV	packed cell volume (hematocrit)
LPN	Licensed Practical Nurse	PD	peritoneal dialysis
LRQ	lower right quadrant	PE	physical examination
LUQ	left upper quadrant	PET	positron emission tomography
LV	left ventricle	PGH	pituitary growth hormone
lymphs	lymphocytes	pH	hydrogen ion concentration
MCH	mean corpuscular hemoglobin	PID	pelvic inflammatory disease
MCHC	mean corpuscular hemoglobin concentration	PKU	phenylketonuria
		PMN	polymorphonuclear neutrophil
MCV	mean corpuscular volume	PMP	previous menstrual period
MD	Medical Doctor	PND	paroxysmal nocturnal dyspnea
mets	metastases	PNS	peripheral nervous system
mg	milligram (1/1000 gram)	PO	orally
MH	marital history	poly	polymorphonuclear neutrophil
MI	myocardial infarction; mitral insufficiency	pp	postprandial (after meals)
		prn	as required
mix. astig	mixed astigmatism	PT	prothrombin time; Physical Therapy
ml	milliliter (1/1000 liter)	PTH	parathyroid hormone
mm	millimeter (1/1000 meter; 0.039 inch)	PTT	partial thromboplastin time
mono	monocyte	PVC	premature ventricular contraction
MRI	magnetic resonance imaging	q	every
MS	mitral stenosis; multiple sclerosis	qam	every morning
MSH	melanocyte-stimulating hormone	qd	every day (quaque die)
MVP	mitral valve prolapse	qh	every hour
Myop	myopia	q2h	every two hours
Na	sodium	qid	four times a day
NB	newborn	qpm	every night
NPH	neutral protamine Hagedorn (insulin)	qns	quantity not sufficient
NPO	nothing by mouth (nulla per os)	R, rt	right
NSAID	nonsteroidal anti-inflammatory drug	RA	right atrium, rheumatoid arthritis
O_2	oxygen		

Abbreviation	Meaning
rad	radiation absorbed dose
RAI	radioactive iodine
RBC	red blood cell; red blood count
RD	respiratory disease
REM	rapid eye movement
RLQ	right lower quadrant
R.N.	registered nurse
RNA	ribonucleic acid
R/O	rule out
ROM	range of motion
RP	retrograde pyelogram
RU	routine urinalysis
RUQ	right upper quadrant
RV	right ventricle
Rx	prescription, treatment, therapy
s	without
S1, S2 to S5	first sacral vertebra, second sacral vertebra through fifth sacral vertebra
SA	sinoatrial node
SC	subcutaneous
SCD	sudden cardiac death
SD	shoulder disarticulation
seg	polymorphonuclear neutrophil
SGOT	serum glutamic-oxaloacetic transminase
SGPT	serum glutamic-pyruvic transaminase
SH	serum hepatitis
SLE	systemic lupus erythematosus
SOB	shortness of breath
sos	if necessary
sp. gr.	specific gravity
SR	sedimentation rate
St	strabismus (esotropia)
staph	staphylococcus
stat	immediately
STD	sexually transmitted disease
strep	streptococcus
subcu, subq	subcutaneous
SVC	superior vena cava
SVD	spontaneous vaginal delivery
T	temperature
T1, T2 to T12	first thoracic vertebra, second thoracic vertebra through twelfth thoracic vertebra
T_3	triiodothyronine
T_4	thyroxine

Abbreviation	Meaning
TAH	total abdominal hysterectomy
T&A	tonsillectomy and adenoidectomy
TB	tuberculosis
THA	total hip arthroplasty
THR	total hip replacement
TIA	transient ischemic attack
tid	three times a day
TKA	total knee arthroplasty
TKR	total knee replacement
TNM	tumor, nodes, metastasis
top	topically
TPN	total parenteral nutrition
TPR	temperature, pulse, and respiration
TPUR	transperineal urethral resection
TSH	thyroid-stimulating hormone
TSS	toxic shock syndrome
TTH	thyrotrophic hormone
TUR, TURP	transurethral resection of the prostate
Tx	tumor cannot be assessed
U	units
UA	urinalysis
UC	uterine contractions
UGI	upper gastrointestinal
ULQ	upper left quadrant
ung	ointment
URI	upper respiratory infection
URQ	upper right quadrant
UTI	urinary tract infection
UV	ultraviolet
VA	visual acuity
VC	vital capacity
VD	venereal disease
VF	visual field
VHD	ventricular heart disease
VLDL	very-low-density lipoprotein
VSD	ventricular septal defect
WBC	white blood cell (count); white blood count
wt	weight
w/v	weight by volume
×	multiplied by
XP	xeroderma pigmentosa
XT	exotropia
XX	female sex chromosomes
XY	male sex chromosomes

Medical Specialties

Medical Specialist	Medical Specialty	Description of Specialties
Allergist or immunologist	Allergy or immunology	Diagnosis and treatment of body reactions resulting from hypersensitivity to foods, pollens, dusts, medicines, or other substances that do not normally cause a reaction.
Anesthesiologist	Anesthesiology	Administration of a drug or gas to induce partial or complete loss of sensation with or without loss of consciousness.
Cardiologist	Cardiology or cardiovascular disease	Diagnosis and treatment of diseases of the heart, arteries, veins, and capillaries.
Dermatologist	Dermatology	Diagnosis and treatment of diseases of the skin.
Endocrinologist	Endocrinology	Diagnosis and treatment of the endocrine glands and their internal secretions.
General practitioner	General practice or family practice	Diagnosis and treatment of disease by both medical and surgical methods, without limitation to organ systems or body regions, to all members of a family regardless of age or sex.
Geriatrician or gerontologist	Geriatrics or gerontology	Diagnosis and treatment of diseases of the aged.
Gynecologist	Gynecology	Diagnosis and treatment of diseases of the female reproductive organs.
Hematologist	Hematology	Diagnosis and treatment of diseases of the blood and blood-forming tissues.
Internist	Internal medicine	Diagnosis and treatment of internal organs by other than surgical means.
Neonatologist	Neonatology	Study and care of newborn infants.
Neurologist	Neurology	Diagnosis and treatment of the nervous system and its diseases.
Neurosurgeon	Neurological surgery	Surgery of the nervous system.
Obstetrician	Obstetrics	Care of women during pregnancy, childbirth, and a short period after childbirth.
Oncologist	Oncology	Diagnosis and treatment of tumors; the physician is a cancer specialist.
Ophthalmologist	Ophthalmology	Diagnosis and treatment of eye diseases, including prescribing glasses.
Orthopedist	Orthopedics	Prevention and correction of disorders involving locomotor structures of the body, especially the skeleton, joints, muscles, fascia, and other supporting structures such as ligaments and cartilage.
Otolaryngologist	Otolargyngology	Diagnosis and treatment of diseases of the ear, nose, and throat.
Pathologist	Pathology	Science that studies the nature and cause of disease and the resulting changes in structure and function.
Pediatrician	Pediatrics	Diagnosis and treatment of children's diseases.
Plastic surgeon	Plastic surgery	Surgery for the restoration, repair, or reconstruction of body structures.

Medical Specialist	Medical Specialty	Description of Specialties
Physiatrist	Physiatrics	Treatment of disease by natural methods, especially physical therapy.
Pulmonologist	Pulmonology	Diagnosis and treatment of diseases of the lungs.
Psychiatrist	Psychiatry	Diagnosis, treatment, and prevention of mental illness.
Radiologist	Radiology	Prevention, diagnosis, and treatment of diseases with radioactive substances, including x-rays.
Rheumatologist	Rheumatology	Diagnosis and treatment of rheumatic diseases.
Surgeon	Surgery	Treatment of deformities, injury, and diseases with manual and operative procedures.
Thoracic surgeon	Thoracic surgery	Surgery involving the rib cage and structures contained within the thoracic cage.
Urologist	Urology	Diagnosis and treatment of the urinary tract in both sexes and of the male genital tract.

Index

An "f" following a page number indicates a figure; a "t" following a page number indicates a table.